Acute Coronary Syndrome

Acute Coronary Syndrome

Editor: Mia Dunn

AMERICAN
MEDICAL PUBLISHERS
www.americanmedicalpublishers.com

AMERICAN
MEDICAL PUBLISHERS
www.americanmedicalpublishers.com

Cataloging-in-Publication Data

Acute coronary syndrome / edited by Mia Dunn.
p. cm.
Includes bibliographical references and index.
ISBN 978-1-63927-011-8
1. Coronary heart disease. 2. Heart--Diseases. 3. Acute diseases. I. Dunn, Mia.
RC685.C6 A28 2022
616.123--dc23

American Medical Publishers,
41 Flatbush Avenue,
1st Floor, New York,
NY 11217, USA

ISBN 978-1-63927-011-8 (Hardback)

Contents

Contents

Preface

Acute coronary syndrome (ACS) is a clinical condition in which there is a decreased blood flow in the coronary arteries. Thus, a part of the heart muscle fails to function properly and dies. The distinguishing feature of an acute coronary syndrome is chest pain radiating to the angle of the jaw or the left shoulder. It is often accompanied by nausea and sweating. ACS is associated with a set of three clinical manifestations- unstable angina, non ST elevation myocardial infarction and ST elevation myocardial infarction. An electrocardiogram is the first line of diagnosis that should be performed in case of acute chest pain. If the electrocardiogram indicates acute heart damage, the heart attack should be immediately addressed by performing angioplasty or thrombolysis. People presumed to have ACS are often prescribed aspirin, nitroglycerin or ticagrelor. This book contains some path-breaking studies in acute coronary syndrome. Also included in this book is a detailed explanation of the various diagnostic and therapeutic techniques in the management of acute coronary syndrome. The topics covered herein offer the readers new insights in this condition.

After months of intensive research and writing, this book is the end result of all who devoted their time and efforts in the initiation and progress of this book. It will surely be a source of reference in enhancing the required knowledge of the new developments in the area. During the course of developing this book, certain measures such as accuracy, authenticity and research focused analytical studies were given preference in order to produce a comprehensive book in the area of study.

This book would not have been possible without the efforts of the authors and the publisher. I extend my sincere thanks to them. Secondly, I express my gratitude to my family and well-wishers. And most importantly, I thank my students for constantly expressing their willingness and curiosity in enhancing their knowledge in the field, which encourages me to take up further research projects for the advancement of the area.

Editor

1

Angiotensin converting enzyme DD genotype is associated with acute coronary syndrome severity and sudden cardiac death in Taiwan

Ying-Hsin Chen[1,2†], Jui-Ming Liu[3†], Ren-Jun Hsu[4,5†], Sheng-Chuan Hu[1,6], Horng-Jyh Harn[7], Shee-Ping Chen[8], Jing-Ren Jeng[1,9], Chieh-Lin Wu[4], Jar-Yi Ho[10,11*] and Cheng-Ping Yu[4,5,11*]

Abstract

Background: Angiotensin converting enzyme (ACE) gene insertion/deletion (I/D) polymorphisms have been associated with acute coronary syndrome (ACS); however, several controversial results have also been found in different studied populations. This hospital-based, emergency room, case-control study in Taiwan retrospectively investigated 111 ACS patients, and 195 non-coronary subjects as a control group, to study the effects of ACE I/D polymorphism in the most urgent ACS patients. ACE I/D polymorphisms were determined by polymerase chain reaction-based assays and their associations with ACS risk, severity, and sudden cardiac death were determined.

Results: The ACE DD genotype was associated with ACS incidence. The DD genotype was associated with a significant 4-fold higher risk of ACS in multivariate analysis (odds ratio (OR) = 4.295; 95% confidence interval (CI): 1.436-12.851, p = 0.009), and a 3.35-fold higher risk of acute myocardial infarction. DD genotype carriers also had more than 3-fold higher risks of stenosis in all the three coronary arteries, left anterior descending artery infarction, and anterior wall infarction. In addition, the DD genotype was also associated with a higher risk of sudden cardiac death (OR = 6.484, 95% CI: 1.036-40.598, p = 0.046).

Conclusions: This study demonstrated that the ACE DD genotype is an independent risk factor for ACS, and in particular, for acute myocardial infarction. In addition, the ACE DD genotype is also associated with greater ACS severity and a higher risk of sudden cardiac death. ACE genotyping is recommended for patients with a history of ACS, and more intensive preventive care is suggested for patients with the DD genotype.

Keywords: Acute coronary syndrome, Angiotensin converting enzyme, Genotype, Pharmacogenomics, Sudden cardiac death

Background

Acute coronary syndrome (ACS) is a common disease in the elderly, and a major determinant of morbidity and mortality in all races, ethnicities, and cultures [1]. The epidemic of coronary artery disease (CAD), especially its manifestation as ACS, is a global issue that accounts for more than 80% of the burden of this disease in developing countries [2], and results in approximately 30% of all deaths worldwide each year [3]. The spectrum of ACS disease severity ranges from unstable angina pectoris (UAP) to acute myocardial infarction (AMI), including ST-segment elevation myocardial infarction (STEMI) and non-STEMI (NSTEMI). Sudden cardiac arrest is a major event of heart failure, and sudden cardiac death frequently presents as the first and only manifestation of previously unrecognized ischemic heart disease [4]. The prognosis of AMI-related heart failure

* Correspondence: jaryiho.tw@yahoo.com.tw; cpyupath@yahoo.com.tw
† Contributed equally
[4]Department of Pathology, and Graduate Institute of Pathology and Parasitology, Tri-Service General Hospital, National Defense Medical Center, Taipei, Taiwan
[10]Graduate Institutes of Life Sciences, National Defense Medical Center, Taipei, Taiwan
Full list of author information is available at the end of the article

depends on the extent and severity of ventricular dysfunction and morbidity [5]. Clinically, heart failure usually results in a 20-25% reduction in left ventricular contractility, and a reduction of more than 40% leads to cardiogenic shock [6].

Angiotensin converting enzyme (ACE) is a membranous zinc-containing decarboxy-peptidase that catalyzes the conversion of angiotensin I to angiotensin II and the inactivation of bradykinin via the kallikrein-kininogen system [6]. The insertion (I)/deletion (D) polymorphism in intron 16 of the ACE gene is designated as the presence or absence of a 287 bp Alu repeat [7,8]. The D allele is associated with high serum ACE in the order homozygote deletion (DD) > heterozygote (ID) > homozygote insertion (II) [7,8]. Cardiac ACE activity is also higher in DD homozygote carriers [9]. Treatment with ACE inhibitors after MI has been found to attenuate pathologic left ventricle remodeling, the incidence of heart failure, and mortality [10,11]. The ACE DD genotype or D allele has been associated with MI by increasing the risk of left ventricular enlargement or remodeling [12] and ischemic or idiopathic dilated cardiomyopathy [13,14], though there are also several reports which found no association [15-17]. Genetic polymorphisms in ACE-related pathways, including the angiotensin II type 1 receptor (AT1R) and AT2R, have been associated with MI-related arrhythmias and risk of sudden cardiac arrest [18]. ACE DD and AT1R 1166 CC genotypes have been linked with a greater risk of diastolic heart failure [19].

The DD genotype or D allele has been most associated with increased risk of ACS, ACS severity and cardiovascular death. However, inconsistencies in the clinical significance in previous reports suggested that the influence of the ACE I/D genotypes may differ across the ACS spectrum. For this reason, we carried out a retrospective emergency room-based case-control study to evaluate the association of the ACE I/D polymorphism with the most urgent ACS events. Therefore, this study addressed ACE genotypes and ACS incidence, severity, and sudden cardiac death within the recruited population.

Methods

Subjects

This retrospective case-control study included 111 acute coronary syndrome (ACS) patients and 195 non-coronary subjects (NCS) who were treated in the emergency room of Tri-Service General Hospital (TSGH) between July 2005 and June 2010. The subjects in this study were all Taiwanese and 20 years of age or older. The study was approved by the institutional review board. Clinical and follow-up information were obtained from the patients' medical records, and peripheral blood samples were obtained from the Biobank of TSGH. Peripheral blood samples of each patient were collected by the Biobank during the follow-up with informed consent; two of the blood samples of each patient were used to confirm the ACE genotype. Among the ACS patients, 91 were identified with ACS by coronary angiography (defined by > 75% stenosis in any major coronary artery), while 20 ACS patients did not receive coronary angiography because of their condition [20]. Fifty four ACS patients experienced STEMI, with cardiac chest pain, serologic evidence of myonecrosis, and persistent (> 20 min) ST-segment elevation. The other 57 ACS patients had either UAP or NSTEMI, that was clinically documented as: (1) UAP when cardiac chest pain was new or worsening without serologic evidence of myonecrosis (i.e., no elevation of serum troponin or creatine kinase MB isoenzyme concentration), or dynamic eletrocardiographic (ECG) changes (i.e., ST depression and/or T wave inversion); (2) NSTEMI when the patient had cardiac chest pain and serologic evidence of myocardial necrosis in the absence of ST-segment elevation on the ECG [21]. The NCS had no clinical evidence of CAD including: (1) no history of typical angina pectoris; (2) no abnormal Q wave or ST-T changes in the resting electrocardiogram; and (3) a negative Master exercise test. The NCS constituted the control group and included 135 men and 60 women. The presence of hypertension, diabetes mellitus, hypercholesterolemia or smoking was obtained from the patients' charts or from the records of examination during follow-up medication or hospitalization. In this study, hypercholesterolemia was defined as a serum total cholesterol level of 200 mg/dl or more. Diagnosis of hypertension and diabetes mellitus were performed according to World Health Organization criteria. A smoking habit was defined as a daily intake of > 10 cigarettes. Sudden cardiac death was defined as death within 24 hours of registration in the emergency room, and ACS was recorded as the cause of death after failure of standard cardiac arrest treatment. Other risk factors were stratified as indicated in each table.

Polymerase chain reaction (PCR) for detection of ACE Insert/Delete (I/D) polymorphism

Genomic DNA was extracted from peripheral blood using the Qiagen PureGene DNA Purification Kit according to the manufacturer's protocol. The presence of the I and D alleles of the ACE gene was detected according to the method in Tiret et al [8]. The sequence of the sense primer was 5'-CTGGAGACCACTCCCATCCTTTCT-3', and the antisense primer was 5'-GATGTGGCCATCACATTCGTCAGAT-3'. PCR was carried out with 80 ng genomic DNA in a final volume of 50 µl containing 3 mmol/l magnesium chloride, 50 mmol/l potassium chloride, 10 mmol/l Tris-HCl (pH8.4), 0.1 mg/dl gelatin, 10 pmol of each primer, 200 μmol of each dNTP and 1 unit Taq-DNA polymerase (Promega, Madison, WI, USA). Amplification was performed in a DNA thermal cycler 480 (Perkin-Elmer, Norwalk, CT, USA) involving 1 minute of denaturation at 94°C, 1 minute of annealing at 55°C and 2 minutes of extension at 72°C for 35 cycles. In the last cycle, the extension step was carried out for 10 minutes. Thereafter, 10 μl of amplified product was electrophoresed in a 2% agarose gel containing 0.5 μg/ml of ethidium bromide and was subsequently visually inspected under ultraviolet light for appropriately sized bands of DNA. The I allele manifested as a 490 bp band, and the D allele was seen as a 190 bp band of DNA. Besides, all DD genotype samples were confirmed using the primers: forward, 5'-TCGGACCACAGCGCCCGCCACTAC-3'; and reverse, 5'-TCGCCAGCCCTCCCATGCCCATAA-3' with identical PCR conditions except for an annealing temperature of 67°C, that produced a 335-bp product only in the presence of the I allele [22].

Data analysis

Patient age at diagnosis was recorded as a continuous variable and shown as mean ± standard deviation. The odds ratios (ORs) and corresponding 95% confidence intervals (CIs) for assessing the effect of the ACE I/D genotype distribution and allele frequencies on ACS were calculated by logistic regression analysis with adjustment for relevant significant variables. All the statistical analyses were performed using SPSS 16.0 and Excel 2007. For all statistical tests, p values were two-sided and the level of significance was set at 0.05.

Results

Risk factors for ACS

Comparisons of the distributions of demographic and relevant clinical risk factors between ACS patients and NCS controls and the estimated OR for each risk factor are listed in Table 1. Patients diagnosed as ACS were significantly older than control NCS (mean age 64.99 ± 13.85 years and 42.44 ± 11.91 years, respectively). ACS patients were also more likely to have higher systolic or diastolic blood pressure and diabetes mellitus than NCS. The groups were similar with respect to gender and body mass index. In the univariate logistic regression model, older age, higher systolic blood pressure or diastolic blood pressure and the presence of diabetes mellitus were found to be significant risk factors for ACS.

ACE DD genotype as an independent risk factor for ACS

Table 1 illustrates that ACS patients demonstrated a lower proportion of II genotypes (33.33%) and ID

Table 1 Univariate and multivariate analyses of ACS risk factors

Subject characteristics	ACS (n = 111)	NCS (n = 195)	Univariate		Multivariate	
			OR (95%CI)	p*	OR (95% CI)	P*
ACE-genotypes						
II	37	78	1 (ref.)		1 (ref.)	
ID	51	99	1.086 (0.648-1.821)	0.754	1.284 (0.595-2.773)	0.524
DD	23	18	**2.694 (1.298-5.592)**	**0.008**	**4.295 (1.436-12.851)**	**0.009**
Demographic factors						
Age	64.99 ± 13.85	42.44 ± 11.91	**1.127 (1.099-1.156)**	**< 0.001**	**1.114 (1.082-1.147)**	**< 0.001**
Sex -Female	25	60	1 (ref.)			
Male	86	135	1.529 (0.892-2.622)	0.123	-	-
Clinical risk factors						
BMI (kg/m^2) < 27	99	174	1.004 (0.474-2.128)	0.991	-	-
≥ 27	12	21				
Systolic blood pressure	73	181	1 (ref.)		1 (ref.)	
< 140 mmHg						
≥ 140 mmHg	38	14	**6.730 (3.443-13.156)**	**< 0.001**	1.765 (0.525-5.934)	0.358
Diastolic blood pressure	88	179	1 (ref.)		1 (ref.)	
< 90 mmHg						
≥ 90 mmHg	23	16	**2.924 (1.471-5.813)**	**0.002**	1.425 (0.497-4.089)	0.510
Diabetes Mellitus - No	75	187	1 (ref.)		1 (ref.)	
Yes	36	8	**11.220 (4.983-25.261)**	**< 0.001**	2.396 (0.869-6.610)	0.091

On the basis of logistic regression, with statistical significance (p < 0.05) shown in bold *ACS*: acute coronary syndrome, *NCS*: non-coronary subjects, *BMI*: body mass index

genotypes (45.95%) but higher proportions of DD genotypes (20.72%) than the control population (II, 40.00%; ID, 50.77%; DD, 9.23%). The ACE DD genotype conferred a 2.69-fold higher risk of ACS compared with the II genotype (95% CI: 1.298-5.592, p = 0.008, logistic regression). After controlling for other risk factors, the DD genotype was still significantly associated with ACS, conferring a 4-fold higher risk (OR = 4.295; 95% CI: 1.436-12.851). Age was the only other independent risk factor under multivariate logistic regression, which was in accordance with other studies [1,23].

ACE DD genotype associated with ACS type, severity and mortality

To further evaluate the etiologic effects of ACE I/D polymorphisms in ACS, we analyzed the association between ACE genotypes and different ACS manifestations (UAP and AMI), complications (hypertension, diabetes mellitus, hypercholesterolemia), relevant clinical risk factors (systolic blood pressure, diastolic blood pressure, total blood cholesterol and triglyceride and body mass index), clinical history (heart failure, CAD, MI and family history) and history of smoking. As shown in Table 2, the DD genotype conferred a significant 3.35-fold higher risk of AMI (Table 2, 95% CI: 1.111-10.115, p = 0.032, logistic regression), however there was no significant association between ACE I/D polymorphisms and any other risk factor among the recruited ACS group. A multivariate analysis was not performed as only ACS was significantly associated with ACE I/D polymorphisms. The foregoing results also supported previous studies that the ACE D allele was associated with higher ACE activity [7-9], converting more angiotensin II and thus stimulating inflammatory/fibrogenic responses and scar formation during myocardial infarction, or inducing reactive oxygen species to cause myocardial damage in the border zones and enlargement of the infarct size [24].

Subsequent analyses evaluated the possible influence of ACE I/D polymorphisms on final ACS clinical outcome, and the association between ACE I/D polymorphisms and ACS severity and mortality was determined. Interestingly, ACS patients with the DD genotype had a significantly higher risk of presenting with a greater number of stenosed vessels, with a 3.87-fold increased risk of stenosis in all three coronary arteries (Table 3, 95% CI: 1.085-13.812, p = 0.037, logistic regression). In addition, the DD genotype was also associated with a 3.08-fold higher risk of left anterior descending artery infarction (Table 3, 95% CI: 1.041-9.118, p = 0.042), and a 3.07-fold higher risk of anterior wall infarction (Table 3, 95% CI: 1.039-9.091, p = 0.043). Previous epidemiological data showed that an anterior wall myocardial infarction is usually caused by an occlusion of the left anterior descending coronary artery [25,26], and the DD genotype is highly associated with those ACS symptoms. We also found that the DD genotype was independently associated with sudden cardiac death (Table 4, OR = 6.484, 95% CI: 1.036-40.598, p = 0.046, logistic regression). This effect seemed more obvious in AMI patients (sudden cardiac death in AMI patients: genotype II = 2, ID = 2, DD = 5; and in UAP patients: genotype II = 0, ID = 2, DD = 1), but there was no statistical significance between ACE I/D polymorphism and sudden cardiac death across the ACS spectrum. A history of heart failure also conferred a 9.69-fold increased risk of sudden cardiac death which was similar to that found in previous epidemiological studies [4,5].

Discussion

The renin-angiotensin system (RAS) has been recognized for many years as a critical pathway for blood pressure control and kidney function [27]. This 5-year period emergency room-based study clearly demonstrates that the ACE DD genotype acts as an independent risk factor for ACS requiring emergency treatment (Table 1), and in particular for AMI (Table 2). In addition, the ACE DD genotype is also associated with greater ACS severity, including more stenosed vessels greater occlusion of the left anterior descending branch and a greater risk of anterior wall myocardial infarction (Table 3) and also of sudden cardiac death (Table 4).

The ACE DD genotype was reported to be associated with CAD risk in several studies including ECTIM [7], INSERM [8], ISIS [10] and CORGENE [28] cohorts, and subsequent studies revealed that the D allele or DD genotype may confer effects mainly on the onset of ACS or MI [29] by modifying ACE abundance or activity, and contributing to increases in plaque instability, ulceration and thrombosis [30]. The ACE D allele was correlated with an increase in serum or cardiac ACE, thus increasing the conversion of angiotensin I to the peptide precursor angiotensin II which induces aldosterone production [7-9]. Elevation of circulating aldosterone increases the risk of arterial hypertension and cardiac fibrosis thus inducing diastolic dysfunction, ventricular remodeling and even atherosclerosis [31]. Similar results were also found in this case-control study, with DD genotype carriers having about a four-fold higher risk of ACS than ID or II genotype carriers. In addition, age of diagnosis, systolic blood pressure, diastolic blood pressure and diabetes mellitus were also identified as ACS risk factors in univariate analyses, though only the ACE DD genotype and age of diagnosis were found to be independent risk factors. Older age is a well-documented risk factor for CAD or its manifestation as ACS [1,23], and the ACE DD genotype or D allele had been found in most studies to be a risk factor for CAD or ACS [12,28,29]. Within the ACS groups, we also compared disease type, complications,

Table 2 Association between ACE I/D polymorphisms and ACS risk factors

ACE genotypes	II (n = 37)		ID (n = 51)			DD (n = 23)		
ACS risk factors				Univariate			Univariate	
	n		n	OR (95%CI)	p*	n	OR (95%CI)	p*
ACS spectrum								
UAP (n = 57)	22	1 (ref.)	28			7		
AMI (n = 54)	15		23	1.205 (0.511-2.839)	0.670	16	**3.352 (1.111-10.115)**	**0.032**
Demographic factors								
Age (mean)	67.7 ± 11.1	1 (ref.)	64.2 ± 13.5	0.981 (0.949-1.013)	0.232	62.4 ± 18.1	0.972 (0.935-1.010)	0.149
Sex -female	10	1 (ref.)	8			7		
male	27		43	2.352 (0.733-7.543)	0.150	16	1.181 (0.375-3.719)	0.776
Complications								
Hypertension- No	10	1 (ref.)	20			11		
- Yes	27		31	0.574 (0.229-1.437)	0.236	12	0.404 (0.135-1.206)	0.104
Diabetes Mellitus-No	25	1 (ref.)	33			17		
- Yes	12		18	0.880 (0.359-2.157)	0.780	6	1.360 (0.427-4.328)	0.603
Hypercholesterolemia-No	31	1 (ref.)	39			19		
- Yes	6		12	0.629 (0.212-1.866)	0.403	4	0.919 (0.229-3.684)	0.905
Other clinical risk factors								
Systolic blood pressure	22	1 (ref.)	38			13		
< 140 mmHg								
≥ 140 mmHg	15		13	0.502 (0.202-1.246)	0.137	10	1.128 (0.393-3.236)	0.822
Diastolic blood pressure	27	1 (ref.)	45			16		
< 90 mmHg								
≥ 90 mmHg	10		6	0.360 (0.118-1.102)	0.074	7	1.181 (0.375-3.719)	0.776
Total cholesterol < 200 mg/dl	31	1 (ref.)	46			17		
≥ 200 mg/dl	6		5	0.562 (0.158-2.002)	0.374	6	1.824 (0.509-6.538)	0.356
Triglyceride < 150 mg/dl	34	1(ref.)	42			17		
≥ 150 mg/dl	3		9	1.768 (0.500-6.251)	0.377	6	2.912 (0.722-11.736)	0.133
BMI (kg/m^2) < 27	35	1 (ref.)	43			21		
≥ 27	2		8	3.256 (0.649-16.328)	0.151	2	1.667 (0.218-12.732)	0.622
History								
Heart failure history-No	29	1 (ref.)	41			16		
-Yes	8		10	0.884 (0.311-2.512)	0.817	7	1.586 (0.485-5.181)	0.445
CAD history -No	22	1 (ref.)	32			17		
-Yes	15		19	0.871 (0.366-2.074)	0.755	6	0.518 (0.166-1.617)	0.257
MI history -No	34	1 (ref.)	46			21		
-Yes	3		5	1.232 (0.275-5.512)	0.785	2	1.079 (0.166-7.004)	0.936
Family history of ACS	35	1 (ref.)	50			22		
-Yes	2		1	0.350 (0.031-4.012)	0.399	1	0.795 (0.068-9.301)	0.855
Smoking	20	1 (ref.)	29			11		
-Yes	17		22	0.892 (0.381-2.091)	0.793	12	1.283 (0.452-3.641)	0.639

On the basis of logistic regression, with statistical significance ($p < 0.05$) shown in bold. Multivariate analyses were not performed as only the DD genotype was significantly associated with AMI

ACE, angiotensin converting enzyme, *UAP*: unstable angina pectoris; *AMI*: acute myocardial infarction, *CAD*: coronary artery disease; *MI*: myocardial infarction.

clinical history, and other relevant clinical risk factors. Interestingly, only the ACE DD genotype conferred about 3-fold risk for AMI compared with UAP and this result was also similar to most studies in different population or study cohorts [32], although some studies found no association [14,25]. There was no significance between any other analyzed risk factor and ACE I/D polymorphisms; even though DD genotype had been

Table 3 Association between ACE I/D polymorphisms and ACS clinical severity

ACE genotypes	II (n = 37)		ID (n = 51)			DD (n = 23)		
Clinical symptoms				**Univariate**			**Univariate**	
	n		**n**	**OR (95%CI)**	**p***	**n**	**OR (95%CI)**	**p***
Stenosis numbers								
0 or 1 vessel	19	1 (ref.)	20			6		
2 vessels	9		12	1.267 (0.435-3.686)	0.665	6	2.006 (0.729-5.515)	0.178
3 vessels	9		19	2.111 (0.530-8.407)	0.289	11	**3.870 (1.085-13.812)**	**0.037**
Infarcted artery (yes vs. no)								
left anterior descending -No	23	1(ref)	22			8		
-Yes	14		29	2.166 (0.912-5.144)	0.080	15	**3.080 (1.041-9.118)**	**0.042**
left circumflex -No	21	1(ref)	24			14		
-Yes	16		27	1.477 (0.630-3.460)	0.370	9	0.844 (0.292-2.436)	0.753
right coronary -No	17	1(ref)	21			12		
-Yes	20		29	1.174 (0.498-2.764)	0.714	11	0.779 (0.275-2.211)	0.639
Infarction locus (yes vs. no)								
anterior wall -No	26	1(ref)	39			10		
-Yes	11		12	0.727 (0.279-1.893)	0.514	13	**3.073 (1.039-9.091)**	**0.043**
inferior wall -No	34	1(ref)	42			19		
-Yes	3		9	2.429 (0.609-9.679)	0.208	4	2.386 (0.482-11.803)	0.286
right ventricle myocardial -No	36	1(ref)	48			22		
-Yes	1		3	2.250 (0.225-22.533)	0.490	1	1.636 (0.097-27.511)	0.732
others -No	35	1(ref)	50			22		
-Yes	2		1	0.350 (0.031-4.012)	0.399	1	0.795 (0.068-9.301)	0.855

* On the basis of logistic regression, with statistical significance ($p < 0.05$) shown in bold.

reported to be associated with hypertension [33] and/or diabetes mellitus [34]. Patients with the ACE DD genotype appeared to have earlier onset of ACS, with a younger mean age than ID or II carriers, but there was no statistical significance among those groups (analysis of variance p = 0.307).

Although ACE I/D polymorphisms have been comprehensively studied in CAD or ACS, there are only a few studies addressing the clinical significance of ACE genotypes on the severity of coronary lesions. In this emergency room-based, case-control study, we enrolled the most urgent ACS cases who required immediate treatment, and we found that DD genotype carriers were likely to have the most severe ACS, including stenosis in all three coronary arteries, left anterior descending artery infarction and also anterior wall infarction (Table 3). Similarly, a previous study found that DD genotype carriers had a greater number of stenosed arteries and/or dangerous infarction loci [26].

Finally, we focused this study on the effects of ACE I/D polymorphisms on sudden cardiac death within 24 hours of the ACS patients being registered in the emergency room. ACE DD genotype carriers also had a higher mortality risk than ID or II carriers. Genetic polymorphisms in ACE-related genes have been associated with risk of MI-related sudden cardiac arrest [18], and the ACE DD genotype was found to confer an increased risk of diastolic heart failure [19,33], ACS recurrence and cardiovascular mortality [19], although controversial and negative [12,17] results have also been reported.

Polymorphisms of ACE and its related genes have also been highly associated with the efficiency of ACE inhibitor treatment and the role of ACE I/D polymorphisms are particularly well documented [35,36].

Conclusions

In summary, this case-control study has demonstrated that the ACE DD genotype is an independent risk factor for ACS incidence, and especially for AMI. In addition, the ACE DD genotype is associated with greater ACS severity and greater risk of sudden cardiac death. This emergency room experience of patients requiring urgent ACS treatment suggests that ACE DD genotype carriers should be followed-up and treated especially carefully because of the higher relative risk of more severe ACS and sudden cardiac death. Further studies are necessary to evaluate the personal pharmacogenomic and pharmacogenetic effects of ACE I/D polymorphisms to improve ACS therapeutic strategies and prognosis.

Table 4 Association between ACE I/D polymorphisms and ACS sudden cardiac death

Subject characteristics	Survival	Expired	Univariate		Multivariate	
	(n = 99)	(n = 12)	OR (95%CI)	p*	OR (95% CI)	p*
ACE-genotypes						
II	35	2	1 (ref.)		1 (ref.)	
ID	47	4	1.489 (0.258-8.595)	0.656	1.659 (0.264-10.427)	0.589
DD	17	6	**6.176 (1.126-33.876)**	**0.036**	**6.484 (1.036-40.598)**	**0.046**
ACS spectrum						
UAP (n = 57)	54	3	1 (ref.)			
AMI (n = 54)	45	9	3.600 (0.919-14.100)	0.066		
Demographic factors						
Age	65.02 ± 13.40	64.85 ± 17.90	0.999 (0.956-1.043)	0.949	-	-
Sex -Female	21	4	1 (ref.)			
Male	78	8	1.857 (0.510-6.769)	0.348	-	-
Complications						
Hypertension- No	36	5	1 (ref.)		-	-
- Yes	63	7	0.800 (0.237-2.706)	0.720		
Diabetes Mellitus-No	68	7	1 (ref.)		-	-
- Yes	31	5	1.567 (0.461-5.327)	0.472		
Hypercholesterolemia-No	78	11			-	-
- Yes	21	1	0.338 (0.041-2.766)	0.312		
Other clinical risk factors						
Systolic blood pressure	67	6	1(ref.)		-	-
< 140 mmHg						
≥ 140 mmHg	32	6	2.094 (0.626-7.003)	0.230		
Diastolic blood pressure	78	10	1 (ref.)		-	-
< 90 mmHg						
≥ 90 mmHg	21	2	0.743 (0.151-3.653)	0.715		
Total cholesterol	83	11	1 (ref.)	-	-	
< 200 mg/dl						
≥ 200 mg/dl	16	1	0.472 (0.057-3.913)	0.486		
Triglyceride < 150 mg/dl	81	11	1 (ref.)	-	-	
≥ 150 mg/dl	18	1	0.409 (0.050-3.374)	0.406		
BMI (kg/m^2) < 27	88	11	1 (ref.)	-	-	
≥ 27	11	1	0.727 (0.085-6.187)	0.771		
History						
Heart failure history-No	82	4	1 (ref.)			
-Yes	17	8	**9.647 (2.606-35.716)**	**0.001**	**9.698 (2.468-38.106)**	**0.001**
CAD history -No	63	8	1 (ref.)	-	-	
-Yes	36	4	0.875 (0.246-3.110)	0.836		
MI history -No	91	10	1 (ref.)	-	-	
-Yes	8	2	2.275 (0.423-12.224)	0.338		
Family history of ACS	96	11	1 (ref.)	-	-	
-Yes	3	1	2.909 (0.278-30.430)	0.373		
Smoking	53	7	1 (ref.)	-	-	
-Yes	46	5	0.823 (0.245-2.770)	0.753		

*On the basis of logistic regression, with statistical significance ($p < 0.05$) shown in bold.

Acknowledgements
This work was supported by the National Science Council (NSC 88-2314-B-016-062, NSC100-2320-B-016-010-) and the Tri-Service General Hospital (TSGH-C98-04, TSGH-C99-004, TSGH-C100-003, and TSGH-C101-003).

Author details
[1]Institute of Medical Sciences, Tzu-Chi University, Hualien, Taiwan. [2]Department of Emergency Medicine, Tri-Service General Hospital, National Defense Medical Center, Taipei, Taiwan. [3]Division of Urology, Department of Surgery, Chang Gung Memorial Hospital and Graduate Institute of Clinical Medical Sciences, Taoyuan, Taiwan. [4]Department of Pathology, and Graduate Institute of Pathology and Parasitology, Tri-Service General Hospital, National Defense Medical Center, Taipei, Taiwan. [5]Biobank Management Center of Tri-Service General Hospital, National Defense Medical Center, Taipei, Taiwan. [6]Department of Emergency Medicine, Buddhist Tzu-Chi General Hospital, Tzu-Chi University, Hualien, Taiwan. [7]Department of Pathology, China Medical University Hospital, China Medical University, Taichung, Taiwan. [8]Tzu-Chi Stem Cell Centre, Buddhist Tzu-Chi General Hospital, Hualien, Taiwan. [9]Division of Cardiology, Buddhist Tzu-Chi General Hospital, Tzu-Chi University, Hualien, Taiwan. [10]Graduate Institutes of Life Sciences, National Defense Medical Center, Taipei, Taiwan. [11]Department of Pathology, Tri-Service General Hospital, 114 No.161, Sec. 6, Minquan E. Rd, Neihu Dist, Taipei City 114, Taiwan.

Authors' contributions
YHC, JML and RJH designed the research plan and study. YHC, JYH, RJH, SCH and CLW carried out all experiments. HJH and YHC provided clinical specimens. JYH, RJH and CPY drafted and edited the manuscript. All authors read and approved the final manuscript.

Competing interests
The authors declare that they have no competing interests.

References

1. Ruff CT, Braunwald E: **The evolving epidemiology of acute coronary syndromes.** *Nat Rev Cardiol* 2011, **8**:140-147.
2. Yusuf S, Reddy S, Ounpuu S, Anand S: **Global burden of cardiovascular diseases: part I: general considerations, the epidemiologic transition, risk factors, and impact of urbanization.** *Circulation* 2001, **104**:2746-2753.
3. In *Global Burden of Disease and Risk Factors.* Edited by: Lopez AD, Mathers CD, Ezzati M, Jamison DT, Murray CJ. New York: Oxford University Press and The World Bank; 2006.
4. Friedlander Y, Siscovick DS, Arbogast P, Psaty BM, Weinmann S, Lemaitre RN, *et al*: **Sudden death and myocardial infarction in first degree relatives as predictors of primary cardiac arrest.** *Atherosclerosis* 2002, **162**:211-216.
5. Antman EM: **General hospital management.** In *Management of acute myocardial infarction.* Edited by: Julian D, Braunwald E. London: W.B. Saunders; 1994:29-70.
6. Ganz P, Ganz W: **Coronary blood flow and myocardial ischemi.** In *Braunwald's heart disease: a textbook of cardiovascular medicine.* 6 edition. Edited by: Braunwald E, Zipes DP, Libby P. Philadelphia: Saunders Elsevier; 2001:1118-1144.
7. Rigat B, Hubert C, Alhenc-Gelas F, Cambien F, Corvol P, Soubrier F: **An insertion/deletion polymorphism in the angiotensin I-converting enzyme gene accounting for half the variance of serum enzyme levels.** *J Clin Invest* 1990, **86**:1343-1346.
8. Tiret L, Rigat B, Visvikis S, Breda C, Corvol P, Cambien F, *et al*: **Evidence, from combined segregation and linkage analysis, that a variant of the angiotensin I-converting enzyme (ACE) gene controls plasma ACE levels.** *Am J Hum Genet* 1992, **51**:197-205.
9. Danser AHJ, Schalekamp MADH, Bax WA, Van den-Brink AM, Saxena PR, Riegger GAJ, *et al*: **Angiotensin-converting enzyme in the human heart: effect of the deletion/insertion polymorphism.** *Circulation* 1995, **92**:1387-1388.
10. Keavney B, McKenzie C, Parish S, Palmer A, Clark S, Youngman L, *et al*: **Large-scale test of hypothesised associations between the angiotensin-converting-enzyme insertion/deletion polymorphism and myocardial infarction in about 5000 cases and 6000 controls. International Studies of Infarct Survival (ISIS) Collaborators.** *Lancet* 2000, **355(9202)**:434-442.
11. Køber L, Torp-Pedersen C, Carlsen JE, Bagger H, Eliasen P, Lyngborg K, *et al*: **A clinical trial of the angiotensin-converting-enzyme inhibitor trandolapril in patients with left ventricular dysfunction after myocardial infarction. Trandolapril Cardiac Evaluation (TRACE) Study Group.** *N Engl J Med* 1995, **333(25)**:1670-1676.
12. Zintzaras E, Raman G, Kitsios G, Lau J: **Angiotensin-converting enzyme insertion/deletion gene polymorphic variant as a marker of coronary artery disease: a metaanalysis.** *Arch Intern Med* 2008, **168**:1077-1089.
13. Harn HJ, Chang CY, Ho LI, Liu CA, Jeng JR, Lin FG, *et al*: **Evidence that polymorphism of the angiotensin I converting enzyme enzyme gene may be raleted to idiopathic dilated cardiomyopathy in the Chinese population.** *Biochem Mol boil Int* 1995, **35**:1175-1181.
14. Lindpaintner K, Pfeller A, Kreutz R, Stampfer MJ, Grodstein F, LaMotte F, *et al*: **A prospective evluation of an angiotensin-converting-enzyme gene polymorpohism and the risk of ischemic heart disease.** *N Engl J Med* 1995, **332**:706-711.
15. Samani NJ, Martin DS, Brack M, Cullen J, Chauhan A, Lodwich D, *et al*: **Insertion/deletion polymorphism in the angiotensin-converting enzyme gene and risk of restenosis after coronary angioplasty.** *Lancet* 1995, **345**:1013-1016.
16. Zee RYL, Solomon SD, Ajani UA, Pfeffer MA, Lindpaintner K: **A prospective evaluation of the angiotensin-converting enzyme D/I polymorphism and left ventricular remodeling in the 'Healing and Early Afterload Reducing Therapy' Study.** *Clin Genet* 2002, **61**:21-25.
17. Keavney B, McKenzie C, Parish S, Palmer A, Clark S, Youngman L, *et al*: **International Studies of Infarct Survival (ISIS) Collaborators. Large-scale test of hypothesized associations between the angiotensin-converting-enzyme insertion/deletion polymorphism and myocardial infarction in about 5000 cases and 6000 controls.** *Lancet* 2000, **355**:434-442.
18. Sotoodehnia N, Li G, Johnson CO, Lemaitre RN, Rice KM, Rea TD, Siscovick DS: **Genetic variation in angiotensin-converting enzyme-related pathways associated with sudden cardiac arrest risk.** *Heart Rhythm* 2009, **6**:1306-1314.
19. Wu CK, Luo JL, Wu XM, Tsai CT, Lin JW, Hwang JJ, *et al*: **A propensity score-based case-control study of renin-angiotensin system gene polymorphisms and diastolic heart failure.** *Atherosclerosis* 2009, **205**:497-502.
20. American Heart Association: **Committee Report: a reporting system on patients evaluated for coronary artery disease.** *Circulation* 1975, **51**:7.
21. Trost JC, Lange RA: **Treatment of acute coronary syndrome: Part 1: Non-ST-segment acute coronary syndrome.** *Crit Care Med* 2011, **39**:2346-2353.
22. Namazi S, Monabati A, Ardeshir-Rouhani-Fard S, Azarpira N: **Association of angiotensin I converting enzyme (insertion/deletion) and angiotensin II type 1 receptor (A1166C) polymorphisms with breast cancer prognostic factors in Iranian population.** *Mol Carcinog* 2010, **49**:1022-1030.
23. Lau JF, Weinberg MD, Olin JW: **Peripheral artery disease. Part 1: clinical evaluation and noninvasive diagnosis.** *Nat Rev Cardiol* 2011, **8**:405-418.
24. Yao S: **Myocardial repair/remodeling following infarction: roles of local factors.** *Cardiovasc Res* 2009, **81**:482-490.
25. Pfohl M, Koch M, Prescod S, Haase KK, Häring HU, Karsch KR: **Angiotensin I converting enzyme gene polymorphism, coronary artery disease and myocardial infarction. An angiographically controlled study.** *Eur Heart J* 1999, **20**:1318-1325.
26. Linhart A, Sedlácek K, Jáchymová M, Jindra A, Beran S, Vondrácek V, *et al*: **Lack of association of angiotensin-converting enzyme and angiotensinogen genes polymorphisms with left ventricular structure in young normotensive men.** *Blood Press* 2000, **9**:47-51.
27. Zucker IH, Zimmerman MC: **The renin-angiotensin system in 2011: new avenues for translational research.** *Curr Opin Pharmacol* 2011, **11**:101-104.
28. Jeunemaitre X, Ledru F, Battaglia S, Guillanneuf MT, Courbon D, Dumont C, *et al*: **Genetic polymorphisms of the renin-angiotensin system and angiographic extent and severity of coronary artery disease: the CORGENE study.** *Hum Genet* 1997, **99**:66-73.
29. Vaisi-Raygani A, Ghaneialvar H, Rahimi Z, Nomani H, Saidi M, Bahrehmand F, *et al*: **The angiotensin converting enzyme D allele is an independent risk factor for early onset coronary artery disease.** *Clin Biochem* 2010, **43**:1189-1194.
30. Igić R, Behnia R: **Properties and distribution of angiotensin I converting enzyme.** *Curr Pharm Des* 2003, **9**:697-706.

31. Yang Q, Khoury MJ: **Evolving methods in genetic epidemiology III. Gene-environment interaction in epidemiologic research.** *Epidemiol Rev* 1997, **19**:33-43.
32. Parenica J, Goldbergova MP, Kala P, Jarkovsky J, Poloczek M, Manousek J, *et al*: **ACE gene insertion/deletion polymorphism has a mild influence on the acute development of left ventricular dysfunction in patients with ST elevation myocardial infarction treated with primary PCI.** *BMC Cardiovasc Disord* 2010, **10**:60.
33. Mondry A, Loh M, Liu P, Zhu AL, Nagel M: **Polymorphisms of the insertion/deletion ACE and M235T AGT genes and hypertension: surprising new findings and meta-analysis of data.** *BMC Nephrol* 2005, **6**:1.
34. Niu W, Qi Y, Gao P, Zhu D: **Angiotensin converting enzyme D allele is associated with an increased risk of type 2 diabetes: evidence from a meta-analysis.** *Endocr J* 2010, **57**:431-438.
35. Scharplatz M, Puhan MA, Steurer J, Bachmann LM: **What is the impact of the ACE gene insertion/deletion (I/D) polymorphism on the clinical effectiveness and adverse events of ACE inhibitors?-Protocol of a systematic review.** *BMC Med Genet* 2004, **5**:23.
36. Kessels AG, Severens JL: **Cost-effectiveness of pharmacogenetic testing to predict treatment response to angiotensin-converting enzyme inhibitor.** *Pharmacogenet Genomics* 2007, **17**:359-368.

2

Association between the docosahexaenoic acid to arachidonic acid ratio and acute coronary syndrome

Yuji Nishizaki[1], Kazunori Shimada[1], Shigemasa Tani[2], Takayuki Ogawa[3], Jiro Ando[4], Masao Takahashi[4], Masato Yamamoto[5], Tomohiro Shinozaki[6], Tetsuro Miyazaki[1], Katsumi Miyauchi[1], Ken Nagao[2], Atsushi Hirayama[7], Michihiro Yoshimura[3], Issei Komuro[4], Ryozo Nagai[8] and Hiroyuki Daida[1*]

Abstract

Background: A low eicosapentaenoic acid (EPA) to arachidonic acid (AA) ratio is a known risk for acute coronary syndrome (ACS). However, the association between the docosahexaenoic acid (DHA) to AA ratio and ACS remains unclear. This study aimed to assess the association between the DHA/AA ratio and ACS by patient characteristics.

Methods: We enrolled 1733 patients and evaluated the serum levels of polyunsaturated fatty acids in 5 cardiology departments in a metropolitan area of Japan. We assessed the relationship between the DHA/AA ratio (median cut-off value: 0.903) and ACS according to the following 10 subgroups: sex, age, diabetes mellitus, hypertension, dyslipidemia, smoking history, family history of ischemic heart disease, chronic kidney disease, obesity, and history of coronary revascularization.

Results: Interaction tests in the 10 subgroup analyses revealed a significant difference for adjusted log odds ratios between male and females ($p = 0.01$), and those with and without hypertension ($p = 0.06$). Especially in the subgroup based on sex difference, a high DHA/AA ratio was significantly associated with a low risk of ACS among men (adjusted odds ratio = 0.389; 95 % confidence interval: 0.211–0.716). In contrast, a reverse association was found among women, although this was not statistically significant (adjusted odds ratio = 3.820; 95 % confidence interval: 0.718–20.325).

Conclusions: The association between the DHA/AA ratio and ACS differed by clinical characteristic. Notably, patients with a low DHA/AA ratio had a higher risk of ACS than those with a high DHA/AA ratio, and this was significant for men in particular.

Keywords: Acute coronary syndrome, Arachidonic acid, Docosahexaenoic acid, Eicosapentaenoic acid, DHA/AA ratio, EPA/AA ratio, Polyunsaturated fatty acids

* Correspondence: daida@juntendo.ac.jp
[1]Department of Cardiology, Juntendo University Graduate School of Medicine, 2-1-1 Hongo Bunkyo-ku, Tokyo 113-8421, Japan
Full list of author information is available at the end of the article

Background

Previous studies have demonstrated the beneficial effect of omega-3 polyunsaturated fatty acids (PUFAs) for preventing coronary events [1, 2]. In particular, several studies have reported that the eicosapentaenoic acid (EPA) to arachidonic acid (AA) ratio is a useful marker for estimating the risk of coronary events [3–5]. We recently reported that a low EPA/AA ratio was significantly associated with acute coronary syndrome (ACS) in a cohort of 1119 participants without any history of coronary revascularization or myocardial infarction [6]. However, the association between the docosahexaenoic acid (DHA) to AA ratio and coronary artery disease (CAD), particularly ACS, remains unclear. Although EPA and DHA are both omega-3 PUFAs, each may have different physiological and pharmacological effects [7]. We hypothesized that the effect of DHA/AA ratio for ACS could differ by patient characteristics, and that this difference might attenuate the association between the DHA/AA ratio and ACS when conducting analyses by ignoring the statistical interaction of the characteristics.

Methods

Study population

The present study was a multicenter observational cross-sectional study performed at four university hospitals and one community hospital located in Tokyo, Japan [6]. We enrolled 1733 patients who had their serum PUFA levels evaluated at these five centers from January 2004 to May 2011. The cohort included 151 patients with ACS and 1582 patients without ACS. Acute myocardial infarction was defined as an increase in the creatine kinase MB fraction or troponin T in patients with ischemic symptoms and/or typical electrocardiographic ST elevation. Unstable angina was defined as angina at rest or accelerated exertional angina combined with typical electrocardiographic ST-changes and an increased requirement for anti-ischemic therapy [8]. Patients were excluded if they were receiving hemodialysis or were currently taking EPA, and if they had concomitant congestive heart failure, severe liver dysfunction, or other systemic diseases, including malignancy and collagen disease. This study was approved by the Institutional Ethics Committees of each hospital, and all subjects gave informed consent.

Measurements

We assessed the coronary risk factors and evaluated serum EPA, DHA, dihomo-gamma-linolenic acid (DGLA), and AA levels. We also measured the following laboratory parameters: total cholesterol, triglycerides (TG), low-density lipoprotein (LDL)-cholesterol, high-density lipoprotein (HDL)-cholesterol, hemoglobin A1c, serum creatinine (Cr), and estimated glomerular filtration rate (eGFR). The eGFR was calculated on the basis of the Japanese equation that utilizes serum Cr, age, and sex, as follows: $\text{eGFR (ml/min/1.73 m}^2) = 194 \times \text{Cr}^{-1.094} \times \text{age}^{-0.287}$ (female × 0.739) [9]. Serum EPA, DHA, DGLA, and AA levels were measured at an external laboratory (SRL, Inc., Tokyo, Japan). Blood samples were obtained from patients either during admission or at the laboratory of the outpatient clinic.

Statistical analyses

We assessed the relationship between the DHA/AA ratio (at a median cut-off value of 0.903) and ACS in 10 different subgroups as follows: sex, age, diabetes mellitus (DM), hypertension (HT), dyslipidemia (DL), smoking history, family history of ischemic heart disease (IHD), chronic kidney disease (CKD), obesity defined as body mass index (BMI) ≥25, and history of coronary revascularization (percutaneous coronary intervention or coronary artery bypass grafting). To adjust for clinical characteristics other than the stratification variable for each subgroup, we fitted multivariable logistic regression models that included the following variables: age, BMI, serum Cr (continuous covariates), sex, smoking history, family history of IHD, HT, DM, or DL, a history of coronary revascularization (binary covariates), and the EPA/AA ratio. The EPA/AA ratio was divided into three tertiles for the present study, in line with our previous report that analyzed data extracted from the same study population [6]. Patients with missing data for any variable were excluded from the multivariable analysis. The alpha level for statistical tests was set at 0.05 and all confidence intervals were presented with their 95 % confidence levels.

The differences in associations (adjusted log odds ratios) between DHA/AA ratio and ACS from different subgroups were evaluated by the approximate formula for testing interaction [10]. Because of the limited power of the interaction test [11] and its nature as a preliminary test for statistical modeling [12], we considered a significance level of 0.10 to reflect a significant difference between subgroups. All analyses were performed with SAS version 9.2 (Cary, NC, USA).

Results

Tables 1 shows the clinical characteristics and laboratory data for all patients by high and low DHA/AA ratios (≥0.903 and <0.903, respectively). Among the high DHA/AA ratio group ($n = 867$), the incidence of ACS was 7.50 % (65/867), compared with 9.93 % (86/866) in the low DHA/AA ratio group ($n = 866$). The crude odds ratio for ACS was 0.735 [95 % confidence interval (CI): 0.525, 1.030, $p = 0.07$] based on a DHA/AA ratio ≥0.903 versus <0.903. The adjusted odds ratio from the multivariable

Table 1 Baseline clinical characteristics and laboratory data

	All patients ($n = 1733$)	High DHA/AA ≥0.903 ($n = 867$)	Low DHA/AA <0.903 ($n = 866$)	P-value
Age (years)	64.5 ± 11.3	67.1 ± 9.2	61.8 ± 12.5	<0.01[a]
Male	77.8 %	79.4 %	76.2 %	0.11
Body mass index (kg/m^2)	24.4 ± 3.5	24.4 ± 3.1	24.4 ± 3.8	0.97
Hypertension	73.1 %	75.7 %	70.6 %	0.01[a]
Diabetes mellitus	39.2 %	39.8 %	38.7 %	0.63
Dyslipidemia	70.4 %	70.6 %	70.2 %	0.86
Family history of ischemic heart disease	18.5 %	19.1 %	17.9 %	0.50
Smoking	45.1 %	47.6 %	42.5 %	0.03[a]
History of coronary revascularization (PCI or CABG)	27.7 %	26.8 %	28.6 %	0.38
Total cholesterol (mg/dl)	190.7 ± 35.8	190.7 ± 34.2	190.7 ± 37.4	0.98
Triglycerides (mg/dl)	146.8 ± 95.5	155.4 ± 100.2	138.4 ± 90.1	<0.01[a]
Low-density lipoprotein cholesterol (mg/dl)	111.2 ± 30.8	111.1 ± 29.9	111.2 ± 31.8	0.94
High-density lipoprotein cholesterol (mg/dl)	51.7 ± 16.5	50.0 ± 15.1	53.4 ± 17.6	<0.01[a]
Hemoglobin A1c (%)	6.3 ± 1.1	6.2 ± 0.9	6.3 ± 1.2	0.44
Serum creatinine (mg/dl)	0.88 ± 0.29	0.88 ± 0.27	0.87 ± 0.31	0.41
Estimated glomerular filtration rate (ml/min/1.73 m^2)	68.7 ± 17.7	67.0 ± 16.4	70.2 ± 18.7	<0.01[a]
EPA (μg/dl)	73.9 ± 44.0	93.5 ± 47.9	54.2 ± 28.5	<0.01[a]
EPA/AA				<0.01[a]
Mean	0.49 ± 0.30	0.66 ± 0.32	0.32 ± 0.17	
Median	0.425	0.588	0.290	
DHA (μg/dl)	143.4 ± 52.8	170.9 ± 53.0	115.9 ± 35.3	<0.01[a]
DHA/AA				<0.01[a]
Mean	0.95 ± 0.38	1.22 ± 0.36	0.68 ± 0.15	
Median	0.903	1.143	0.706	
DGLA (μg/dl)	33.2 ± 12.3	30.8 ± 11.5	35.6 ± 12.6	<0.01[a]
AA (μg/dl)	157.4 ± 49.5	142.1 ± 33.8	172.8 ± 57.4	<0.01[a]
Statins	53.1 %	48.7 %	57.5 %	<0.01[a]
Antiplatelet agents	62.7 %	67.5 %	58.0 %	<0.01[a]
Renin angiotensin system inhibitor (ACE-I and ARB)	50.7 %	50.1 %	51.4 %	0.59
Calcium channel blockers	45.6 %	47.8 %	43.5 %	0.08
Beta blockers	38.6 %	39.6 %	37.6 %	0.43
Hypoglycemic agents	21.1 %	21.0 %	21.1 %	0.95

Values are mean ± standard deviation, or percentage, [a]indicates statistical signficance, PCI = Percutaneous coronary intervention, *CABG* coronary artery bypass grafting, *EPA/AA* eicosapentaenoic acid to arachidonic acid ratio, *DHA/AA* docosahexaenoic acid to arachidonic acid ratio, *DGLA* dihomo-gamma-linolenic acid, *ACE-I* angiotensin converting enzyme inhibitor, *ARB* angiotensin II receptor blocker

logistic model including all variables as regression covariates was 0.523 (95 % CI: 0.300, 0.910, $p = 0.022$).

In the high DHA/AA ratio group, the patient age, TG levels, and the prevalence of HT and smoking were significantly higher than in the low DHA/AA ratio group, whereas, the opposite was found in these groups regarding the HDL-cholesterol levels. In addition, the use of statins was significantly lower, and the use of antiplatelet agents was significantly higher in the high DHA/AA ratio group than in the low DHA/AA ratio group.

Serum AA level was significantly higher in patients with statin treatment than in patients without statin treatment (160.3 ± 40.9 vs. 154.1 ± 57.6 μg/dl, P = 0.01). Conversely, serum AA level was significantly lower in patients with antiplatelet agent treatment (152.5 ± 38.4 vs. 165.7 ± 63.2 μg/dl, $P < 0.01$), beta blocker treatment (152.9 ± 39.6 vs. 160.3 ± 54.7 μg/dl, $P < 0.01$), and hypoglycemic agent treatment (151.9 ± 40.1 vs. 158.9 ± 51.7 μg/dl, $P = 0.01$) than in patients without these treatments.

Table 2 shows the baseline clinical characteristics according to gender. The patient age, the levels of total cholesterol, LDL-cholesterol, and HDL-cholesterol were significantly higher in the female group than in the male group. The prevalence of DM, smoking, and family history of CAD as well as the use of antiplatelet agents and beta blockers was significantly lower in the female group than in the male group. The levels of BMI, TG, hemoglobin A1c, and Cr were significantly lower in the high DHA/AA ratio group than in the low DHA/AA ratio group.

Table 3 shows the relationship between the DHA/AA ratio (≥0.903/<0.903) and ACS in the various subgroups. From interaction tests in 10 different subgroup analyses, the most significant difference in the adjusted log odds ratios was between men and women ($p = 0.01$), followed by the difference between those with and without HT ($p = 0.06$). A high DHA/AA ratio was significantly associated with a low risk of ACS among men in particular (adjusted odds ratio = 0.389; 95 % CI: 0.211–0.716), whereas it was associated with a high risk of ACS in women, although this latter result was not statistically significant (adjusted odds ratio = 3.820; 95 % CI: 0.718–20.325). These associations were in opposite directions, but of similar magnitude (i.e., 1/0.389 = 2.57). In all of the other groups, except for the female subgroup and the subgroup without DL, a high DHA/AA ratio (≥0.903) tended to have a negative association for ACS (Table 3).

Figure 1 shows the prevalence of ACS by a quartile of DHA/AA ratio in all patients. The prevalence of ACS in quartile 1 was 9.5 % (41/433), in quartile 2 was 10.4 % (45/433), in quartile 3 was 8.6 % (38/434), and in

Table 2 Baseline clinical characteristics according to gender

	Male ($n = 1348$)	Female ($n = 385$)	P-value
Age (years)	63.6 ± 11.1	67.5 ± 11.5	<0.01[a]
Body mass index (kg/m^2)	24.5 ± 3.2	24.0 ± 4.3	0.02[a]
Hypertension	72.6 %	75.1 %	0.36
Diabetes mellitus	41.5 %	31.4 %	<0.01[a]
Dyslipidemia	70.5 %	70.1 %	0.89
Family history of ischemic heart disease	20.0 %	13.2 %	<0.01[a]
Smoking	53.6 %	47.6 %	<0.01[a]
History of coronary revascularization (PCI or CABG)	31.2 %	15.6 %	<0.01[a]
Total cholesterol (mg/dl)	187.1 ± 34.8	202.7 ± 36.8	<0.01[a]
Triglycerides (mg/dl)	151.8 ± 99.9	130.3 ± 77.6	<0.01[a]
Low-density lipoprotein cholesterol (mg/dl)	109.8 ± 30.3	115.6 ± 32.2	<0.01[a]
High-density lipoprotein cholesterol (mg/dl)	48.8 ± 14.3	61.3 ± 19.4	<0.01[a]
Hemoglobin A1c (%)	6.3 ± 1.1	6.1 ± 1.0	0.02[a]
Serum creatinine (mg/dl)	0.93 ± 0.29	0.71 ± 0.23	<0.01[a]
Estimated glomerular filtration rate (ml/min/1.73 m^2)	68.8 ± 17.4	68.4 ± 18.7	0.72
EPA (μg/dl)	73.7 ± 43.2	74.4 ± 47.0	0.76
EPA/AA	0.50 ± 0.31	0.46 ± 0.29	0.01[a]
DHA (μg/dl)	141.8 ± 52.5	149.0 ± 53.2	0.01[a]
DHA/AA	0.96 ± 0.40	0.92 ± 0.33	0.06
DGLA (μg/dl)	32.7 ± 12.5	35.0 ± 11.5	<0.01[a]
AA (μg/dl)	154.4 ± 51.3	167.8 ± 41.3	<0.01[a]
Statins	53.0 %	53.2 %	0.95
Antiplatelet agents	67.9 %	44.7 %	<0.01[a]
Renin angiotensin system inhibitors (ACE-I and ARB)	50.7 %	50.6 %	1.00
Calcium channel blockers	44.4 %	50.1 %	0.04[a]
Beta blockers	41.7 %	27.8 %	<0.01[a]
Hypoglycemic agents	22.0 %	17.9 %	0.08

Values are mean ± standard deviation, or percentage, [a]indicates significance, *PCI* Percutaneous coronary intervention, *CABG* coronary artery bypass grafting, *EPA/AA* eicosapentaenoic acid to arachidonic acid ratio, *DHA/AA* docosahexaenoic acid to arachidonic acid ratio, *DGLA* dihomo-gamma-linolenic acid, *ACE-I* angiotensin converting enzyme inhibitor, *ARB* angiotensin II receptor blocker

Table 3 Relationship between DHA/AA (≥0.903) and ACS, subgroup analysis

Subgroup	DHA/AA	ACS	N	Prevalence	Crude OR (95 % CI)	Adjusted OR(95 % CI)	P-value for interaction
Male	≥0.903	47	688	6.8 %	0.572 (0.391, 0.838)	0.389 (0.211, 0.716)	0.01[a]
	<0.903	75	660	11.4 %			
Female	≥0.903	18	179	10.1 %	1.982 (0.910, 4.317)	3.820 (0.718, 20.325)	
	<0.903	11	206	5.3 %			
Age ≥65	≥0.903	43	539	8.0 %	0.842 (0.528, 1.343)	0.658 (0.329, 1.317)	0.23
	<0.903	35	375	9.3 %			
Age <65	≥0.903	22	328	6.7 %	0.620 (0.368, 1.044)	0.312 (0.115, 0.846)	
	<0.903	51	491	10.4 %			
Diabetes mellitus, yes	≥0.903	25	345	7.2 %	0.576 (0.341, 0.973)	0.424 (0.197, 0.915)	0.31
	<0.903	40	335	11.9 %			
Diabetes mellitus, no	≥0.903	40	522	7.7 %	0.875 (0.562, 1.361)	0.758 (0.338, 1.700)	
	<0.903	46	531	8.7 %			
Hypertension, yes	≥0.903	51	656	7.8 %	0.819 (0.552, 1.216)	0.706 (0.377, 1.320)	0.06[a]
	<0.903	57	611	9.3 %			
Hypertension, no	≥0.903	14	211	6.6 %	0.554 (0.285, 1.078)	0.162 (0.039, 0.670)	
	<0.903	29	255	11.4 %			
Dyslipidemia, yes	≥0.903	46	612	7.5 %	0.656 (0.443, 0.973)	0.447 (0.237, 0.845)	0.15
	<0.903	67	608	11.0 %			
Dyslipidemia, no	≥0.903	19	255	7.5 %	1.013 (0.523, 1.961)	1.139 (0.368, 3.527)	
	<0.903	19	258	7.4 %			
Smoking history, yes	≥0.903	40	413	6.8 %	0.652 (0.420, 1.010)	0.475 (0.218, 1.031)	0.68
	<0.903	52	368	14.1 %			
Smoking history, no	≥0.903	25	454	5.5 %	0.795 (0.467, 1.355)	0.598 (0.265, 1.350)	
	<0.903	34	498	6.8 %			
Family history of IHD, yes	≥0.903	9	166	5.4 %	0.298 (0.134, 0.661)	0.621 (0.174, 2.219)	0.76
	<0.903	25	155	16.1 %			
Family history of IHD, no	≥0.903	56	701	8.0 %	0.925 (0.633, 1.351)	0.499 (0.266, 0.939)	
	<0.903	61	711	8.6 %			
Chronic kidney disease, yes	≥0.903	18	236	7.6 %	0.607 (0.317, 1.161)	0.738 (0.277, 1.963)	0.40
	<0.903	23	192	12.0 %			
Chronic kidney disease, no	≥0.903	21	439	4.8 %	0.582 (0.337, 1.002)	0.439 (0.219, 0.880)	
	<0.903	40	503	8.0 %			
Obesity (BMI ≥25), yes	≥0.903	23	319	7.2 %	0.707 (0.402, 1.242)	0.909 (0.376, 2.196)	0.19
	<0.903	31	313	9.9 %			
Obesity (BMI <25), no	≥0.903	42	516	8.1 %	0.777 (0.508, 1.189)	0.425 (0.206, 0.877)	
	<0.903	53	518	10.2 %			
History of coronary revascularization, yes	≥0.903	32	232	13.8 %	0.742 (0.452, 1.217)	0.488 (0.243, 0.979)	0.84
	<0.903	44	248	17.7 %			
History of coronary revascularization, no	≥0.903	33	635	5.2 %	0.752 (0.470, 1.203)	0.554 (0.211, 1.454)	
	<0.903	42	618	6.8 %			

[a]indicates statistical signficance for interaction ($P < 0.10$), OR = odds ratio, CI = confidence interval, ACS = acute coronary syndrome, DHA/AA = docosahexaenoic acid to arachidonic acid ratio, IHD = ischemic heart disease, BMI = body mass index

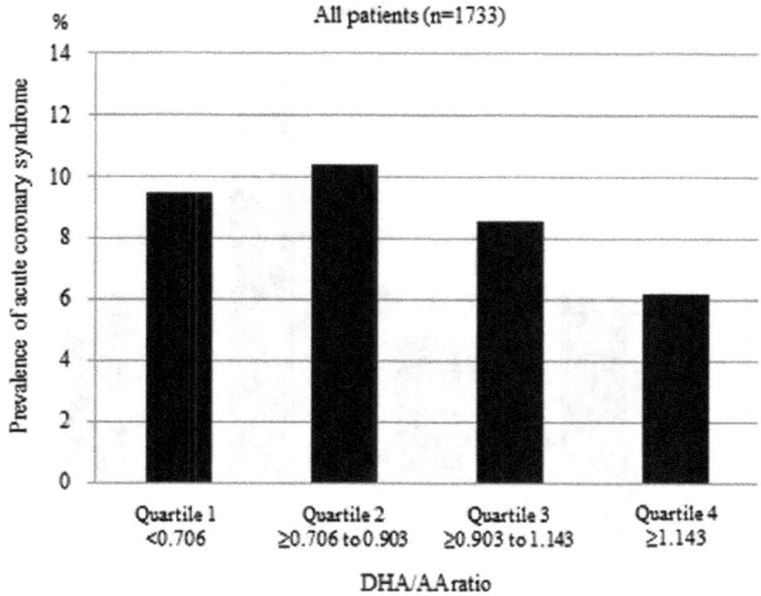

Fig. 1 The prevalence of acute coronary syndrome by DHA to AA ratio quartile in all patients. DHA = docosahexaenoic acid, AA = arachidonic acid

quartile 4 was 6.3 % (27/433). Figure 2 shows the prevalence of ACS by a quartile of DHA/AA ratio for men, revealing a prevalence of ACS in quartile 1 of 10.5 % (35/333), in quartile 2 of 12.2 % (40/327), in quartile 3 of 7.4 % (25/338), and in quartile 4 of 6.3 % (22/350). Figure 3 then shows the prevalence of ACS by a quartile of DHA to AA ratio for women, revealing a prevalence of ACS in quartile 1 of 6.0 % (6/100), in quartile 2 of 4.7 % (5/106), in quartile 3 of 13.5 % (13/96), and in quartile 4 of 6.0 % (5/83). Thus, there were clearly different trends of ACS risk for the DHA/AA ratio between men and women.

Discussion

Previous studies have demonstrated that treatment with EPA can reduce the risk of CAD [1, 2]. The Japan EPA Lipid Intervention Study (JELIS) proved that EPA administration could reduce residual risk in statin-treated

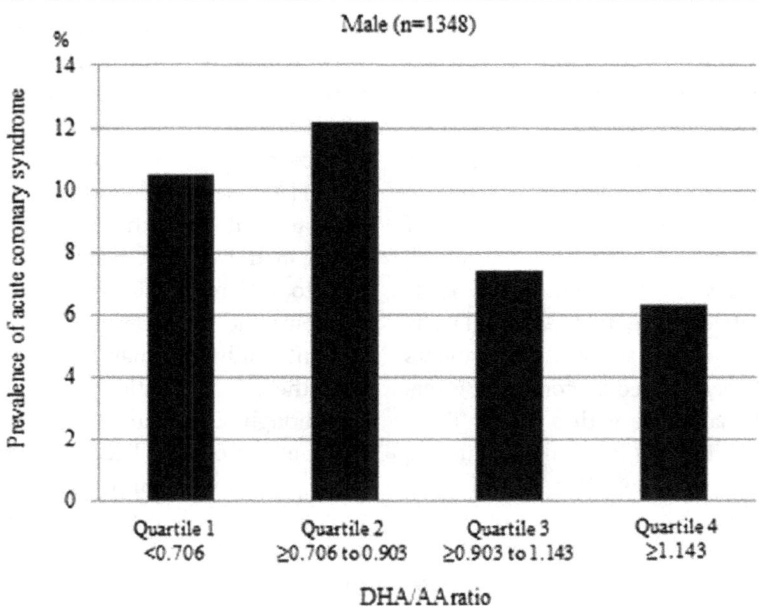

Fig. 2 The prevalence of acute coronary syndrome DHA to AA ratio quartile in men. DHA = docosahexaenoic acid, AA = arachidonic acid

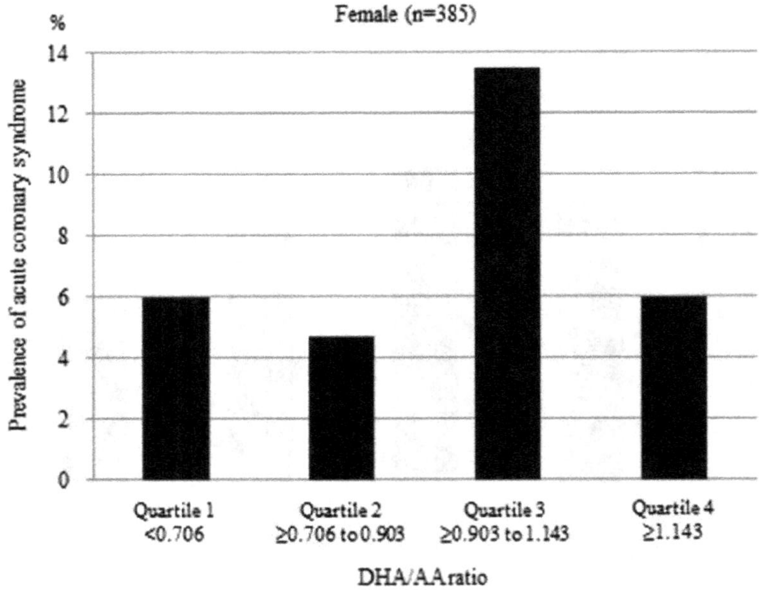

Fig. 3 The prevalence of acute coronary syndrome by DHA to AA ratio quartile in women. DHA = docosahexaenoic acid, AA = arachidonic acid

patients [1]. In a sub-analysis of the JELIS, EPA administration had a beneficial effect for coronary or cerebrovascular events, particularly in statin-treated patients with abnormal TG and HDL- cholesterol levels, as well as in patients with glucose intolerance, a history of stroke, and those with CAD [13–16]. These data suggested the importance of supplemental EPA for reducing any residual risk after statin treatment. However, the clinical usefulness of DHA treatment remains unclear, partially because no purified DHA-only agent has been launched in the clinical setting.

We report that a low EPA/AA ratio is associated with CAD and ACS, which is consistent with previous reports [3–6]. Therefore, an imbalance in the ratio of omega-3 to omega-6 PUFAs in the serum might be one of the residual risks. Several studies have reported the association between coronary events and the EPA/AA and DHA/AA ratios. Ninomiya et al. showed that a low EPA/AA ratio but not the DHA/AA ratio was associated with a risk of cardiovascular disease in subjects with higher levels of high-sensitivity C-reactive protein [4]. Domei et al. evaluated the relationship between the EPA/AA or DHA/AA ratios and major adverse cardiac events in patients who underwent elective percutaneous coronary intervention. They concluded that those with a higher EPA/AA ratio (>0.4037) had significantly lower major adverse cardiac events than those with a low EPA/AA ratio, but not DHA/AA, ratio [5]. Lee et al. demonstrated that high EPA levels rather than DHA were significantly associated with cardiovascular mortality [17]. EPA biologically competes with AA and works as a central substance for anti-inflammation reducing prostaglandins or leukotrienes, which are induced by AA. We believe that the clinical assessment of DHA/AA is also important because DHA and EPA have anti-inflammatory effects.

In contrast, a previous study has reported that high plasma DHA is associated with reduced progression of coronary atherosclerosis in patients with CAD [18]. In a clinical study using virtual histology intravascular ultrasound, the DHA/AA ratio had a stronger negative relationships with changes in plaque volume than the EPA/AA ratio in statin-treated patients with CAD [19]. Previous studies have also reported that the DHA level has a strong inverse association with intima-media thickness when compared with the EPA level [20, 21]. DHA rather than EPA has also been shown to lower ambulatory blood pressure and heart rate [22]. Moreover, other studies have demonstrated numerous beneficial effects of DHA, including microcirculation [23], antiplatelet [24], and anti-inflammation effects [25]. However, differences in the current results for EPA and DHA may be due to differences in participants, ethnic groups, and concomitant medications. As demonstrated in the present study, we may need to focus on the levels of both the EPA/AA ratio and the DHA/AA ratio.

Although EPA and DHA are both omega-3 PUFAs, more attention has been focused on the differences in their physiological and pharmacological effects [7]. Although the detailed mechanisms are yet to be clarified, both EPA and DHA have anti-inflammatory, antithrombotic, TG-lowering, inhibition of platelet aggregation, improvement of endothelial function, and plaque stabilization effects [26–29]. These beneficial effects might be additive for anti-atherogenesis in patients with high EPA/AA and DHA/AA ratios. Further investigation is needed to clarify these issues.

Several clinical studies have previously reported gender differences in the relationship between omega-3 PUFAs and cardiovascular mortality [17, 30, 31]. In 2013, The Risk and Prevention Study Collaboration Group conducted a double-blind, placebo-controlled clinical trial to evaluate the preventive effects of omega-3 PUFAs (EPA and DHA) on cardiovascular mortality in 12,513 patients with multiple cardiovascular risk factors [30]. Although null results were observed for the primary and secondary endpoints, a gender difference was observed in a subgroup analysis. Omega-3 PUFAs showed preventive effects for cardiovascular events in women (hazard ratio, 0.82; 95 % CI, 0.67–0.99) but not in men (hazard ratio, 1.04; 95 % CI, 0.92–1.17). Lee et al. reported a stronger association between high plasma EPA level and mortality reduction among women with acute myocardial infarction than among men [17]. In a Finnish study, higher fish consumption was related to a decreased risk of coronary heart disease among women, but no significant relationship was observed among men [31]. Although previous studies have reported that omega-3 PUFAs were significantly associated with cardiovascular events and mortality in women, we found a significant relationship between the DHA/AA ratio and ACS events in men. While gender differences can partially be explained by the effects of sex hormones, the precise mechanisms that lead to gender differences are not fully understood. It is also not clear whether gender altered the effects of omega-3 PUFAs on cardiovascular mortality. In particular, reports that focus on gender differences in the relationship between the DHA/AA ratio and cardiovascular events are rare.

We also assessed the association between serum AA level and medications and found that the administration of statins, antiplatelet agents, beta blockers, and hypoglycemic agents was significantly associated with serum AA levels. The relationship between statin administration and AA cascade has already been reported [32], and it is well known that aspirin prevents antithrombotic events through affecting the AA cascade; [33] thus, it could reduce serum AA levels. The relationships between beta blocker, hypoglycemic agents, and AA have still not been clarified and need further studies.

It has been reported that human immunodeficiency virus (HIV) infection is a prognostic indicator for recurrent thrombotic events [34]. However, we believe that it has a relatively low impact on the results of our study because the incidence of HIV infection is quite low in Japan.

There are several limitations of the present study. First, because it was conducted in the metropolitan Tokyo area, the results are not necessarily applicable to patients living in rural areas or foreign countries. Second, we were unable to prove a cause-effect relationship because of the cross-sectional design of our study. Third, as the duration of the study was over 7 years, medical advances during this period might have affected the study results. Fourth, assessment of dietary habits is important because plasma fatty acid profile depends upon their dietary habits. The assessment was not conducted in this study. However, PUFAs, such as EPA and DHA, are not sufficiently produced in the human body. We believe that the levels of essential plasma fatty acids, such as EPA and DHA, must be influenced by dietary habits. Fifth, fatty acid profiles were assessed only in four subsets (EPA, DHA, DGLA, and AA), and complete fatty acid profiles were not presented. Sixth, we have not conducted an assessment of inflammatory cytokines in this study. Inflammatory cytokines reduction in the plasma was observed. Dietary intake of omega-3 fatty acids correlates with the decrease in inflammatory cytokines in the plasma [35]. Seventh, the red blood cell lipid profile is known to have a significant correlation between serum lipid profile and ACS [36]. We should have evaluated between them. Eighth, because the data in the present study is male dominant (close to 80 %), a bias from the patient cohort or study design might be associated with these results. Ninth, in the present study, fasting blood samples from patients with ACS were collected during admission. In the early stage of ACS, the serum fatty acid profiles would possibly be altered [37]. Finally, we also enrolled the patients who had any coronary intervention and/or coronary artery bypass grafting due to stable angina. These patients may have less incidence of ACS because of their medical therapy. A large-scale multicenter prospective study is necessary to validate the results of this study.

The present study showed that the DHA/AA ratio was more effective for risk stratification due to the ACS events and that the relationship of EPA/AA ratio with ACS events was not significant. In our previous report [6], patients with a medical history of percutaneous coronary intervention, coronary artery bypass grafting, and myocardial infarction were excluded, whereas those with past coronary revascularization were included in the present study. In a meta-analysis of randomized placebo-controlled trials of EPA vs DHA intervention, both EPA and DHA reduced TG, with a greater reduction seen with DHA. DHA, but not EPA, also raised HDL-cholesterol [38]. There are several reported mechanisms by which the differences between EPA and DHA treatment may affect lipid metabolism. EPA induces the reduction of hepatic lipogenesis with a more potent peroxisome proliferator-activated receptor-alpha effect, whereas DHA enhances very-low-density lipoprotein

(VLDL) lipolysis and increases HDL and large LDL particles [39]. Several studies demonstrate that DHA, but not EPA, reduces the apolipoprotein C-III concentration [40, 41]. Apolipoprotein C-III particularly inhibits the actions of lipoprotein lipase and hepatic lipase, which slow TG hydrolysis [42]. By regulating different hepatic transcription factors than EPA, DHA reduces apolipoprotein C-III production, resulting in enhanced conversion of VLDL to LDL to reduce TG [39, 43]. However, until now, there was no study that investigated the difference between EPA alone and EPA/DHA combination on clinical outcomes, including cardiovascular events and total mortality. The bio-reactive function of EPA or DHA may be different among the characteristically different groups of patients. In addition, the data of EPA/AA and DHA/AA ratio was not strongly, but moderately correlated (data not shown) in the present study. EPA and DHA may show a parallel function in the body, but data collected from a real clinical setting, as the present study, do not necessarily show a notable correlation. Further studies should be conducted to clarify these mechanisms. In the near future, we believe that EPA or DHA will be appropriately administered to patients, depending on their clinical background.

Conclusions

The present study showed that the relationship between the DHA/AA ratio and ACS differed with the sex of participants who evaluated the serum levels of PUFAs in cardiology departments. Those men with low DHA/AA ratios had 2.57 times more ACS than those with a high DHA/AA ratio. In contrast, a reverse association of similar magnitude was found among women, although this was not statistically significant. In the present study, healthy subjects were not the focus of attention. Further studies are needed to clarify the association between DHA/AA ratio and the risk of ACS in apparently healthy subjects.

Abbreviations

AA, arachidonic acid; ACS, acute coronary syndrome; BMI, body mass index; CAD, coronary artery disease; CI, confidence interval; CKD, chronic kidney disease; Cr, creatinine; DGLA, dihomo-gamma-linolenic acid; DHA, docosahexaenoic acid; DL, dyslipidemia; DM, diabetes mellitus; eGFR, estimated glomerular filtration rate; EPA, eicosapentaenoic acid; HDL, high-density lipoprotein; HIV, human immunodeficiency virus; HT, hypertension; IHD, ischemic heart disease; JELIS, Japan EPA Lipid Intervention Study; LDL, low-density lipoprotein; PUFAs, polyunsaturated fatty acids; TG, triglycerides; VLDL, very-low-density lipoprotein.

Acknowledgements

The authors thank Takeshi Asakura, LLB, for help in translating this report into English.

Authors' contributions

YN and KS have designed this study in whole and drafted this manuscript. ST, TO, JA, MT, MY, KM, and KN have contributed to collect data. TS has contributed to statistical analyses in this study. AH, MY, IK, and RN have contributed to provide advice on interpretation of the results. HD has revised this manuscript critically for important intellectual content and approved finally the manuscript submitted. All authors read and approved the final manuscript.

Competing interests

KS, ST, and KM received lecture fees from Mochida Pharmaceutical Company and Takeda Pharmaceutical Company. MY received scholarship funds and lecture fees from Mochida Pharmaceutical Company and Takeda Pharmaceutical Company. IK received lecture fees and scholarship funds from Takeda Pharmaceutical Company. RN received consultation and lecture fees from Mochida Pharmaceutical Company. HD received scholarship funds and lecture fees from Mochida Pharmaceutical Company and Takeda Pharmaceutical Company. The other authors report no conflicts.

Author details

[1]Department of Cardiology, Juntendo University Graduate School of Medicine, 2-1-1 Hongo Bunkyo-ku, Tokyo 113-8421, Japan. [2]Department of Cardiology, Nihon University Hospital, 1-6 Kanda Surugadai Chiyoda-ku, Tokyo 101-8309, Japan. [3]Divison of Cardiology, Department of Internal Medicine, The Jikei University School of Medicine, 3-25-8, Nishi-Shimbashi Minato-ku, Tokyo 105-8461, Japan. [4]Department of Cardiovascular Medicine, Graduate School of Medicine, The University of Tokyo, 7-3-1 Hongo Bunkyo-ku, Tokyo 113-8655, Japan. [5]Department of Internal Medicine, Tokyo Takanawa Hospital, 3-10-11, Takanawa Minato-ku, Tokyo 108-8606, Japan. [6]Department of Biostatistics, School of Public Health, The University of Tokyo, 7-3-1 Hongo Bunkyo-ku, Tokyo 113-0033, Japan. [7]Division of Cardiology, Department of Medicine, Nihon University School of Medicine, 30-1 Ohyaguchi Kamichou Itabashi-ku, Tokyo 173-8610, Japan. [8]Jichi Medical University, 3311-1 Yakushiji, Shimotsuke-shi, Tochigi-ken 329-0498, Japan.

References

1. Yokoyama M, Origasa H, Matsuzaki M, Matsuzawa Y, Saito Y, Ishikawa Y, et al. Japan EPA lipid intervention study (JELIS) Investigators. Effects of eicosapentaenoic acid on major coronary events in hypercholesterolaemic patients (JELIS): a randomised open-label, blinded endpoint analysis. Lancet. 2007;369:1090–8.
2. Dietary supplementation with n-3 polyunsaturated fatty acids and vitamin E after myocardial infarction: results of the GISSI-Prevenzione trial. Gruppo Italiano per lo Studio della Sopravvivenza nell'Infarto miocardico. Lancet. 1999;354:447–455.
3. Itakura H, Yokoyama M, Matsuzaki M, Saito Y, Origasa H, Ishikawa Y, et al. Relationships between plasma fatty acid composition and coronary artery disease. J Atheroscler Thromb. 2011;18:99–107.
4. Ninomiya T, Nagata M, Hata J, Hirakawa Y, Ozawa M, Yoshida D, et al. Association between ratio of serum eicosapentaenoic acid to arachidonic acid and risk of cardiovascular disease: The Hisayama Study. Atherosclerosis. 2013;231:261–7.
5. Domei T, Yokoi H, Kuramitsu S, Soga Y, Arita T, Ando K, et al. Ratio of serum n-3 to n-6 polyunsaturated fatty acids and the incidence of major adverse cardiac events in patients undergoing percutaneous coronary intervention. Circ J. 2012;76:423–9.
6. Nishizaki Y, Shimada K, Tani S, Ogawa T, Ando J, Takahashi M, et al. Significance of Imbalance in the Ratio of Serum n-3 to n-6 Polyunsaturated Fatty Acids in Patients With Acute Coronary Syndrome. Am J Cardiol. 2014; 113:441–5.
7. Mozaffarian D, Wu JH. Omega-3 fatty acids and cardiovascular disease: effects on risk factors, molecular pathways, and clinical events. J Am Coll Cardiol. 2011;58:2047–67.
8. Braunwald E. Unstable angina: a classification. Circulation. 1989;80:410–4.

9. Matsuo S, Imai E, Horio M, Yasuda Y, Tomita K, Nitta K, et al. Collaborators developing the Japanese equation forestimated GFR. Revised equations for estimated GFR from serum creatinine in Japan. Am J Kidney Dis. 2009;53: 982–92.
10. Altman DG, Bland JM. Interaction revisited: the difference between two estimates. BMJ. 2003;326:219.
11. Greenland S. Basic problems in interaction assessment. Environ Health Perspect. 1993;101:59–66.
12. Greenland S. Modeling and variable selection in epidemiologic analysis. Am J Public Health. 1989;79:340–9.
13. Saito Y, Yokoyama M, Origasa H, Matsuzaki M, Matsuzawa Y, Ishikawa Y, et al. Effects of EPA on coronary artery disease in hypercholesterolemic patients with multiple risk factors: sub-analysis of primary prevention cases from the Japan EPA Lipid Intervention Study (JELIS). Atherosclerosis. 2008; 200:135–410.
14. Oikawa S, Yokoyama M, Origasa H, Matsuzaki M, Matsuzawa Y, Saito Y, et al. Suppressive effect of EPA on the incidence of coronary events in hypercholesterolemia with impaired glucose metabolism: Sub-analysis of the Japan EPA Lipid Intervention Study (JELIS). Atherosclerosis. 2009;206:535–9.
15. Tanaka K, Ishikawa Y, Yokoyama M, Origasa H, Matsuzaki M, Saito Y, et al. Reduction in the recurrence of stroke by eicosapentaenoic acid for hypercholesterolemic patients: subanalysis of the JELIS trial. Stroke. 2008;39:2052–8.
16. Matsuzaki M, Yokoyama M, Saito Y, Origasa H, Ishikawa Y, Oikawa S, et al. Incremental effects of eicosapentaenoic acid on cardiovascular events in statin-treated patients with coronary artery disease. Circ J. 2009;73:1283–90.
17. Lee SH, Shin MJ, Kim JS, Ko YG, Kang SM, Choi D, et al. Blood eicosapentaenoic acid and docosahexaenoic acid as predictors of all-cause mortality in patients with acute myocardial infarction–data from Infarction Prognosis Study (IPS) Registry. Circ J. 2009;73:2250–7.
18. Erkkilä AT, Matthan NR, Herrington DM, Lichtenstein AH. Higher plasma docosahexaenoic acid is associated with reduced progression of coronary atherosclerosis in women with CAD. J Lipid Res. 2006;47:2814–9.
19. Nozue T, Yamamoto S, Tohyama S, Fukui K, Umezawa S, Onishi Y, et al. Effects of Serum n-3 to n-6 Polyunsaturated Fatty Acids Ratios on Coronary Atherosclerosis in Statin-Treated Patients With Coronary Artery Disease. Am J Cardiol. 2013;111:6–11.
20. Sala-Vila A, Cofán M, Pérez-Heras A, Núñez I, Gilabert R, Junyent M, et al. Fatty acids in serum phospholipids and carotid intima-media thickness in Spanish subjects with primary dyslipidemia. Am J Clin Nutr. 2010;92:186–93.
21. Sekikawa A, Kadowaki T, El-Saed A, Okamura T, Sutton-Tyrrell K, Nakamura Y, et al. Differential association of docosahexaenoic and eicosapentaenoic acids with carotid intima-media thickness. Stroke. 2011;42:2538–43.
22. Mori TA, Bao DQ, Burke V, Puddey IB, Beilin LJ. Docosahexaenoic acid but not eicosapentaenoic acid lowers ambulatory blood pressure and heart rate in humans. Hypertension. 1999;34:253–60.
23. Mori TA, Watts GF, Burke V, Hilme E, Puddey IB, Beilin LJ. Differential effects of eicosapentaenoic acid and docosahexaenoic acid on vascular reactivity of the forearm microcirculation in hyperlipidemic, overweight men. Circulation. 2000;102:1264–9.
24. Woodman RJ, Mori TA, Burke V, Puddey IB, Barden A, Watts GF, et al. Effects of purified eicosapentaenoic acid and docosahexaenoic acid on platelet, fibrinolytic and vascular function in hypertensive type 2 diabetic patients. Atherosclerosis. 2003;166:85–93.
25. Weldon SM, Mullen AC, Loscher CE, Hurley LA, Roche HM. Docosahexaenoic acid induces an anti-inflammatory profile in lipopolysaccharide-stimulated human THP-1 macrophages more effectively than eicosapentaenoic acid. J Nutr Biochem. 2007;18:250–8.
26. Einvik G, Klemsdal TO, Sandvik L, Hjerkinn EM. A randomized clinical trial on n-3 polyunsaturated fatty acids supplementation and all-cause mortality in elderly men at high cardiovascular risk. Eur J Cardiovasc Prev Rehabil. 2010; 17:588–92.
27. Witte KK, Clark AL. Fish oils–adjuvant therapy in chronic heart failure? Eur J Cardiovasc Prev Rehabil. 2004;11:267–74.
28. Kromhout D, Yasuda S, Geleijnse JM, Shimokawa H. Fish oil and omega-3 fatty acids in cardiovascular disease: do they really work? Eur Heart J. 2012; 33:436–43.
29. Yasuda S, Shimokawa H. Potential usefulness of fish oil in the primary prevention of acute coronary syndrome. Eur Heart J. 2010;31:15–6.
30. Fisk and Prevention Study Collaborative Group, Roncaglioni MC, Tombesi M, Avanzini F, Barlera S, Caimi V, et al. n-3 fatty acids in patients with multiple cardiovascular risk factors. N Engl J Med. 2013;368:1800–8.
31. Järvinen R, Knekt P, Rissanen H, Reunanen A. Intake of fish and long-chain n-3 fatty acids and the risk of coronary heart mortality in men and women. Br J Nutr. 2006;95:824–9.
32. Jula A, Marniemi J, Rönnemaa T, Virtanen A, Huupponen R. Effects of diet and simvastatin on fatty acid composition in hypercholesterolemic men: a randomized controlled trial. Arterioscler Thromb Vasc Biol. 2005;25:1952–9.
33. Antithrombotic Trialists' Collaboration. Collaborative meta-analysis of randomized trials of antiplatelet therapy for prevention of death, myocardial infarction, and stroke in high-risk patients. BMJ. 2002;324:71–86.
34. D'Ascenzo F, Cerrato E, Appleton D, Moretti C, Calcagno A, Abouzaki N, et al. Percutaneous coronary intervention and surgical revascularization in HIV Database (PHD) Study Investigators. Prognostic indicators for recurrent thrombotic events in HIV-infected patients with acute coronary syndromes: use of registry data from 12 sites in Europe, South Africa, and the United States. Thromb Res. 2014;134:558–64.
35. Lopez-Garcia E, Schulze MB, Manson JE, Meigs JB, Albert CM, Rifai N, et al. Consumption of (n-3) fatty acids is related to plasma biomarkers of inflammation and endothelial activation in women. J Nutr. 2004;134:1806–11.
36. Yanagisawa N, Shimada K, Miyazaki T, Kume A, Kitamura Y, Ichikawa R, et al. Polyunsaturated fatty acid levels of serum and red blood cells in apparently healthy Japanese subjects living in an urban area. J Atheroscler Thromb. 2010;17:285–94.
37. Sakamoto A, Saotome M, Hosoya N, Kageyama S, Yoshizaki T, Takeuchi R, et al. Aberrant serum polyunsaturated fatty acids profile is relevant with acute coronary syndrome. Heart Vessels. 2015, in press.
38. Wei MY, Jacobson TA. Effects of eicosapentaenoic acid versus docosahexaenoic acid on serum lipids: a systematic review and meta-analysis. Curr Atheroscler Rep. 2011;13:474–83.
39. Davidson MH. Omega-3 fatty acids: new insights into the pharmacology and biology of docosahexaenoic acid, docosapentaenoic acid, and eicosapentaenoic acid. Curr Opin Lipidol. 2013;24:467–74.
40. Buckley R, Shewring B, Turner R, Yaqoob P, Minihane AM. Circulating triacylglycerol and apoE levels in response to EPA and docosahexaenoic acid supplementation in adult human subjects. Br J Nutr. 2004;92:477–83.
41. Homma Y, Ohshima K, Yamaguchi H, Nakamura H, Araki G, Goto Y. Effects of eicosapentaenoic acid on plasma lipoprotein subfractions and activities of lecithin:cholesterol acyltransferase and lipid transfer protein. Atherosclerosis. 1991;91:145–53.
42. Kawakami A, Yoshida M. Apolipoprotein CIII links dyslipidemia with atherosclerosis. J Atheroscler Thromb. 2009;16:6–11.
43. Tatsuno I. Omega-3 polyunsaturated fatty acids and cardiovascular disease: an emphasis on omega-3-acid ethyl esters 90 for the treatment of hypertriglyceridemia. Expert Rev Cardiovasc Ther. 2014;12:1261–8.

3

Management of acute coronary syndromes in a developing country

Arjuna Medagama[1*], Ruwanthi Bandara[2], Chinthani De Silva[1] and Manoj Prasanna Galgomuwa[1]

Abstract

Background: There are limited contemporary data on the presentation, management and outcomes of acute coronary syndromes (ACS) in Sri Lanka. We aimed to identify the critical issues that limit optimal management of ACS in Sri Lanka.

Methods: We performed a prospectively observational study of 256 consecutive patients who presented with ACS between November 2011 and May 2012 at a tertiary care general medical unit in Sri Lanka.

Results: We evaluated data on presentation, management, in-hospital mortality, and major adverse cardiovascular events (MACE) of participants. Smoking, alcohol abuse, and obesity were more common in patients with ST elevation myocardial infarction (STEMI) ($P < 0.05$). Discharge diagnoses were STEMI in 32.8 % (84/256) and unstable angina (UA)/non-ST elevation myocardial infarction [NSTEMI] in 67.1 % (172/256) of participants. The median time (IQR) from onset of pain to presentation was 60 (319) minutes for STEMI and 120 (420) for UA/NSTEMI ($P = 0.058$). A median delay of 240 min was noted in patients who had presented initially to smaller hospitals. Cardiac markers were assessed in only 35 % of participants. In-hospital anti-platelet use was high (>92 %). Only 70.2 % of STEMI patients received fibrinolytic therapy. Fewer than 20 % of patients were received fibrinolytic therapy within 30 min of arrival. Major adverse cardiac events (MACE) were recorded in 11.9 % of subjects with STEMI and 11.6 % of those with UA/NSTEMI ($P = 0.5$). According to logistic regression analysis, body mass index ($P = 0.045$) and duration of diabetes ($P = 0.03$) were significant predictors of in-hospital MACE. On discharge, aspirin, thienopyridine, and statins were prescribed to more than 90 % of patients. Only one patient underwent coronary angiography during the index admission.

Conclusions: Delays in presentation and in initiation of thrombolytic therapy and coronary interventions are key hurdles that need attention to optimize ACS care in Sri Lanka.

Keywords: Acute coronary syndrome, Sri Lanka, Thrombolysis

Background

Sri Lanka, a developing Asian country, has a population of 21 million and a rapidly increasing burden of non-communicable diseases. South Asians experience higher fatality rates and premature death attributable to cardiovascular disease (CVD) (deaths occurring at least 10–15 years before expected) than do persons in Western countries [1, 2]. Cardiovascular deaths and disease incidence have increased at an alarming rate in low and middle-income countries [3].

In 2005, the prevalences of hypertension, diabetes, and dysglycemia in Sri Lanka were 20, 11, and 20 %, respectively [4]. Mortality from CVD in Sri Lanka is recognized to be one of the highest causes of death worldwide [5]. Ischemic heart disease (IHD) is the leading cause of death in Sri Lanka, accounting for 27.6 deaths per 100,000 people. Data from 2004–2012 show a steady increase in mortality from IHD in hospitals; in 2012 IHD accounted for 14.4 % of all deaths in hospitals in Sri Lanka [6]. This high mortality rate remains unexplained,

* Correspondence: arjuna.medagama@gmail.com
[1]Department of Medicine, Faculty of Medicine, University of Peradeniya, Galaha Rd, Peradeniya 20400, Sri Lanka
Full list of author information is available at the end of the article

but may be attributable in part to a combination of modifiable and non-modifiable cardiovascular risk factors. Previous research has shown that management of CVD in Sri Lanka [7–9], regionally [10], and in developing countries is generally suboptimal compared to Western developed countries [11].

The term acute coronary syndrome (ACS) encompasses a spectrum of coronary artery diseases, including unstable angina (UA), ST-segment-elevation myocardial infarction (STEMI), and non-ST elevation myocardial infarction (NSTEMI). While clinical trials have provided clinicians with evidence for many interventions and medications for ACS, observational studies provide useful information on differences and shortcomings in management practices among countries as well as within different regions of the same country [12, 13].

Treatment with aspirin for patients experiencing ACS and post discharge treatment with aspirin, statins, and blood pressure lowering drugs are cost-effective strategies and considered "best practice" by the World Health Organization [14].

Previous published studies in Sri Lanka have highlighted the following issues in management of ACS: late presentation [8, 9], time delays between presentation and arrival to out-patient departments and wards [9], and less than optimal adherence to current ACS guidelines [7].

The aim of the current study was to gain insights into the following aspects of ACS: epidemiology, presentation, in-ward management, and adherence to current management guidelines, for patients admitted to a tertiary care hospital in Sri Lanka.

Methods

This prospective observational study was carried out at the Professorial Medical Unit of Teaching Hospital, Peradeniya, Sri Lanka over a 6-month period beginning in November 2011. The hospital is a busy, state-run, tertiary-care institution with nonselective intake of acute patients.

All patients presenting to the out-patients' department with chest pain within the preceding 24 h and fulfilling ECG criteria for acute STEMI, NSTEMI and UA were included in the study. Such patients were recruited consecutively to avoid selection bias. A diagnosis of STEMI was made in subjects with electrocardiographic (ECG) changes that fulfilled current ECG criteria for the diagnosis of acute STEMI or new-onset left bundle-branch block, and increased serum concentrations of biochemical markers of myocardial necrosis where these measurements were available. Diagnoses of UA and NSTEMI were made in the presence of ischemic type chest pain and ECG changes of ST segment depression more than 1 mm and T wave inversion greater than 1 mm in contiguous leads. Troponin concentrations are not checked routinely at most government hospitals; when required, the test is performed in a private laboratory at the patient's expense. The distinction between UA and NSTEMI is therefore not routinely made because troponin concentrations are assessed only for patients with uncertain diagnoses or for those who are willing to pay for the test to be performed. The initial diagnosis of ACS was made by a senior house officer or registrar on admission and later confirmed by a consultant physician.

Every patient presenting with chest pain underwent assessment of their history, physical examination, and ECG; those fulfilling the criteria for ACS were included in the present study. Data on pre-hospital and in-ward management were collected from patient records and clarifications were made when necessary by the authors interviewing the patients.

All participants received standard care, that is, their participation in the study did not alter the care they received. Ethical approval for this study was obtained from the Ethics Review Committee of the Faculty of Medicine of the University of Peradeniya, Sri Lanka (2011/EC/22). Informed written consent was obtained from all participants prior to collecting data and was formally recorded.

Statistical analysis

Continuous variables are presented in means (standard deviation) or median (inter quartile range), when skewed in distribution. Categorical variables are presented as proportions or percentages. ACS types were compared via analysis for variance for continuous variables and the χ^2 test for categorical variables. A two-sided P value <0.05 was defined as statistically significant. Univariate and multivariate logistic regression was used to assess possible predictors of death and in-hospital major cardiovascular events (MACE being defined as death, re-infarction, stroke, heart failure, or cardiogenic shock).

Results

Study subjects

The study group comprised 256 patients with confirmed ACS, 115 (44.9 %) men and 141 (55.1 %) women. The mean age was 63.2 (STD 11.1) years. Most patients were in the 51–70 year age group (145, 57 %), followed by those aged over 70 years (77, 30 %) and then by those aged less than 50 years (34, 13.3 %). There were no significant age variations between STEMI and UA/NSTEMI patients. The socio-demographic profile of the subjects is summarized in Table 1.

Discharge diagnoses were STEMI in 32.8 % (84/256) and UA/NSTEMI in 67.1 % (172/256). The troponin concentrations of 19 of the 84 STEMI patients were measured and all were positive. Troponin concentrations were measured in only 70 (40.6 %) of the remaining 172

Table 1 Patient baseline characteristics according to discharge diagnosis and overall

Variable	STEMI ($n = 84$)	ACS ($n = 172$)	Total ($n = 256$)	P value
Sex Male	22 (26.2 %)	93 (54.1 %)	115 (44.9 %)	
Female	62 (73.8 %)	79 (45.9 %)	141 (55.1 %)	
Age (Y)-mean	62.19 (SD = 11.4)	63.7 (SD = 11.1)	63.2 (SD = 11.2)	0.316
Age Strata <50 year	13 (15.5 %)	21 (12.2 %)	34 (13.3 %)	0.564
51–70 year	49 (58.3 %)	96 (55.8 %)	145 (56.6 %)	
>70 year	22 (26.2 %)	55 (31.9 %)	77 (30.1 %)	
Race Sinhala	61 (72.6 %)	151 (87.8 %)	212 (82.8 %)	
Muslim	15 (17.9 %)	17 (9.9 %)	32 (12.5 %)	
Tamil	8 (9.5 %)	4 (2.3 %)	12 (4.7 %)	
Presentation				
Chest pain	75 (89.3 %)	149 (86.6 %)	224 (87.5 %)	0.546
Shortness of breath	1 (1.2 %)	6 (3.5 %)	7 (2.7 %)	0.290
Median time to present (minutes)	60	120	120	0.058
Presenting time >6 h	12 (14.3 %)	34 (19.8 %)	46 (18 %)	0.480
Delay at transfer in minutes (median)	120, IQR = 397.2	240, IQR = 720	180, IQR = 634.8	0.334
Risk Factors				
Coronary artery disease/MI	7 (8.3 %)	46 (26.7 %)	53 (20.7 %)	0.001
Heart Failure	7 (8.3 %)	19 (11.2 %)	26 (10.2 %)	0.059
Stroke	0 (0 %)	7 (4.1 %)	7 (2.8 %)	0.158
Family History Of Cardio Vascular Disease	19 (22.6 %)	32 (18.9 %)	51 (20.1 %)	0.355
History of PCI or CABG	1 (1.2 %)	0 (0 %)	1 (0.4 %)	0.155
Hypertension	26 (31 %)	99 (57.6 %)	125 (48.8 %)	0.001
Dyslipidemia	7 (8.3 %)	12 (7 %)	19 (7.4 %)	0.726
Diabetes Mellitus	27 (32.1 %)	64 (37.2 %)	91 (35.5 %)	0.371
BMI mean	24.63 (SD = 5.287)	23 (SD = 3.687)	23.51 (SD = 4.312)	0.018
Normal BMI (<23 kg/m2)	34 (40.5 %)	86 (50 %)	120 (46.9 %)	
Over Weight (BMI 23–27 kg/m2)	31 (36.9 %)	61 (35.5 %)	92 (35.9 %)	
Obese (BMI >27 kg/m2)	19 (22.6 %)	25 (14.5 %)	44 (17.2 %)	
Waist circumference (mean) in cm	85.61	83.54	84.23	0.092
Current Smoker	17 (20.2 %)	12 (7 %)	29 (11.3 %)	0.001
Alcohol Misuse	23 (27.4 %)	25 (14.5 %)	48 (18.8 %)	0.035

patients with ACS and 42 of those were positive, confirming a diagnosis of NSTEMI. Troponin concentrations were negative in 28 of this group, so they were categorized as having UA. Because a distinction between UA and NSTEMI was not made in most patients in this group, they were considered as having UA/NSTEMI.

Sixty-seven percent of patients came directly to our center, whereas the remainder (33 %) first visited either a general practitioner (GP) or other hospitals in which ACS was not managed. Only 15 % of these patients were transported to our center by ambulance, the remainder had to provide their own transport. The median delay during transfer was 4 h.

The median (interquartile range) delay from symptom onset to hospital admission was shorter for STEMI patients at 60 (319) minutes than for UA/NSTEMI patients at 120 (420) minutes ($P = 0.058$); this difference was not statistically significant. For patients initially presenting to a GP or other hospital for either STEMI or UA/NSTEMI, there was a median delay of 240 (IQR 480) minutes from symptom onset to hospital admission.

Baseline characteristics of the study subjects are shown in Table 1. The body mass index (BMI) and waist circumference of patients with STEMI were higher than those of patients with UA/STEMI. Smoking and alcohol abuse was more common among patients with STEMI than among those with UA/NSTEMI. Generally patients with UA/NSTEMI had a worse medical history and more risk factors than those with STEMI (Table 1).

Management in hospital and at discharge

Interventions and in-hospital treatments are shown in Table 2. The most commonly used medications were aspirin (95.3 %), clopidogrel (98 %), statins (96.1 %), angiotensin-converting enzyme (ACE)/angiotensin II receptor blockers (ARB) (87 %), and beta blockers (68.7 %) with little differences in the medications administered between patients with STEMI and those with UA/NSTEMI. However, only 16 % those presenting initially to a GP or other hospital received aspirin, compared with 95.3 % at our center ($P < 0.01$). Aspirin was the commonest medication to be withheld, either because of presumed gastric bleeding or epigastric pain. Beta blockers were more commonly given to patients with STEMI (75 %) than to those with UA/NSTEMI (65.7 %, $P = 0.07$) Enoxaparin or unfractionated heparin was given to 87.8 % of patients with UA/NSTEMI and 62 % of those with STEMI.

Fifty-nine patients (70.2 %) with STEMI underwent fibrinolytic therapy with streptokinase. Thirteen of the 84

Table 2 Selected in-hospital management, medications, and interventions according to discharge diagnosis

		STEMI ($n = 84$)	ACS ($n = 172$)	Whole population ($n = 256$)	*P* value
Aspirin		(78) 92.9 %	(166) 96.5 %	(244) 95.3 %	0.194
Clopidogel		(82) 97.6 %	(169) 98.3 %	(251) 98.0 %	0.464
Statins		(81) 96.4 %	(165) 95.9 %	(246) 96.1 %	0.987
Beta blockers	Atenolol	(6) 7.1 %	(23) 13.4 %	(29) 11.3 %	0.073
	Carvedilol	(10) 11.9 %	(11) 6.4 %	(21) 8.2 %	
	Metaprolol	(47) 56.0 %	(79) 45.9 %	(126) 49.2 %	
	Total	(63) 75 %	(113) 65.7 %	(176) 68.7 %	
ACEI, ARB	Captopril	(2) 2.4 %	(21) 12.2 %	(23) 9.0 %	0.946
	Enalapril	(66) 78.6 %	(101) 58.7 %	(167) 65.2 %	
	Losartan	(5) 6 %	(28) 16.3 %	(33) 12.9 %	
	Total	(73) 87 %	(150) 87.2 %	(223) 87.1 %	
Nitrates		(31) 36.9 %	(72) 41.9 %	(103) 40.9 %	0.145
Heparin		(20) 23.8 %	(28) 16.3 %	(48) 18.8 %	0.167
Enoxaparin		(52) 61.9 %	(151) 87.8 %	(203) 79.3 %	0.001
Diuretics		(18) 21.4 %	(25) 14.6 %	(43) 16.9 %	0.209
Troponin done		19 (22.6 %)	70 (41.7 %)	89 (35.3 %)	0.004
Troponin positive in		19 (100 %)	42 (60 %)	61 (23.8 %)	-
Fibrinolysis		(59) 72.8 %	(0) 0 %	-	-
Door to needle time: median (IQR) min		64 (55)			
<30 min		(10) 16.9 %			
30–60 min		(18) 30.5 %			
>60 min		(31) 52.5 %			
Transferred to Ward		36 (43.3 %)	129 (78.2 %)	165 (67.6 %)	0.001
HDU		43 (58.1 %)	31 (19.3 %)	74 (30.3 %)	0.001
ICU		4 (4.8 %)	1 (0.6 %)	5 (2 %)	0.028
MACE		10 (11.9 %)	20 (11.6 %)	30 (11.7 %)	0.948
Echocardiography performed in		71 (84.5 %)	164 (95.3 %)	235 (91.8 %)	0.003
EF mean (%)		43.38 (SD 18.7)	52.65 (SD 13.6)	49.65 (SD 16.0)	0.001
Stress Test planned on discharge		19 (24.1 %)	44 (26.5 %)	63 (25.7 %)	0.866
Referred for	PCI	1 (1.2 %)	0 (0 %)	1 (0.39 %)	
	Angiogram	9 (11.5 %)	11 (6.9 %)	20 (8.4 %)	
	CABG	0 (0 %)	1 (0.6 %)	1 (0.4 %)	
Mean duration of hospital stay		5.12 (SD = 1.430)	4.33 (SD = 2.089)	4.57 (SD = 1.946)	0.001

(15.4%) patients with STEMI were not eligible for thrombolytic therapy because of their late presentation. The remaining 12 patients were eligible on the basis of arrival time; however, three of these (3.7 %) had absolute or relative contraindications to thrombolytic therapy; the reasons for the remaining nine (11.1 %) eligible patients not undergoing this treatment were unknown. Median door-to-needle time was 64 (IQR 55) minutes. Only 10 patients (16.9 %) received thrombolytic therapy within 30 min, 28 (47.4 %) within 60 min, and 39 (66 %) within 90 min. Twenty (33.9 %) received thrombolytic therapy more than 90 min after arriving at the hospital.

Mean duration of in-hospital stay was 5.12 (1.4) days for patients with STEMI, which was greater than the mean of 4.3 (2.0) days for patients with UA/NSTEMI ($P < 0.01$). Overall, only 32.3 % of patients were managed in an intensive care or high dependency unit.

There were no reported deaths in patients with STEMI and two in those with UA/NSTEMI. Thirty (11.7 %) patients developed MACE, which was defined as death, reinfarction, stroke, heart failure, or cardiogenic shock occurring during their hospital stays (Table 2). One patient with STEMI had major non-fatal bleeding.

During the index admission, 84.5 % of patients with STEMI and 95.3 % of those with UA/NSTEMI had transthoracic echocardiography performed. The mean ejection fraction of patients with STEMI was 43.38 % (18.7), which was significantly lower than the mean ejection fraction 52.6 % (13.6) for those with UA/STEMI ($P < 0.001$). Coronary angiography was performed on only one patient during the index admission. At discharge, coronary angiography was planned for 20 patients (8.4 %) and cardiac stress testing for 63 (25.7 %).

At discharge, medications prescribed included aspirin (94.8 %), clopidogrel (97.8 %), statins (96.1 %), ACEI/ARB (82 %), and beta-blockers (72.6 %).

Predictors of in-hospital mortality and morbidity

During the index admission, MACE occurred in 30 (11.7 %) of patients. Logistic regression showed BMI ($P = 0.045$) and duration of diabetes ($P = 0.03$) were significant predictors of MACE. Patients presenting with STEMI did not have a higher risk of MACE than UA/STEMI patients. Time to presentation, presence of hypertension, diabetes, and previous cardiac disease were not significant predictors of MACE.

Discussion

In this study, ACS was diagnosed with reasonable accuracy using clinical and ECG criteria. Troponin concentrations were measured only in a minority of patients because of the non-availability of this test in the state sector and its high cost in private-sector laboratories.

Teaching Hospital, Peradeniya is one of the two largest tertiary-care institutions in the area; many smaller hospitals redirect patients with ACS to our unit. Thus, we believe that our sample can be considered representative of patients with ACS in this region.

The management of patients presenting with ACS in Sri Lanka has not been well documented. Previous studies have explored the time delay to initiation of thrombolytic therapy and adherence to guidelines [7–9]. Sri Lanka still relies heavily on medical management of ACS as opposed to primary coronary intervention. At present, few centers have commenced treating patients with primary percutaneous coronary intervention (PCI) [3].

There was no significant difference in age distribution between patients with STEMI and those with UA/NSTEMI, the majority of patients were in the 51–70 year age range in both groups. Patients with STEMI tended to have fewer risk factors and less frequently had a history of previous cardiac disease; they were however, more often smokers and had higher BMI. Hypertension and previous cardiac disease were notably more prevalent in the UA/NSTEMI group. The prevalence of risk factors among patients in Sri Lanka with ACS has not been reported previously. The prevalences of hypertension, diabetes, and previous cardiac disease (48.8, 35.5 and 20.7 %, respectively) found in this study are comparable to those reported for India (48.4, 37.6 and 14.2 %, respectively) [10]. However, the Acute Coronary Events – a Multinational Survey of Current Management Strategies (ACCESS) investigators reported a higher prevalence of hypertension (STEMI 78 %, NSTE-ACS 87 %) among ACS patients in other developing countries compared to Sri Lanka and India [11].

The types of ACS diagnosed in the current study were broadly similar to those reported for other observational studies conducted locally and globally. Rajapakse et al. [7] reported that 33.6 % of ACS patients in Sri Lanka had STEMI. Mohanan and colleagues reported a similar rate of 37 % in India. The ACCESS group of investigators reported that in developing countries 46 % of ACS patients had STEMI and 54 % NSTEMI-ACS. Our finding of 32.8 % for STEMI is marginally lower than previously reported figures.

The median time delay from symptom onset to presentation was shorter in patients with STEMI than in those with UA/NSTEMI (60 min vs. 120 min, $P = 0.058$); this difference was not statistically significant. Previously reported median pre-hospital delays for Sri Lankan patients with STEMI were 130 [8] and 720 min [9]; our results show a considerable improvement over these previous findings. The median in-hospital delay in admitting patients to an acute care unit was 5 min in the current study compared with previously reported figures of 70 [8] and 20 min [9]. Pre-hospital delays were longer for those who sought pre-hospital care than for those who presented directly to our institution. In previous studies, the reported average symptom onset to treatment time has ranged from 1.5–6 h globally [15]. The ACCESS study reported median delays of 4.0 and 6.0 h for patients with STEMI and NSTEMI-ACS, respectively [11]. The European Society of Cardiology has identified that the pre-hospital period is the most critical phase for reducing mortality and reiterated that efforts should be made to shorten this delay [16].

The overall use of aspirin, thienopyridines, and statins on admission, in-ward and at discharge were satisfactory [greater than 92 % (Table 2)]. The use of these medications did not differ significantly between patients with STEMI and those with UA/NSTEMI. Beta blockers were underutilized at admission (30.1 %), during hospital stay (68.7 %), and at discharge (72.6 %). The World Health Organization considers the use of aspirin, statins, and blood pressure-reducing agents post discharge to be a cost-effective strategy for patients with ACS; these medications are considered *best buys* [14].

In the present study, 83 % of eligible patients received thrombolytic therapy, a result consistent with the findings of Rajapakse et al., who reported that thrombolytic therapy was administered in 84.6 % of patients with STEMI [7]. Both figures show a tremendous improvement from the 17 % reported in Sri Lanka in 1999 [9]. However, in our study, a considerable proportion of patients with STEMI (30 %) received neither thrombolytic therapy nor PCI. Reported rates of thrombolytic therapy are 24.7 % in Kerala, India [10] and 39 % in the ACCESS study, which was performed in developing countries besides India and Sri Lanka [11]. However the overall rates of reperfusion therapy (PCI and coronary artery bypass graft surgery [CABG]) in both these studies were considerably higher (14 and 43.8 %, respectively) than in the present study.

Only 1 % of our study subjects underwent an interventional reperfusion procedure during the index admission. This largely reflects the current management of patients with ACS in the state sector, which caters to over 90 % of the population. At present, primary PCI is being introduced in few state-run cardiology units in the country. This probably reflects the limited resources of a state run, free health care system prevalent in Sri Lanka. However, coronary angiography and primary PCI are available in Sri Lanka in fee levying centers [3]. Rates of coronary angiography rates in Kerala, India were 19.6 and 18.6 % for patients with STEMI and NSTEMI-ACS, respectively, [10], 56 and 59 %, respectively, in the ACCESS study [11] and 62–63 and 70–80 %, respectively, in the second Euro Heart Survey (EHS-ACS-II) [17] and Global Registry of Acute Coronary Events (GRACE) [18]. The rates of PCI in the ACCESS, EHS-ACS-II, and GRACE studies for NSTEMI/ACS and STEMI were 31 and 41 %, 35 and 58 %, and 47 and 64 % respectively [8].

There is global evidence for favoring early coronary angiography and intervention following ACS [19, 20]. A recent meta-analysis has shown that complete revascularization (as opposed to culprit-only revascularization) during primary PCI may have beneficial outcomes at one year [21]. This largely reflects the non-critical atherosclerotic disease burden in coronary arteries, which unfortunately is not addressed by medical revascularization. We believe that the available evidence strongly favors an urgent transition from medical revascularization to PCI in Sri Lanka.

Median door-to-needle time in our study was 64 min; the mean of 96 min was attributable to late initiation of thrombolytic therapy in some patients. The recommended door to needle time of 30 min was achieved in only 16.9 % of study subjects. A previous study reported a median door-to-needle time of 70 min [8]. In Malaysia the median door-to-needle time is reportedly 48–54 min [22]. In India, the door to needle time exceeded 30 min in only 31 % of patients with STEMI [10].

During the index admission, MACE was observed in 11.7 % of patients; this incidence did not differ significantly between STEMI and UA/NSTEMI groups. Two deaths occurred in the UA/NSTEMI group and none in the STEMI group; however, the small sample size prevents drawing any definite conclusions from these findings. The in-hospital mortality rates for patients with STEMI is reportedly 8.2 % in the Kerala registry in India, 7 % in the GRACE study and 4.3 % in the ACTION study [23]. The in-hospital mortality for patients with UA/NSTEMI in our study (1.1 %) is low compared with reported mortality rates of 1.8 % in India [10], 3 % in the Euro heart survey ACS II [17], and 3.9 % in the ACTION study [23] for patients with NSTEMI.

Because Sri Lanka does not currently have a cardiac registry, the outcomes of ACS following the index admission are not known. This study attempts to highlight this deficiency and express the urgent need for better record keeping and registration of ACS patients. With the phased-in introduction of primary PCI in selected centers, it would be interesting to compare treatment and outcomes of ACS a few years in the future, just as previous studies [7–9] have paved the way for the current comparisons.

Implications for quality improvement

Higher BMI and duration of diabetes were significant predictors of in-hospital MACE in the current study. Although we failed to demonstrate time to treatment, and door to needle time as significant predictors of MACE, previous studies have shown that these factors are significant predictors of adverse cardiac outcomes [10]. However, delayed presentation (STEMI, median 60 min and UA/NSTEMI, median 120 min) remains a critical factor in the deployment of effective treatment. Late presentation resulted in 12.3 % of patients with STEMI not receiving fibrinolytic therapy.

Transfer of patients between GPs, smaller hospitals, and ACS treatment facilities remain a hurdle in Sri Lanka's emergency response system. The observed median delay of 240 min is considerable and largely attributable to most patients having to find their own transport. Educating the public on early warning symptoms, streamlining emergency services at smaller hospitals and GP centers, and developing outreach and emergency cardiac response teams are critical for improving cardiac services in Sri Lanka.

The emergency care provided was minimal in smaller hospitals and at GP practices; only 16 % of patients with ACS receiving aspirin or a thienopyridine. Furthermore, only 16.9 % of patients with STEMI received thrombolytic therapy within the recommended 30 min of admission. Fibrinolytic therapy was not administered to 11 % of eligible patients for unknown reasons, implying both deficiencies in cardiac response team training and poor record keeping.

At the time of this study, PCI was heavily underutilized in the management of ACS in Sri Lanka. Over the last 3 years, significant efforts have been taken to train health workers and increase the use of PCI in treating ACS. Although the use of aspirin, thienopyridines, and statins was satisfactory, beta blocker use was suboptimal in our study sample. Poor utilization of beta blockers has been reported in earlier studies [7] and clearly needs to be addressed.

Limitations

This study is the first to compare demographic characteristics, presentation and management of patients with STEMI and NSTEMI/UA at a tertiary care center in Sri Lanka. Because of limited resources, cardiac markers were not measured in all patients, preventing further characterization of the NSTEMI/UA group. The relatively small sample size of 256 patients and the absence of post discharge follow up are additional limitations of this study.

Conclusions

The use of aspirin, thienopyridines, and statins on admission, in ward, and on discharge was satisfactory. Only 72.8 % of STEMI patients received thrombolytic therapy and there was significant delay in initiating fibrinolysis. Emergency care at smaller hospitals was suboptimal and transfer of patients between hospitals was unsafe. PCI was minimally utilized at presentation and thereafter. Instituting safe and effective patient transfer to hospitals, improving the training of first contact doctors, and increasing the use of current PCI practices are key areas that need to be urgently addressed.

Abbreviations

ACCESS: Acute Coronary Events—Multinational Survey of Current Management Strategies; ACE: Angiotensin-converting enzyme; ACS: Acute coronary syndrome; ARB: Angiotensin II receptor blocker; BMI: Body mass index; CVD: Cardiovascular disease; EHS-ACS: Second Euro Heart Survey; GP: General practitioner; GRACE: Global Registry of Acute Coronary Events; IHD: Ischemic heart disease; MACE: Major adverse cardiac events; STEMI: ST segment elevation myocardial infarction; NSTEMI: Non ST segment elevation myocardial infarction; PCI: Percutaneous coronary intervention; UA: Unstable angina.

Competing interests

None of the authors have any competing interests to declare.

Authors' contributions

AM conceptualized the project, reviewed the literature, analyzed the data, and wrote the manuscript. RB conceptualized the project and collected the data.CD and MG analyzed the data and helped with writing of the manuscript. All authors read and approved the final manuscript.

Acknowledgements

We wish to thank Dr. Sampath Tennakoon, Department of Community Medicine, University of Peradeniya for his assistance with the statistical analysis and Drs. Ruwan Munasinghe, NP Dinamithra, Amila Subasinghe and Jayantha Herath of the Teaching Hospital Peradeniya for their assistance with data collection.

Author details

[1]Department of Medicine, Faculty of Medicine, University of Peradeniya, Galaha Rd, Peradeniya 20400, Sri Lanka. [2]Professorial Medical Unit, Teaching Hospital, Peradeniya, Sri Lanka.

References

1. Hughes LO, Raval U, Raftery EB. First myocardial infarctions in Asian and white men. BMJ. 1989;298(6684):1345–50.
2. Ghaffar A, Reddy KS, Singhi M. Burden of non-communicable diseases in South Asia. BMJ. 2004;328(7443):807–10.
3. Abeysuriya V, Chandrasena LG, Kasturiratne A, Hettiarachchi VS, Wickramasinghe AR. Outcome of patients with ST segment elevation myocardial infarction (STEMI) following percutaneous transluminal coronary angioplasty: a retrospective study. Ceylon Med J. 2014;59(4):118–23.
4. Wijewardene K, Mohideen MR, Mendis S, Fernando DS, Kulathilaka T, Weerasekara D, et al. Prevalence of hypertension, diabetes and obesity: baseline findings of a population based survey in four provinces in Sri Lanka. Ceylon Med J. 2005;50(2):62–70.
5. Abeywardena MY. Dietary fats, carbohydrates and vascular disease: Sri Lankan perspectives. Atherosclerosis. 2003;171(2):157–61.
6. Medical Statistics Unit. Ministry of Health Sri Lanka, Annual Health Bulletin 2012: Colombo, Ministry of Health Sri Lanka: 2012.
7. Rajapakse S, Rodrigo PC, Selvachandran J. Management of acute coronary syndrome in a tertiary care general medical unit in Sri Lanka: how closely do we follow the guidelines? J Clin Pharm Ther. 2010;35(4):421–7.
8. Constantine GR, Thenabadu PN. Time delay to thrombolytic therapy–a Sri Lankan perspective. Postgrad Med J. 1998;74(873):405–7.
9. Constantine GR, Herath JI, Chang AA, Suganthan P, Hewamane BS, Thenabadu PN. Management of acute myocardial infarction in general medical wards in Sri Lanka. Postgrad Med J. 1999;75(890):718–20.
10. Mohanan PP, Mathew R, Harikrishnan S, Krishnan MN, Zachariah G, Joseph J, et al. Presentation, management, and outcomes of 25 748 acute coronary syndrome admissions in Kerala, India: results from the Kerala ACS Registry. Eur Heart J. 2013;34(2):121–9.

11. Investigators A. Management of acute coronary syndromes in developing countries: acute coronary events-a multinational survey of current management strategies. Am Heart J. 2011;162(5):852–9. e22.
12. Eagle KA, Goodman SG, Avezum A, Budaj A, Sullivan CM, Lopez-Sendon J. Practice variation and missed opportunities for reperfusion in ST-segment-elevation myocardial infarction: findings from the Global Registry of Acute Coronary Events (GRACE). Lancet. 2002;359(9304):373–7.
13. Fox KA, Goodman SG, Anderson FA, Granger CB, Moscucci M, Flather MD, et al. From guidelines to clinical practice: the impact of hospital and geographical characteristics on temporal trends in the management of acute coronary syndromes. The Global Registry of Acute Coronary Events (GRACE). Eur Heart J. 2003;24(15):1414–24.
14. World Health Organization, Global Status Report on Noncommunicable Diseases 2010. World Health Organization 2011, Geneva, Switzerland.
15. O'Donnell S, McKee G, Mooney M. Slow-onset and fast-onset symptom presentations in Acute Coronary Syndrome (ACS): new perspectives on pre-hospital delay in patients with ACS. J Emerg Med. 2014;46:507–15.
16. Tubaro M, Danchin N, Goldstein P, Filippatos G, Hasin Y, Heras M, et al. Pre-hospital treatment of STEMI patients. A scientific statement of the Working Group Acute Cardiac Care of the European Society of Cardiology. Acute Card Care. 2011;13(2):56–67.
17. Mandelzweig L, Battler A, Boyko V, Bueno H, Danchin N, Flippatos G, et al. The second Euro Heart Survey on acute coronary syndromes: Characteristics, treatment, and outcome of patients with ACS in Europe and the Mediterranean Basin in 2004. Eur Heart J. 2006;27(19):2285–93.
18. Fox KA, Goodman SG, Anderson FA, Granger CB, Moscucci M, Flather MD, et al. Management of acute coronary syndromes. Variations in practice and outcome; findings from the Global Registry of Acute Coronary Events (GRACE). Eur Heart J. 2002;23(15):1177–89.
19. A clinical trial comparing primary coronary angioplasty with tissue plasminogen activator for acute myocardial infarction. The Global Use of Strategies to Open Occluded Coronary Arteries in Acute Coronary Syndromes (GUSTO IIb) Angioplasty Substudy Investigators. N Engl J Med. 1997;336(23):16261–1628.
20. Raber L, Windecker S. Primary percutaneous coronary intervention and risk of stent thrombosis: a look beyond the HORIZON. Circulation. 2011;123(16):1709–12.
21. Moretti C, D'Ascenzo F, Quadri G, Omede P, Montefusco A, Taha S, et al. Management of multivessel coronary disease in STEMI patients: a systematic review and meta-analysis. Int J Cardiol. 2015;179:552–7.
22. Loch A, Lwin T, Zakaria IM, Abidin IZ, Wan Ahmad WA, Hautmann O. Failure to improve door-to-needle time by switching to emergency physician-initiated thrombolysis for ST elevation myocardial infarction. Postgrad Med J. 2013;89(1052):335–9.
23. Roe MT, Messenger JC, Weintraub WS, Cannon CP, Fonarow GC, Dai D, et al. Treatments, trends, and outcomes of acute myocardial infarction and percutaneous coronary intervention. J Am Coll Cardiol. 2010;56(4):254–63.

4

Cost-effectiveness of fondaparinux versus enoxaparin in non-ST-elevation acute coronary syndrome in Canada (OASIS-5)

Jorge Alfonso Ross Terres[1,2,4*], G. Lozano-Ortega[2,4], R. Kendall[2,4] and M. J. Sculpher[3,4]

Abstract

Background: Acute coronary syndrome (ACS) refers to a spectrum of life-threatening cardiac diseases usually due to coronary artery plaque rupture, subsequent thrombin generation plaque activation and thrombus formation. To date, no economic analyses have been published about the use of fondaparinux in NSTE-ACS patients in Canada. The purpose of our study is to estimate the lifetime cost-effectiveness of fondaparinux compared to enoxaparin for non-ST-elevation acute coronary syndrome (NSTE-ACS) patients in a Canadian hospital setting.

Methods: As an extension of a previous published economic analysis for US patients, an event-based decision analytic model was constructed using clinical and resource use data from OASIS-5, a randomized trial of 20,078 patients from 41 countries. A public payer perspective in the hospital setting was adopted. Resource use data from the trial were valued using Canadian costs. A cost regression model was developed to estimate the mean cost of managing the clinical events over the 180 day period. Annual costs of long-term care for ACS patients were added after 180 days until death. Long-term survival was incorporated using Canadian life tables with further adjustment for additional risks associated with NSTE-ACS. Quality-of-life (utility) decrements from published sources were applied to clinical events. Lifetime costs (2009 CAD$) and quality-adjusted life-years (QALYs), discounted annually at 5 %, were estimated for the typical patient in OASIS-5 (i.e., at mean covariate values).

Results: The trial data showed that fondaparinux is protective against all clinical events observed in the trial. The model showed that: over 180 days, fondaparinux dominates enoxaparin, producing similar estimates of QALYs gained and saving $439; over a patient's lifetime, fondaparinux yields an ICER of $4293/QALY. Based on PSA, the probabilities that fondaparinux dominates enoxaparin (less costly and more effective) and that is cost-effective at a $50,000 threshold were 42 % and 96 %, respectively.

Conclusions: In the Canadian hospital setting, fondaparinux is cost-effective when compared to enoxaparin for the treatment of NSTE-ACS. This result holds both in the immediate post-event period and over the lifetimes of patients.

Keywords: Acute coronary syndromes, Health economics

Background

Acute coronary syndrome (ACS) refers to a spectrum of life-threatening cardiac diseases usually due to coronary artery plaque rupture, subsequent thrombin generation plaque activation and thrombus formation.

Non-ST-elevation acute coronary syndrome (NSTE-ACS) comprises 2 components: unstable angina (UA) and non-ST-elevation myocardial infarction. Pharmacological recommendations and sequence of therapy will depend on the individual management strategy and treatment guidelines, but for both invasive and conservative strategies, a combination of antiplatelet and anticoagulation agents is recommended. Most commonly, antiplatelet therapy will be comprised of aspirin plus clopidogel and/or a glycoprotein IIb/IIIa (GP) inhibitor, followed by an anticoagulant agent. Options for anticoagulation therapy include fondaparinux (Arixtra), unfractionated heparin (UFH) bivalirubin and low-molecular heparins, such as enoxaparin.

* Correspondence: Jorge.A.Ross@gsk.com
[1]GlaxoSmithKline, Mississauga, ON, Canada
[2]GlaxoSmithKline, 2301 Renaissance Boulevard, King of Prussia, PA 19406, USA
Full list of author information is available at the end of the article

Fondaparinux is a well established synthetic anticoagulant that inhibits thrombus formation by interrupting the blood coagulation cascade through antithrombin IIIA-mediated selective inhibition of factor Xa.

The Fifth Organization to Assess Strategies in Acute Ischemic Syndromes Investigators (OASIS-5) trial randomized 20,078 patients with NSTE-ACS to fondaparinux or enoxaparin [1].

Patients were randomly assigned to a study group within 24 h after the onset of symptoms and were eligible if they met at least two of the three following criteria: an age of at least 60 years, an elevated level of troponin or creatine kinase MB isoenzyme, or electrocardiographic changes indicative of ischemia. Patients with contraindications to low-molecular-weight heparin, recent hemorrhagic stroke, indications for anticoagulation other than an acute coronary syndrome, or a serum creatinine level of at least 3 mg per deciliter (265 μmol per liter) were excluded [2]. The study protocol was approved by the respective ethics committees and regulatory bodies (ClinicalTrials.gov number, NCT00139815) Additional file 1.

The Trial showed similar rates of ischemic events at 9 days but, by 180 days, fondaparinux reduced major bleeding and improved mortality and morbidity.

To date, no economic analyses have been published about the use of fondaparinux in NSTE-ACS patients in Canada. As an extension of a previous published analysis based on US patients [1], this article reports on an evaluation of the costs and benefits of fondaparinux and enoxaparin, in order to determine which one is more cost-effective, both in short term (180 days) and in the long term, using a life-time model in a Canadian hospital setting.

Methods

This cost-effectiveness analysis was based on a published and well-established methodology applied to estimate the cost-effectiveness of fondaparinux versus enoxaparin in the United States hospital setting [1]. Briefly, the analysis consisted of 2 phases. First phase estimates the differential cost of fondaparinux and enoxaparin over 180 days (mean OASIS-5 follow-up). The analysis relates to a public-payer perspective in the Canadian hospital setting. The second phase assessed long-term cost-effectiveness in terms of costs and quality-adjusted life years (QALYs). Costs and QALYs are discounted at 5 % per annum.

An event-based decision analytical model was constructed using clinical and resource use data from OASIS-5 and was previously published by Sculpher et al [1]. The probabilities of death, non-fatal myocardial infarction (MI), non-fatal stroke, and major and minor bleeds over a period of 180 days, for both treatment strategies, were estimated using a set of risk equations derived from OASIS-5 data. Bleeding events are included in the cost analysis but they are assumed not to affect long-term prognosis.

In the short-term cost analysis, the differential cost of each therapy was calculated by multiplying the estimated cost of each event by the relevant event risk and summing all the products. Decrements in health-related quality of life (HRQoL) and long-term prognoses estimates were used for the long-term cost-effectiveness analysis. A 5 % annual discount rate was applied to all costs and QALYs.

Clinical events and resource use over a mean follow-up of 173 days (range, 90–180 days) where used from the OASIS-5 trial. This trial involved 20,078 patients with NSTE-ACS which were randomized to either fondaparinux (2.5 mg daily) or enoxaparin (1 mg per kg twice daily) for a mean of 5 days. This was a global study in which 41 countries participated including multiples hospitals Canada. The primary end point of death, MI or refractory ischemia at 9 days, was similar between treatments, but major bleeding at 9 days was lower with fondaparinux [1]. The trial found significantly lower rates of death and nonfatal events with fondaparinux at 180 days [1].

The differential cost of fondaparinux and enoxaparin was based on the acquisition costs of the 2 therapies and the product of 2 sets of estimates from the trial (i) risks of key clinical events: death, nonfatal MI, nonfatal stroke, a combination of MI and stroke and major and minor bleeds (ii) the mean costs of these events. The 180-day probabilities of clinical events used OASIS-5 data and were based on parametric survival modeling using a Weibull [3] distribution. The hazard of each event is estimated as a function of treatment and baseline covariates. The choice of covariates has been based on the clinical judgment of and variables used in the TIMI [4] and GRACE [4] risk scoring systems.

Key resource use data in OASIS-5 included study drugs, concomitant medications, and inpatient days. The base-case analysis uses resource use data from the 1403 Canadian patients valued using Canadian costs (2009 $CAD), largely based on data obtained through the Ontario Health Insurance Program (OHIP) [5–7]. These costs include: medications, laboratory and diagnostic procedures, therapeutic services, and primary and secondary diagnoses, total costs (fixed and variable) to the hospital. Daily room costs are included for inpatient interventions. In the case of procedures and interventions, fees to medical professionals are estimated using the Ontario Case Costing Initiative (OCCI), OHIP and the published literature [8–10]. Drug costs are derived from the Ontario Drug Benefit (ODB) formulary. Blood transfusion costs are from ODB formulary and published sources [11].

Table 1 Summary of key resource use observed in the OASIS-5 trial patients randomized in Canada (n = 1.403) within the 180-day follow-up period together with associated unitcosts (adapted from Table 2 in US analysis')

Item of resource use	Fondaparinux (n = 701)	Enoxaparin (n = 7 02)	Unit cost (CAD 2009 S)
Sudy drugs (mean (SD) days)	4.10 (2.28)	3.65 (2.11)	Enoxaparin: 15 per day [a] Fondaparinux: 15 per day [b]
Days in hospital (mean (SD))			
ICU	3.54 (5.07)	3.57 (3.83)	1433 per day
General ward	4.64 (10.13)	4.46 (9.61)	547 per day
Step down	2.98 (5.01)	2.85 (5.28)	547 per day
Selected concomitant medicines			
Clopidcgrel (mean (SD) days)	105.25 (77.18)	106.07 (77.69)	2.58 per day
Ticlopidine (mean (SD) days)	0.08 (1.75)	1.04 (12.14)	0.55 per day
Glycoprotein IIb/IIIa antagonists (n (%))	201 (28.67)	212 (30.20)	1094
Selected procedures (n (%) with one or more)	47 (6.70)	39 (5.56)	543 per procedure
Blood transfusion	603 (86.02)	607 (86.47)	5401 per procedure
Coronary angiography	298 (42.51)	335 (47.72)	10,543 per procedure
Percutaneous coronary intervention	143 (20.40)	134 (19.09)	21,286 per procedure
Coronary artery bypass graft			

SD Standard deviation, *n* Number, *ICU* Intensive care unit
[a]Based on 80 mg injection
[b]Based on 2.5 mg injection

In order to estimate the mean cost over 180 days of: (i) patients without clinical events, and (ii) the additional cost associated with each event, regression modeling was used. An ordinary least squares model was used with a series of dummy variables used to represent events. Concomitant drug costs were based on the mean dosage in OASIS-5 and the mean therapy duration in Canadian trial patients. In the base case, these costs are based on the ODB formulary.

Patients remaining alive at 180 days will survive, though with some decrements to their health, for a time depending on sex, age and health state at 180 days. Patients will also continue incurring costs for the treatment of their heart disease. Long-term cost-effectiveness assumes that the clinical differences between the alternative antithrombotics ceases at 180 days.

Since the OASIS-5 trial did not collect any data on HRQoL, estimates are derived from other published sources and applied to clinical events. Due to the unavailability of Canadian-specific values, estimates were derived from age-and sex-specific "population norms" for the United States (US) based on EQ-5D instrument [12].

Long-term mortality rates are incorporated using Canadian life tables. The additional mortality risk in NSTE-ACS is quantified in terms of a relative risk compared with the general population and distinguishes between patients with a nonfatal MI, a nonfatal stroke of any severity, both types of nonfatal event or neither within 6 months of their ACS episode. This uses data from the United Kingdom UK PRAIS study [13]. Beyond the initial 180-day period, the cost of long-term care for ACS patients was assumed to be $10,783 per annum [14].

Mean (expected) cost-effectiveness of the probability of each therapy being the least costly, and the more cost-effective therapy assuming a cost-effectiveness threshold of $50,000 per QALY gained is presented using probabilistic sensitivity analysis (PSA) [15]. Short-term costs and long-term cost-effectiveness are shown for the "average" trial patient. Also, results are calculated for national patients at high and low risk of the composite event of death and nonfatal MI and stroke with enoxaparin over 180 days, assuming the relative effect of fondaparinux remains unchanged.

Lifetime costs and (QALYs) were estimated for the typical patient in OASIS-5 (i.e., at mean covariate values), as well as for a patient at the 2.5th and 97.5th percentiles of composite risk of death, nonfatal MI or nonfatal stroke. A cost analysis was performed at 180 days, and incremental cost-effectiveness ratios (ICERs) were output over the entire lifetime. PSA was carried out to assess parameter uncertainty.

Results

The risk equations showed consistent results with the clinical analysis [2]. For each type of event over the 180-day follow-up period, fondaparinux was protective compared with enoxaparin, although the effect was not statistically significant for nonfatal MI. (See Table 1 in [1]). Table 1 shows key resource use over the 180-day follow up in OASIS-5 in Canadian patients, together with estimated unit costs. Resource use was very similar between enoxaparin and fondaparinux patients; the main difference between fondaparinux and enoxaparin was in the rate of percutaneous coronary intervention. Also, a higher proportion of Canadian subjects needed blood transfusion under fondaparinux, although this difference was not statistically significant (relative risk (RR) of having a blood transfusion: 1.21; 95 % confidence interval: 0.80, 1.82). When considering all patients randomized in the trial, the RR of having a blood transfusion was 0.75 (0.65 to 0.86).

Table 2 presents the results of the short-term cost analysis. The total expected costs of the two therapies over 180 days shows fondaparinux was associated with potential cost savings, although this finding was not statistically significant.

The long-term cost-effectiveness analysis reported in Table 3 showed that the ICER is well below conventional thresholds for the 3 types of patients considered in the model (patients of average characteristics, and patients at low and high risk of the composite event of death, MI or stroke, respectively). The uncertainty in these results is shown in terms of the probabilities that fondaparinux is cost saving, and cost-effective at a threshold of $50,000 per QALY gained; these probabilities ranged from 34 to 48 % and 83 to 97 %, respectively.

Discussion

After assessing the cost-effectiveness of the alternative therapies reflecting Canadian practice based on resource use, unit costs, age- and sex-specific population, mortality risks and HRQoL data specific to the country, we found that fondaparinux is cost-effective and, under most scenarios, a dominant strategy compared with enoxaparin. In part, this reflects not only the lower acquisition cost of fondaparinux but also the lower rates of clinical events during the 6-month period after treatment.

There are limitations to modeling the cost-effectiveness of products studied in multinational trials because studies are powered on overall event rates, not event rates in individual countries, yet local country resource use and cost data are required for decision making. Therefore, to inform payers in Canada, the model was based on Canadian resource use from the trial, while using whole trial event rates.

At baseline in OASIS-5, Canadian patients were generally similar to those in the overall trial with some differences with the US population which were less likely to have unstable angina (rather than MI), had undergone more revascularization procedures, were more likely to be diabetic, and were less likely to have ST-segment depression. Differences in medical care between Canada and the United States have been reported in the contemporary management of patients with non– ST-elevation MI and UA. Several studies have reported findings in which angiography, angioplasty, and bypass surgery are more common in the United States than in Canada. The differences could be explained in the availability on-site

Table 2 Six-month cost analysis comparison of the expected costs of enoxaparin and fondaparinux over six months (estimates relate to a patient with "average" characteristics [4], adapted from Table 2 in US analysis')

	Cost of event[b] (95 % CI)	Probability of event (95 % CI)		Cost per patient[c] (95 % CI) (2009 CADS)	
Event/resource use	(2009 CAD $)	Enoxaparin	Fondaparinux	Enoxaparin	Fondaparinux
Death	−691 (−4943, 3487)	0.046 (0.042, 0.050)	0.041 (0.038, 0.045)	−28 (−225, 157)	−25 (−203, 141)
Non-fatal MI	15,021 (10,997, 19,053)	0.049 (0.046, 0.055)	0.047 (0.043, 0.052)	752 (527, 978)	712 (505, 927)
Non-fatal stroke	18,755 (10,698, 26,864)	0.011 (0.009, 0.014)	0.007 (0.006, 0.009)	217 (113, 340)	141 (76, 226)
Non-fatal MI & Stroke	3407 (−29,232, 35,980)	0.0006 (0.0005, 0.0007)	0.0003 (0.0003, 0.0005)	2 (−17, 20)	1 (−10, 13)
Major bleed	17,553 (13,827, 21,023)	0.052 (0.048, 0.057)	0.038 (0.034, 0.042)	921 (728, 1126)	665 (524, 823)
Minor bleed	3604 (171, 7182)	0.071 (0.066, 0.077)	0.036 (0.032, 0.040)	257 (10, 521)	129 (5, 254)
Enoxaparin Treatment	60	1	0	60	0
Fondaparinux Treatment	63	0	1	0	63
Other costs[d]	24,143 (22,785, 25,425)	1	1	24,143 (22,785, 25,425)	24,143 (22,785, 25,425)
Total mean cost				26,302 (25,042, 27,473)	25,864 (24,689, 27,025)
Difference in mean costs					*$-439 (−2069, 1322)*

MI Myocardial infarction, *CI* Confidence interval, *CAD* Canadian dollars

[a]Covariates at mean values are Age 67.1; proportion male 0 62; proportion with history of: heart failure 0 14. diabetes 0 25. hypertension 0 67. ST depression 0 51; creatinine quartiles quartile 1 0 26. quartile 2 0 26. quartile 3 0 25. quartile 4 0 23

[b]Results of the cost regression relating to patients randomized in Canada (n = 1.403) (2009 CAD $)

[c]Estimated by multiplying the probability of event times cost of event, when performing the probabilistic sensitivity analysis

[d]Background cost associated with patients who experienced ischemic heart disease

Table 3 Cost-effectiveness results over a lifetime time horizon (adapted from Table 2 in US analysis)

	Enoxaparin	Fondaparinux	ICER
Patient with average characteristics			
Expected cost	$110,477	$110,661	
Expected quality-adjusted life years	6.37	6.42	
Probablity most cost-effective at a threshold of $50,000 per QALY		96 %	$4293
Probability of cost-saving		42 %	
Patient at low risk of composite event over 180 days (2.5th percentile)			
Expected cost	$164,824	$164,836	
Expected quality-adjusted life years	11.01	11.03	
Probability most cost-effective at a threshold of $50,000 per QALY		83 %	$661
Probability of cost-saving		48 %	
Patient at high risk of composite event over 180 days (97.5th percentile)			
Expected cost	$70,846	$71,299	
Expected quality-adjusted life years	3.37	3.47	
Probability most cost-effective at a threshold of $50,000 per QALY		100 %	$4666
Probability of cost-saving		34 %	

facilities in different institutions across Canada which could lead to longer waiting times which could have an impact on long outcome of this population. This could be reflection of longer stay in ICU and general ward [16].

As previously published in the original analysis performed in the US population, fondaparinux resulted in cost savings to the hospital [1]. When 180-day cost and clinical results were extrapolated to long-term cost-effectiveness, fondaparinux was dominant (less costly and more effective in terms of QALYs under most scenarios.

The OASIS-5 trial reported that in the subgroup of patients undergoing percutaneous coronary intervention (PCI), fondaparinux reduced major bleeding by one half while maintaining similar efficacy to enoxaparin. This resulted in superior net clinical benefit of fondaparinux relative to enoxaparin in PCI patients. In this analysis, both enoxaparin and fondaparinux were associated with catheter thrombosis in 1 % of patients. Consequently, it is recommended that, in patients treated with fondaparinux for ACS, adjunctive UFH (50–60 IU/kg bolus) be used in place of an IV fondaparinux bolus just before the PCI procedure. It has been shown in OASIS-5 that, even with the use of supplemental UFH in PCI patients, the reduction in bleeding with fondaparinux appears to be preserved [1].

Given this, and the modest cost of UFH relative to IV fondaparinux, the use of adjunctive UFH can be expected to have little effect on the cost-effectiveness results presented here.

Conclusions

This analysis showed that differences in clinical events over 180 days have long-term prognostic implications. In the Canadian hospital setting, fondaparinux is cost-effective when compared to enoxaparin for the treatment of NSTE-ACS. This result holds both in the immediate post-event period and over the lifetimes of patients.

Abbreviations

ACS: acute coronary syndrome; CAD$: Canadian dollars; GP: glycoprotein IIb/IIIa; HRQoL: health-related quality of life; ICERs: incremental cost-effectiveness ratios; MI: myocardial infarction; NSTE-ACS: non-ST-elevation acute coronary syndrome; OASIS-5: Organization to Assess Strategies in Acute Ischemic Syndromes Investigators; OCCI: Ontario Case Costing Initiative; ODB: Ontario Drug Benefit; OHIP: Ontario Health Insurance Program; PSA: probabilistic sensitivity analysis; QALYs: Quality-adjusted life-years; RR: Relative risk; UA: unstable angina; UFH: unfractionated heparin; US: United States.

Competing interests

JART is an employee of GlaxoSmithKline, and own stock in the company. MS is a former director and shareholder in Oxford Outcomes and has received consulting fees from GSK. All others declare that they have no competing interests.

Authors' contributions

JART – study conception, interpretation of results, drafting manuscript; GLO - data collection, analysis, interpretation; RK – data collection, review manuscript; MS - analysis, interpretation. All authors reviewed and approved the final manuscript.

Acknowledgements

We thank all patients who participated in OASIS-5 and all the investigators and staff at the participating sites. The OASIS-5 study was coordinated by the Population Health Research Institute at McMaster University, Hamilton, Canada, who were responsible for data management and analysis of the data for the main publications. We thank Jennifer Pierrera for providing data on Canadian costs and Kavisha Jayasundara for assistance with drafting the manuscript. GlaxoSmithKline contracted Oxford Outcomes Ltd Canada for this economic analysis. OASIS-5 was funded by Sanofi-Aventis and GSK.

Author details
[1]GlaxoSmithKline, Mississauga, ON, Canada. [2]GlaxoSmithKline, 2301 Renaissance Boulevard, King of Prussia, PA 19406, USA. [3]Oxford Outcomes Ltd, Vancouver, Canada. [4]Center of Helth Economics, University of York, York, UK.

References

1. Sculpher MJ, Lozano-Ortega G, Sambrook J, Palmer S, Ormanidhi O, Bakhai A, et al. Fondaparinux versus Enoxaparin in non-ST-elevation acute coronary syndromes: short-term cost and long-term cost-effectiveness using data from the Fifth Organization to Assess Strategies in Acute Ischemic Syndromes Investigators (OASIS-5) trial. Am Heart J. 2009;157:845–852.
2. The Fifth Organisation to Assess Strategies in Acute Ischemic Syndromes Investigators. Comparison of fondaparinux and enoxaparin in acute coronary syndromes. N Engl J Med. 2006;354:1464–76.
3. Collet D. Modelling survival data in medical research. London: Chapman and Hall; 2012.
4. Antman EM, Cohen M, Bernink PJ, McCabe CH, Horacek T, Papuchis G, et al. The TIMI risk score for unstable angina/non-ST elevation MI: A method for prognostication and therapeutic decision making. JAMA. 2000;284:835–42.
5. Ontario Health Insurance Program. Ontario Physician Fee Schedule. OHIP 2008. 2012. Ref Type: Online Source.
6. Ontario Health Insurance Program. Ontario Drug Benefits Formulary. ODB 2010. 2012. Ref Type: Online Source.
7. Ontario Health Insurance Program. Ontario Lab Fee Schedule. OHIP 1999. 2012. Ref Type: Online Source.
8. Kolm P, Yuan Y, Veledar E, Mehta SR, O'Brien JA, Weintraub WS. Cost-effectiveness of clopidogrel in acute coronary syndromes in Canada: a long-term analysis based on the CURE trial. Can J Cardiol. 2007;23:1037–42.
9. O'Brien BJ, Connolly SJ, Goeree R, Blackhouse G, Willan A, Yee R, et al. Cost-Effectiveness of the Implantable Cardioverter-Defibrillator Results From the Canadian Implantable Defibrillator Study (CIDS). Circulation. 2010;103:1416–21.
10. Lynd LD, Goeree R, Crowther MA, O'Brien BJ. A probabilistic cost-effectiveness analysis of enoxaparin versus unfractionated heparin for the prophylaxis of deep-vein thrombosis following major trauma. Can J Clin Pharmacol. 2007;14:e215–26.
11. Dranitsaris G, Vincent M, Crowther M. Dalteparin versus warfarin for the prevention of recurrent venous thromboembolic events in cancer patients: a pharmacoeconomic analysis. Pharmacoeconomics. 2006;24:593–607.
12. Kind P. The EuroQoL instrument: an index of health-related quality of life. In: Spilker B, editor. Quality of life and pharmacoeconomics in clinical trials. 2nd ed. Philadelphia: Lippincott-Raven; 1996. p. 191–201.
13. Taneja AK, Collinson J, Flather MD, Bakhai A, de Arenaza DP, Wang D, et al. Mortality following non-ST elevation acute coronary syndrome: 4 years follow-up of the PRAIS UK Registry (Prospective Registry of Acute Ischaemic Syndromes in the UK).
Eur Heart J. 2004;25:2013–8.
14. Lamy A, Yusuf S, Pogue J, Gafni A. Cost implications of the use of ramipril in high-risk patients based on the Heart Outcomes Prevention Evaluation (HOPE) study. Circulation. 2003;107:960–5.
15. Briggs A, Claxton K, Sculpher M. Decision Modelling for health economic evaluation. Oxford: Oxford University Press; 2006.
16. Yuling F, Wei-Ching C, Dan M, Califf RM, Brian M, Granger CB, et al. Canadian-American Differences in the Management of Acute Coronary Syndromes in the GUSTO IIb Trial One-Year Follow-Up of Patients Without ST-Segment Elevation. Circulation. 2000;102:1375–81.

5

Relationship and prognostic importance of thyroid hormone and N-terminal pro-B-Type natriuretic peptide for patients after acute coronary syndromes

Julija Brozaitiene, Narseta Mickuviene, Aurelija Podlipskyte, Julius Burkauskas* and Robertas Bunevicius^

Abstract

Background: Altered thyroid function and increased rates of N-terminal pro-B-Type natriuretic peptide (NT-pro-BNP) are highly prevalent in coronary artery disease (CAD) patients with heart failure, and are associated with unfavorable prognosis. This study was undertaken to examine the relationship and prognostic impact of thyroid hormones, inflammatory biomarkers, and NT-pro-BNP on long-term outcomes in patients after acute coronary syndrome (ACS).

Methods: The study comprised of 642 patients (age 58 ± 10 years, 77 % male) attending an in-patient cardiac rehabilitation program after experiencing ACS. Patients were evaluated for demographic, clinical and CAD risk factors as well as thyroid hormones (e.g., fT3, fT4 level, fT3/fT4 ratio), inflammatory biomarkers (hs-CRP, IL-6) and NT-pro-BNP levels. Data on fT3/fT4 ratio and NT-pro-BNP levels were not normally distributed and were natural-log transformed (ln). Both all-cause (cumulative) and cardiac-related mortality were considered the primary outcomes of interest.

Results: According to the Cox model, age, NYHA class, (ln)NT-pro-BNP levels (HR 1.53, 95 % CI 1.13–2.07), fT4 level (HR 1.15, 95 % CI 1.04–1.27), and (ln)fT3/fT4 ratio (HR 0.08, 95 % CI 0.02–0.32) were the most important predictors of all-cause mortality among CAD patients after ACS. Similarly, age, NYHA class, (ln)NT-pro-BNP levels (HR 1.62, 95 % CI 1.11–2.36), fT4 (HR 1.15, 95 % CI 1.02–1.29) and (ln)fT3/fT4 ratio (HR 0.10, 95 % CI 0.02–0.55) independently predicted cardiac-related mortality. Kaplan-Meier analyses provided significant prognostic information with the highest risk for all-cause mortality in the low cut off measures of fT3/fT4 ratio <0.206 and NT-pro-BNP ≥290.4 ng/L (HR 2.03, 95 % CI 1.39–2.96) and fT4 level >12.54 pg/ml (HR = 2.34, 95 % CI 1.05–5.18). There was no association between hs-CRP, IL-6 and mortality in CAD patients after ACS.

Conclusions: Thyroid hormones (i.e., fT4 level and fT3/fT4 ratio) together with NT-pro-BNP level may be valuable and simple predictors of long-term outcomes of CAD patients after experiencing ACS.

Keywords: NT-pro-BNP, Thyroid hormones, Mortality, Coronary artery disease

* Correspondence: julius.burkauskas@lsmuni.lt
^Deceased
Behavioral Medicine Institute, Lithuanian University of Health Sciences, Palanga, Lithuania

Background

Thyroid hormones play a key role in cardiovascular regulation through various physiological and pathological manifestations [1, 2]. In recent years, increased attention has been focused on various circulating biologically active substances, collectively known as plasma biomarkers, and their utility in coronary artery disease (CAD) and heart failure (HF) prognosis [1–4]. Neurohormonal activation of N-terminal pro-B-type natriuretic peptides (NT-pro-BNP) remains one of the established markers for the detection and evaluation of HF severity and is considered a prognostic determinant of disease progression in CAD patients [5–7]. NT-pro-BNP is an important biomarker in patients with acute coronary syndrome (ACS) as it is a marker of myocardial cell necrosis and a strong predictor of morbidity and mortality [7, 8]. Increased NT-pro-BNP levels predict cardiac-related mortality in HF patients [9–11].

Altered thyroid function in the absence of primary thyroid disease is characterized by low total triiodothyronine (T3), free T3 (fT3) levels with normal total thyroxine (T4) and thyroid-stimulating hormone (TSH). This is due to reduced enzyme 5′ monodeiodinase activity, responsible for converting T4 into T3 in the peripheral tissues [12, 13]. It has been established that low circulating T3 levels are common in patients with HF [2, 13, 14], acute myocardial infarction (MI), [3, 15–17] and are linked with poor prognosis [18, 19]. The literature in this area indicates disparate perspectives on the association of thyroid hormones and NT-pro-BNP serum levels; some authors have demonstrated that higher thyroid function is associated with the higher NT-pro-BNP levels. In contrast others have suggested that hypothyroidism alters NT-pro-BNP concentrations [20, 21].

In CAD, the rupturing of a patient's coronary plaque triggers an inflammatory cascade [22]. Studies have reported that interleukin-6 (IL-6) can stimulate BNP expression and that IL-6 has a significant positive association with NT-pro-BNP [23–25]. It has recently been hypothesized that IL-6, a pleiotropic proinflammatory cytokine, may exert an inhibitory effect on thyroid function and suggests the development of euthyroid sick syndrome in patients with systemic diseases [26–28].

Inflammatory marker C-reactive protein (CRP) is mainly produced in response to IL-6 and plays many pathophysiological roles in the inflammatory process in HF. It was shown that IL-6 and CRP are all inversely correlated with fT3 levels in patients with stable HF [29, 30].

Moreover, it has been demonstrated that the relative risk for CAD is higher in people with more inflammatory biomarkers such as CRP and IL-6 and NT-pro-BNP. These biomarkers also have the prognostic value of cardiovascular events in HF patients [22]. NT-pro-BNP, thyroid hormone and inflammatory biomarkers concentrations have also been found to change in patients treated with primary percutaneous coronary intervention following ACS [8, 13, 22]. However, the relationship between NT-pro-BNP, thyroid hormone and inflammatory biomarkers in patients undergoing a cardiac rehabilitation programme following ACS is not well described.

From a clinical perspective, understanding whether thyroid hormones and inflammatory biomarkers play a role in the relationship between NT-pro-BNP and mortality, would assist in greater accuracy with respect to the risk-stratification of CAD patients admitted to rehabilitation program and would also provide the opportunity for early interventions to address clinical risk factors and improve patient prognosis.

The primary objective of this study was to measure the associations between thyroid hormones, inflammatory biomarkers and NT-pro-BNP. The second aim of the study was to examine the potential impact of thyroid hormones, inflammatory biomarkers and NT-pro-BNP on long-term outcomes in patients enrolled in an in-patient cardiac rehabilitation program after ACS.

Methods

Study population

During the period from January 2006 until January 2013 a total of 826 CAD patients consecutively attending an in-patient cardiac rehabilitation program, at the Cardiovascular Rehabilitation Clinic of the Behavioral Medicine Institute of the Lithuanian University of Health Sciences in Palanga, Lithuania, were invited to participate in the study. All patients were admitted to the rehabilitation program after two weeks of in-hospital stationary treatment for ACS. Patients were excluded from the present study if they had history of thyroid or adrenal disease ($n = 74$), were actively taking thyroid medications or amiodarone ($n = 34$), had increased TSH (>3.7 μg/mL) concentrations indicating hypothyroidism ($n = 14$) or decreased TSH (<0.5 μg/mL) concentrations indicating hyperthyroidism ($n = 10$), had high concentrations of anti-thyroid peroxidase antibodies (anti-TPO ≥60 U/mL) indicating autoimmune thyroid disease ($n = 15$) or who declined the opportunity to participate in the study ($n = 37$). The final study population meeting inclusion/exclusion criteria was comprised of 642 CAD patients (77 % men; mean age, 58 ± 9 years) after ACS. All study participants took part in the exercise-based cardiac rehabilitation program and received standard treatment for secondary prevention of CAD according to the existing guidelines of secondary prevention through cardiac rehabilitation [31–33].

Study design

This was a prospective study approved by The Regional Biomedical Research Ethics Committee. More details of study design, recruitment, and procedures have been published elsewhere [34, 35]. In short, the baseline measure was chosen to be patients' assessment within three days of admission to the rehabilitation program, once they signed written informed consent. Eligible participants were evaluated for demographic factors (e.g., age and gender), clinical characteristics (e.g., New York Heart Association [NYHA] functional class, left ventricular ejection fraction [LVEF]), CAD risk factors (e.g., diabetes mellitus, smoking, hypertension, body mass index, and dyslipidemia) and current medication use. Blood samples were drawn for each participant to evaluate individual levels of thyroid hormones, NT-pro-BNP, high-sensitivity CRP (hs-CRP) and IL-6.

Follow-up data on mortality (time and cause of death) was used in the analysis as the primary outcome of interest. The data was primarily obtained from death certificates, post-mortem reports, and medical records. When data could not be obtained from these sources, the study team attempted to conduct telephone interviews with participant family members to obtain self-report mortality data or to contact the Causes of Death Register at the Institute of Hygiene of the Lithuanian Ministry of Health. In some cases, this outcome data was unavailable.

It should be noted that to be classified as a cardiac-related death, documentation of arrhythmias or cardiac arrest, death due to progressive HF or MI in the absence of a precipitating factor was required. Sudden unexpected death was classified as cardiac death when it occurred outside the hospital and was not followed up by autopsy. Death caused by accidents was excluded. Both cardiac-related and all-cause mortality (cumulative – death from any natural cause) were ascertained.

Evaluation thyroid axis hormones, NT-pro-BNP, hs-CRP and IL-6 concentrations

All participants had a blood sample collection on second day after admission to the rehabilitation clinic. Venous blood samples were drawn after a minimum 12 h overnight fast for the evaluation of thyroid axis hormones, NT-pro-BNP, hs-CRP and IL-6 concentrations. Blood was centrifuged and serum was frozen at –40 °C. Serum concentrations of T3, fT3, T4, free T4 (fT4), TSH were analysed using automated enzyme immunoassay analyser AIA 600/21/1800 (Tosoh corporation, US) and radioimmunoassay kit RIA (R-EW-125, Belgium) for reverse T3 (rT3). Normal range for T3, from 70 to 170 ng/dL; fT3, from 2.0 to 4.0 pg/mL; rT3, from 9 to 35 nd/dl; T4, from 4,5 to 12.0 µg/dL; fT4, from 7.0 to 17.0 pg/mL; TSH, from 0.25 to 4.5 µIU/mL. Serum concentration of NT-pro-BNP and IL-6 were assessed using radio-immunoassay method (Roche Cobas analyser, Roche Diagnostics, UK). Normal serum concentration of NT-pro-BNP and IL-6 are <157 ng/L and from 0 to 7 pg/mL, respectively. Serum hs-CRP concentrations were assessed using the chemiluminescent immunoassay method (Beckman Coulter Unicel DXC 600) with normal values of ≤0.3 mg/dL.

Statistical analysis

Data is expressed as mean ± standard deviation (SD) for variables with Gaussian distribution and as median (25th–75th percentile) for variables with non-normal distribution. Distribution of measurements was assessed using Kolmogorov-Smirnov test. Group comparisons were made using Student *t* test, Mann–Whitney *U* test, Fisher's exact test, or chi-square test, as appropriate. Associations between continuous variables were assessed by Pearson product–moment analysis (Pearson r) or Spearman rank correlation analysis (Spearman r), as appropriate. Multivariate regression models were created for NT-pro-BNP, inflammatory biomarkers, and thyroid hormones adjusting for gender, age and body mass index. A two-tailed P value <0.05 was regarded as significant. All variables were examined for normal distribution and natural-log transformed (ln) when necessary. Univariate and multivariate Cox regression analyses were used to determine the relative risks (hazard ratio [HR]) for all-cause and cardiac-related mortality associated with demographic and clinical risk factors, such as age, gender, hypertension, NYHA class, and diabetes mellitus, as well as with NT-pro-BNP, thyroid hormones, thyroid hormones ratios, hs-CRP and IL-6 levels.

We also generated receiver operating characteristic (ROC) curves to assess cut-off values for demographic, clinical, thyroid hormones, inflammatory biomarkers and NT-pro-BNP characteristics that would prognostically discriminate between non-survivors (all-cause mortality) and survivors. We used the approach by DeLong et al. [36] to compare the areas under the ROC curves (AUCs) of demographic and clinical models with AUCs from biomarkers and additive models.

Then, based on the cut-off values patients outcomes were assessed using Kaplan-Meier curves; a log-rank (Mantel-Cox) test was used to compare survival curves and estimate HR. All tests were performed using software SPSS for Windows, version 17.0 (SPSS Inc., Chicago, USA) and MedCalc for Windows, version 12.5 (MedCalc Software, Ostend, Belgium).

Results

Baseline socio-demographic variables, clinical characteristics, CAD risk factors and the mean concentrations of thyroid hormones, NT-pro-BNP, IL-6, hs-CRP and current treatment of 642 patients are shown in Table 1.

During the follow-up period (i.e., maximum of 118 months) there were 23 cardiac-related and 35 all-cause deaths. Death most frequently occurred following MI and the patients who died tended to be older, have a higher NYHA functional class, lower LVEF, have more severe hypertension, were more likely to have used nitrates and to have higher concentrations of NT-pro-BNP, hs-CRP, T4, fT4 and lower concentrations of fT3 during the rehabilitation period at baseline assessment, as compared to survivors (Table 1).

Table 1 Patients characteristics

Characteristics	All	Survived throughout follow-up	Died during follow-up	p-value
	n = 642	n = 607	n = 35	
Age (years), mean ± SD	57.6 ± 9.5	57.4 ± 9.4	62.3 ± 9.2	0.004
Gender, n (%)				0.382
Men	493 (76.8)	464 (76.4)	29 (82.9)	
Women	149 (23.2)	143 (23.6)	6 (17.1)	
Body mass index, mean ± SD	29.8 ± 4.7	29.9 ± 4.7	29.0 ± 5.2	0.355
Diagnosis, n (%)				0.010
Angina pectoris	159 (24.8)	149 (24.6)	10 (28.6)	
Acute myocardial infarction	405 (63.1)	381 (62.8)	24 (68.6)	
Previous myocardial infarction	78 (12.1)	77 (12.7)	1 (2.9)	
Angina pectoris class, n (%)				0.063
I	143 (22.3)	138 (22.8)	5 (14.3)	
II	214 (33.3)	196 (32.3)	18 (51.4)	
III	18 (2.8)	16 (2.6)	2 (5.7)	
NYHA, n (%)				<0.001
I	52 (8.1)	52 (8.6)	-	
II	468 (72.9)	451 (74.2)	17 (48.6)	
III	122 (19.0)	104 (17.2)	18 (51.4)	
Hypertension, n (%)				0.001
Grade 1 (mild)	39 (6.1)	37 (6.1)	2 (5.7)	
Grade 2 (moderate)	354 (55.2)	345 (56.8)	9 (25.7)	
Grade 3 (severe)	109 (17.0)	96 (15.8)	13 (37.1)	
Left ventricular ejection fraction %, mean ± SD	50.2 ± 9.0	50.5 ± 8.9	43.4 ± 8.2	0.001
Diabetes mellitus, n (%)	74 (11.5)	67 (11.1)	7 (20.0)	0.107
Nitrate, n (%)	255 (39.7)	233 (38.4)	22 (62.9)	0.004
Beta-blockers, n (%)	557 (86.8)	529 (87.3)	28 (80.0)	0.214
Angiotensin-converting enzyme inhibitors, n (%)	527 (82.1)	496 (81.8)	31 (88.6)	0.312
Diuretic, n (%)	101 (15.7)	92 (15.2)	9 (25.7)	0.096
N-terminal pro-B-Type natriuretic peptide (ng/L), median (interquartile ranges)	328.3 (120.8–770.5)	303.7 (115.7–709.7)	570.0 (305.5–299.0)	0.001
hs-C-reactive protein (mg/dL), median (interquartile ranges)	0.26 (0.12–0.58)	0.26 (0.12–0.57)	0.47 (0.13–0.88)	0.077
Interleukin-6 (pg/ml), median (interquartile ranges)	3.1 (1.7–5.5)	3.1 (1.7–5.5)	3.7 (2.1–8.0)	0.209
Reverse Triiodothyronine (ng/ml), median (interquartile ranges)	0.27 (0.22–0.37)	0.27 (0.22–0.36)	0.30 (0.20–0.43)	0.375
Free Triiodothyronine (pg/ml), median (interquartile ranges)	2.80 (2.55–3.06)	2.80 (2.56–3.06)	2.72 (2.24–3.00)	0.036
Thyroid-stimulating hormone (μIU/ml), median (interquartile ranges)	1.8 (1.2–2.6)	1.8 (1.2–2.8)	1.7 (1.4–2.5)	0.875
Free Thyroxine (pg/ml), mean ± SD	13.0 ± 2.5	12.9 ± 2.4	14.6 ± 3.9	<0.001
Total Triiodothyronine (ng/dl), mean ± SD	106.7 ± 19.0	106.8 ± 19.0	104.3 ± 18.3	0.519
Total Thyroxine (μg/dl), mean ± SD	7.1 ± 1.5	7.8 ± 1.5	8.4 ± 1.4	0.042
Follow-up (months), mean ± SD	52.0 ± 29.2	52.5 ± 29.1	43.7 ± 30.6	0.029

NYHA New York Heart Association functional class

Associations between thyroid hormones, hs-CRP, IL-6 and NT-pro-BNP

There were significant correlations between (ln)fT3 and fT4 levels ($r = 0.179$, $p < 0.001$), and (ln)fT4 and T3 ($r =$ 0.112, $p = 0.02$). Significant correlations were also found between (ln)rT3 and fT4 ($r = 0.776$, $p < 0.001$). There were also strong correlation between (ln)hs-CRP and (ln)IL-6 serum concentrations ($r = 0.650$, $p < 0.001$) and between (ln)IL-6 and fT4 ($r = 0.091$, $p = 0.03$). The univariate regression analysis indicated that higher (ln)NT-pro-BNP levels were negatively correlated with concentrations of (ln)fT3 ($\beta = -0.112$, $p = 0.005$), positively correlated with concentrations of T4 ($\beta = 0.126$, $p = 0.009$), and (ln)TSH ($\beta = 0.097$, $p = 0.015$). Biomarker (ln)NT-pro-BNP correlated positively with fT4 ($\beta = 0.100$, $p = 0.012$). A lower (ln)fT3/fT4 ratio was associated with higher (ln)NT-pro-BNP ($\beta = -0.112$, $p = 0.004$). The positive association between (ln)hs-CRP and (ln)NT-pro-BNP ($\beta = 0.146$, $p < 0.001$), (ln)IL-6 ($\beta = 0.228$, $p < 0.001$, respectively) was determined.

However, multivariate linear regression models, adjusted for age, gender and body mass index, revealed that (ln)NT-pro-BNP remain associated with hs-CRP ($\beta = 0.59$, $p < 0.001$), (ln)IL6 ($\beta = 0.254$, $p < 0.001$), fT4 ($\beta = 0.100$, $p = 0.011$), and T4 ($\beta = 0.112$, $p = 0.019$).

Prognostic impact of thyroid hormones and NT-pro-BNP

Univariate analysis of data showed that age, NYHA class, (ln)NT-pro-BNP, (ln)rT3, fT4, (ln)fT3, and (ln)fT3/fT4 ratio were associated with all-cause mortality. Moreover age, NYHA class, (ln)NT-pro-BNP, (ln)rT3, fT4, and (ln)fT3/fT4 ratio were associated with cardiac-related mortality (Table 2). A multivariate Cox regression model showed that age (HR 1.06, 95 % CI 1.02–1.11, $p = 0.003$), NYHA class (HR 3.01, 95 % CI 1.44–6.23, $p = 0.003$), (ln)NT-pro-BNP levels (HR 1.53, 95 % CI 1.13–2.07, $p = 0.006$), fT4 level (HR 1.15, 95 % CI 1.04–1.27, $p = 0.005$), and (ln)fT3/fT4 ratio (HR 0.08, 95 % CI 0.02–0.32, $p < 0.001$) were associated with all-cause mortality. However, NYHA class (HR 3.58, 95 % CI 1.43–8.94, $p = 0.006$), (ln)NT-pro-BNP levels (HR 1.62, 95 % CI 1.11–2.36, $p = 0.013$), fT4 level (HR 1.15, 95 % CI 1.02–1.29, $p = 0.018$) and (ln)fT3/fT4 ratio (HR 0.10, 95 % CI 0.02–0.55, $p =$

Table 2 Cox regression analyses for factors associated with all-cause and cardiac-related mortality

Variable	Univariate HR (95 % CI)	p-value	Multivariate[a] HR (95 % CI)	p-value
All-cause mortality				
Age	1.07 (1.03–1.11)	0.001	1.06 (1.02–1.11)	0.003
Gender	0.67 (0.28–1.61)	0.368	0.52 (0.21–1.27)	0.150
Arterial Hypertension	0.98 (0.79–1.21)	0.821	0.97 (0.78–1.20)	0.785
Diabetes mellitus	2.26 (0.98–5.20)	0.055	2.00 (0.85–4.68)	0.111
NYHA class	4.32 (2.23–8.35	<0.001	3.01 (1.44–6.29)	0.003
(ln)NT-pro-BNP	1.56 (1.16–2.11)	0.004	1.53 (1.13–2.07)	0.006
(ln)hs-CRP	1.32 (0.99–1.76)	0.062	1.26 (0.93–1.71)	0.137
(ln)IL-6	1.39 (0.90–2.14)	0.138	1.21 (0.77–1.90)	0.398
fT4	1.17 (1.06–1.28)	0.002	1.15 (1.04–1.27)	0.005
(ln)fT3	0.12 (0.02–0.96)	0.045	0.14 (0.01–1.36)	0.089
(ln)fT3/fT4	0.09 (0.03–0.31)	<0.001	0.08 (0.02–0.32)	<0.001
(ln)rT3	2.29 (1.11–4.73)	0.025	2.15 (1.01–4.58)	0.049
Cardiac-related mortality				
Age	1.06 (1.01–1.11)	0.023	1.05 (1.00–1.10)	0.062
Gender	1.12 (0.44–2.84)	0.815	0.79 (0.30–2.06)	0.623
Arterial Hypertension	1.02 (0.78–1.34)	0.871	1.06 (0.81–1.38)	0.688
Diabetes mellitus	1.35 (0.40–4.56)	0.627	1.08 (0.31–3.76)	0.899
NYHA class	6.01 (3.57–14.05)	<0.001	3.58 (1.43–8.94)	0.006
(ln)NT-pro-BNP	1.65 (1.13–2.41)	0.009	1.62 (1.11–2.36)	0.013
(ln)hs-CRP	1.12 (0.78–1.60)	0.537	1.08 (0.75–1.56)	0.667
(ln)IL-6	1.41 (0.82–2.40)	0.213	1.35 (0.77–2.34)	0.293
fT4	1.17 (1.04–1.31)	0.007	1.15 (1.02–1.29)	0.018
(ln)fT3	0.13 (0.01–1.71)	0.122	0.23 (0.02–3.49)	0.287
(ln)fT3/fT4	0.09 (0.02–0.43)	0.002	0.10 (0.02–0.55)	0.008
(ln)rT3	2.46 (1.02–5.29)	0.045	2.05 (0.81–5.16)	0.128

HR hazard ratio, *CI* confidence interval, *ln* natural logarithm, *hs-CRP* high-sensitivity C-reactive protein, *fT3* Free Triiodothyronine, *fT4* Free Thyroxine, *IL-6* Interleukin-6, *NT-pro-BNP* N-terminal pro-B-Type natriuretic peptide, *rT3* Reverse triiodothyronine, *NYHA* New York Heart Association functional class
[a]Final model: adjusted for age, arterial hypertension, diabetes mellitus, peripheral arterial disease

0.008) remained independent predictors of cardiac-related mortality. The hs-CRP and IL-6 levels were not found to be associated with mortality (Table 2).

Figure 1 shows ROC curves for age and NYHA class. Figures 2 and 3 show ROC curves and Kaplan-Meier survival plots for biomarkers characteristics predicting all-cause mortality. When participants were stratified into high and low NT-pro-BNP level groups (cut-off 290.4 ng/L), the outcome (cumulative survival) for patients with high NT-pro-BNP levels was significantly different in comparison to patients with low NT-pro-BNP levels (HR 3.79, 95 % CI 1.57–9.15, $p = 0.003$) (Fig. 2a). When patients were stratified into high and low fT3/fT4 ratio groups (cut-off of <0.206), the outcome for patients with lower fT3/fT4 ratio was significantly worse than for patients with a higher fT3/fT4 ratio (HR 2.99, 95 % CI 1.43–6.26, $p = 0.004$) (Fig. 2b). ROC analysis was used to assess the best cut-off values for fT4 levels (cut-off 12.54 pg/ml) predicting all-cause mortality (AUC 0.63, 95 % CI 0.53–0.72, $p = 0.013$). When we stratified participants into two groups according to cut-off values, we found that higher fT4 levels were associated with worse outcomes (HR 2.34, 95 % CI 1.05–5.18, $p = 0.036$) (Fig. 2c). When patients were subdivided based on the cut-off values for fT3/fT4 ratio (of <0.206) and NT-pro-BNP (≥290.4 ng/L) levels, the outcomes for patients with a lower fT3/fT4 ratio and higher NT-pro-BNP were worse, as compared with the other groups (HR 2.03, 95 % CI 1.39–2.96, $p < 0.001$) (Fig. 3).

Data on how the AUCs from the demographic and clinical predictors compares with the biomarkers alone or combined models are presented in Table 3 and Fig. 4. Overall, age and NYHA class showed good discriminatory power for predicting all-cause mortality during follow up. The NT-pro-BNP level and fT3/fT4 ratio model had the best AUC of all isolated parameters. A combined model comprising of age, NYHA class, NT-pro-BNP level, and fT3/fT4 ratio showed the highest discriminatory power among other predictors.

Evaluating all-cause mortality, the model comprised of age, NYHA class, NT-pro-BNP level, and fT3/fT4 ratio was significantly better than age (difference between AUC: 0.150, 95 % CI 0.064–0.235, $p < 0.001$), NYHA class (difference between AUC: 0.090, 95 % CI 0.030–0.150, $p = 0.003$), NT-pro-BNP level (difference between AUC: 0.115, 95 % CI 0.023–0.207, $p = 0.014$), and fT3/fT4 ratio (difference between AUC: 0.103, 95 % CI

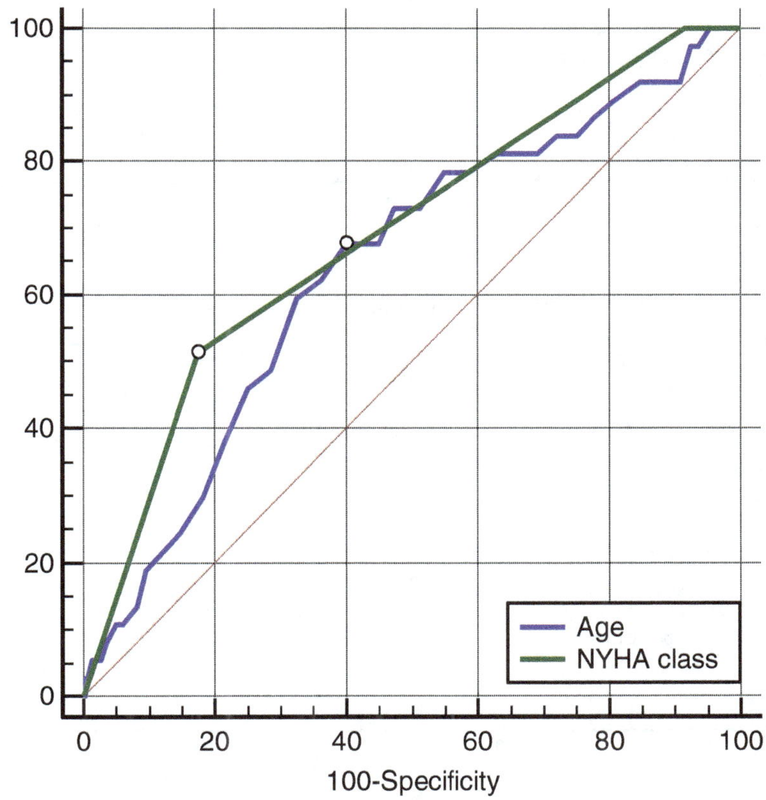

Fig. 1 Receiver operating characteristic curves for age and NYHA class predicting all-cause mortality during follow up. NYHA – New York Heart Association functional class. Area under the curve of age was 0.642 (95 % confidence interval [CI], 0.604–0.678; $p = 0.003$), of NYHA 0.690 (95 % CI, 0.653–0.725; $p < 0.001$)

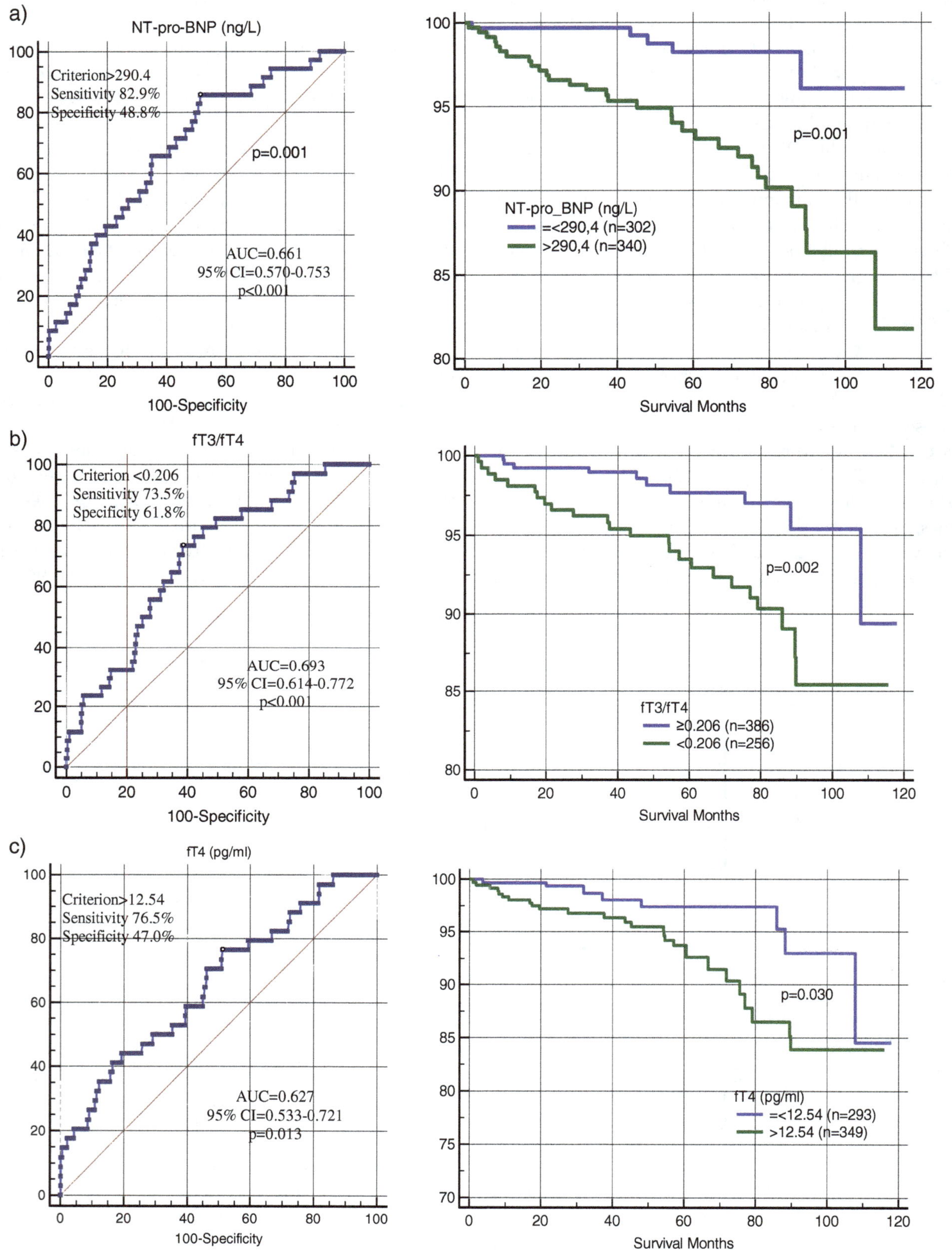

Fig. 2 (See legend on next page.)

(See figure on previous page.)
Fig. 2 Receiver operating characteristics curves and Kaplan-Meier survival plots for **a** NT-pro-BNP, **b** fT3/fT4 ratio, and **c** fT4 values for predicting all-cause mortality during follow-up. Results are the area under the curve (AUC) and associated 95 % confidence interval (CI). The best cut-off values are labeled. A log-rank test was used to compare survival curves. NT-pro-BNP – N-terminal pro-B-Type natriuretic peptide, fT3/fT4 – Free Triiodothyronine/Free Thyroxine ratio, fT4 – Free Thyroxine

0.034–0.173, $p = 0.218$). However, it failed to perform significantly better than NT-pro-BNP level and fT3/fT4 ratio model.

Discussion

Our study demonstrated a significant relationship between the suppression of thyroid axis function, increased inflammation markers and increased NT-pro-BNP levels in CAD patients undergoing rehabilitation after ACS. We have also demonstrated that measures of fT4 and fT3/fT4 ratio together with NT-pro-BNP can be important prognostic markers of negative long-term outcomes (i.e., mortality). We found no association between hs-CRP and IL-6 and mortality among CAD patients.

A positive relationship between hs-CRP, IL-6 and NT-pro-BNP was established in our study indicating that thyroid function disturbances contribute to inflammatory processes even during the rehabilitation period (i.e., after acute coronary events). Numerous studies have confirmed fT3 and low-T3 syndrome as predictors of elevated NT-pro-BNP [7, 37]. The correlation of fT3 and NT-pro-BNP was weaker in our study compared to Pfister et al. [37], which might be due to the dominant influence of cardiac abnormalities on NT-pro-BNP values in our patients' population. However, association of fT4 and NT-pro-BNP was evident in our study. Mayer et al. [38] showed that even mild changes of fT4, still within normal clinically accepted levels, may influence the burden of HF as quantified by its biological surrogates (i.e., natriuretic peptides). Free thyroxine concentrations were significantly positively associated with NT-pro-BNP and BNP in a continuous manner. In this study association was more evident at high-normal fT4 levels, than at low-normal, where only the increase of a more sensitive marker (NT-pro-BNP) was observed. Our findings add to the developing understanding of the relationship between NT-pro-BNP, thyroid hormones and inflammatory biomarkers in CAD patients during rehabilitation after

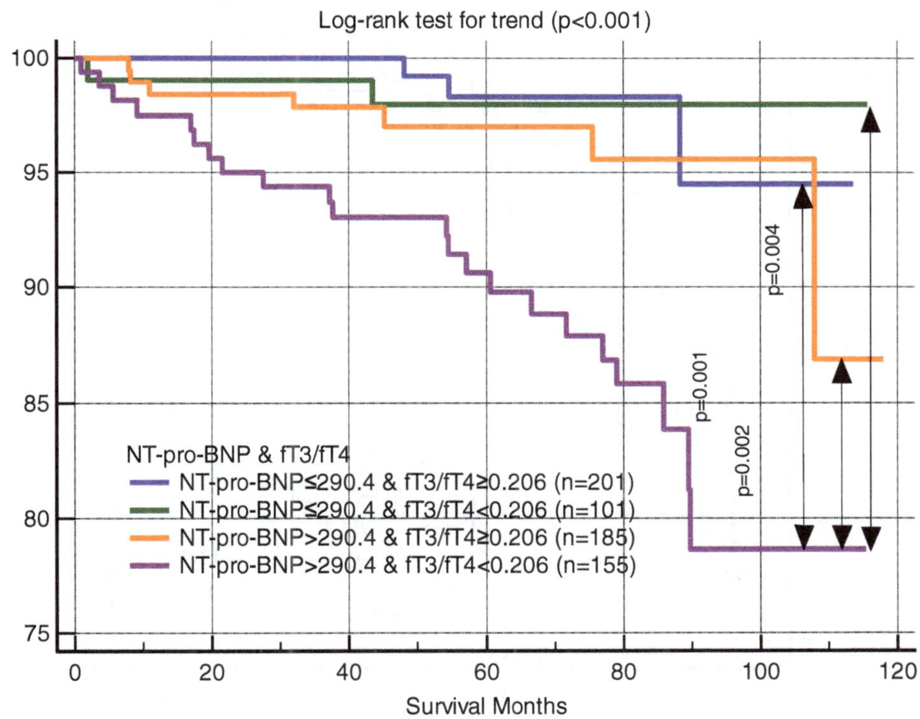

Fig. 3 Kaplan-Meier survival plots for all-cause mortality for 642 CAD patients stratified into 4 groups based on cut-off values for NT-proBNP (290.4 ng/L) and ratio fT3/fT4 (0.206) levels. fT3/fT4 – Free Triiodothyronine/Free Thyroxine ratio; NT-pro-BNP – N-terminal pro-B-Type natriuretic peptide. The group with low fT3/fT4 ratio (<0.206) and high NT-proBNP (>290.4 ng/L) (*bottom line*) had a worse prognosis than others groups ($p < 0.001$; by the log-rank test)

Table 3 Receiver operating characteristic (ROC) curve evaluation for all-cause mortality prediction

Prediction of all-cause mortality: ROC analysis	Area under the curve (AUC)	95 % CI	p
Age	0.642	0.604–0.678	0.003
NYHA class	0.690	0.653–0.725	<0.001
NT-pro- BNP	0.675	0.638–0.711	<0.001
fT3/fT4	0.684	0.647–0.719	<0.001
NT-pro-BNP & fT3/fT4 model	0.732	0.693–0.766	<0.001
Combined model	0.800	0.753–0.817	<0.001
ROC curves comparison – Combined model vs:	AUC (difference)	95 % CI	p
Age	0.150	0.064–0.235	<0.001
NYHA class	0.090	0.030–0.150	0.003
NT-pro-BNP	0.115	0.023–0.207	0.014
fT3/fT4	0.103	0.034–0.173	0.004
NT-pro-BNP & fT3/fT4 model	0.055	0.032–0.142	0.218

CI confidence interval, *NT-pro-BNP* N-terminal pro-B-Type natriuretic peptide, *fT3/fT4* Free Triiodothyronine/Free Thyroxine ratio, *fT4* Free Thyroxine, *NYHA* New York Heart Association functional class; Combined model - composed by parameters of age, NYHA, NT-pro-BNP, and fT3/fT4

ACS. Specifically, that NT-pro-BNP and thyroid hormone level during rehabilitation could be an important predictor of negative outcomes. Determining whether these particular associations remain the same after rehabilitation, and whether changes in these associations are related to long term outcomes of CAD patients is beyond the scope of this study but should be subject of further investigation.

In the numerous prognostic studies, the altered thyroid metabolism assessed by various parameters, indicated

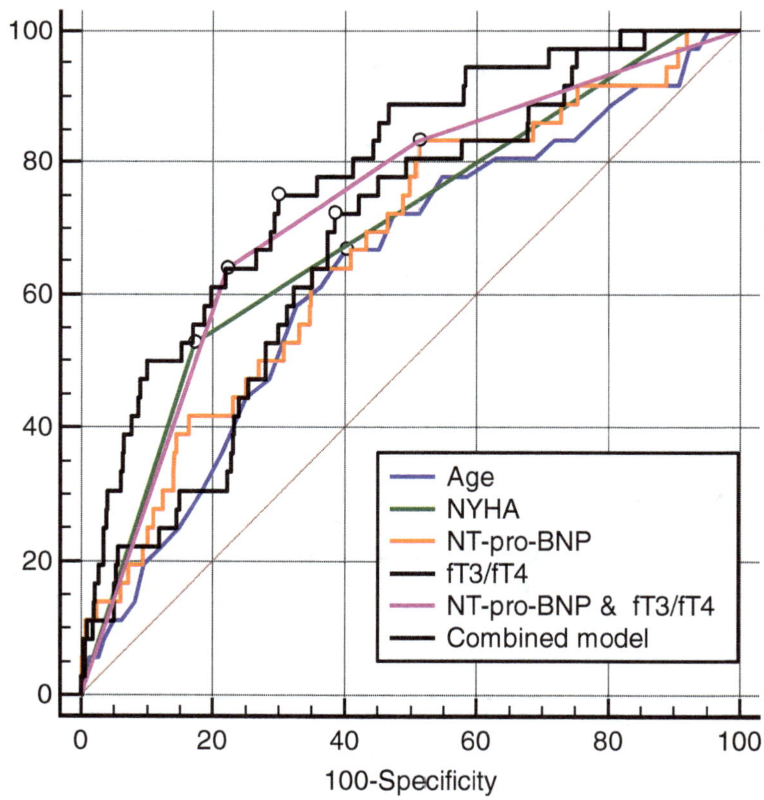

Fig. 4 Receiver operating characteristics curves of different parameters and models for predicting all-cause mortality during follow-up. NT-pro-BNP – N-terminal pro-B-Type natriuretic peptide, fT3/fT4 – Free Triiodothyronine/Free Thyroxine ratio, NYHA – New York Heart Association functional class. Combined model - composed by parameters of age, NYHA class, NT-pro-BNP, and fT3/fT4

disturbed T4 peripheral conversion, such as a reduction in circulating levels of T3 [18, 39, 40], low T3 syndrome [19, 41–44], mild changes of fT4 [45], a high rT3 level [46], a low fT3/rT3 ratio [46] and a low fT3/fT4 ratio in serum [45].

Passino et al. [20] showed that monitoring the combination of low fT3 and high BNP levels is a useful approach for determining long-term prognosis in patients with advanced HF. Irrespective of the parameters used, all these studies showed that altered peripheral thyroid hormones pathways were associated with a high incidence of fatal events (cumulative or cardiac-related death). Low fT3 levels are the most common alternation of thyroid hormones metabolism in patients with HF and are related with the severity of HF. Presently, low fT3 levels are found in approximately 20–30 % of patients with overt HF, 58 % of patients with advanced HF and in less than 10 % of those with early HF [47]. Low T3 reduction is more frequent in patients with NYHA classes III-IV [12]. In the present study with CAD patients group (73 % with a NYHA II functional class, 63 % after acute MI) the fT3 levels have not exposed prognostic impact to the long-term mortality. This might be due to dominant influence of cardiac abnormalities on NT-pro-BNP values in our cohort or to the recovered T3 level after ACS during the rehabilitation period [17]. Friberg et al. [17] showed that patients with poor heart function or who experienced a more intense inflammatory reaction to acute MI, showed more pronounced down-regulation of the thyroid hormones. The mean levels of the T3 declined between the first 6 h and the 24–36 h period after acute MI, although T3 levels were found to recover within 12 weeks [17].

Our study also revealed that age, NYHA class, (ln)NT-pro-BNP, fT4 and (ln)fT3/fT4 ratio were independent predictors of all-cause mortality and that NYHA class, (ln)NT-pro-BNP, fT4, (ln)fT3/fT4 ratio remained independent predictors of cardiac-related mortality. Additionally, it was demonstrated that higher levels of NT-pro-BNP (≥290.4 ng/L) and a lower fT3/fT4 ratio (<0.206) were independent predictors of cumulative mortality. When patients were subdivided based on the cut-off values for fT3/fT4 ratio and NT-pro-BNP levels, the outcome for the patient group with the lower fT3/fT4 ratio and higher NT-pro-BNP were found to be worse, as compared with the other 3 groups.

However, there was no association between inflammatory markers and mortality in our study. Conversely, some authors have suggested that hs-CRP > 3.90 mg/L and NT pro-BNP > 2247 pmol/L are associated with all-cause mortality in dilated cardiomyopathy patients [48, 49] and can be a potential predictors for all-cause mortality [50].

Euthyroid sick syndrome is the most common type of thyroid hormones abnormality where elevation of fT4 levels is frequently found. Friberg et al. [17, 40] showed that rT3, the inactive metabolite of T3, is positively correlated with its precursor fT4, which suggests that fT4 levels can also be used instead of rT3. Higher levels of rT3 and fT4 were associated with worse rates of survival, that is, patients that died within the first week after acute MI had a median free fT4 level of 16 pmol/L as compared with 15 pmol/L in survivors. Similar differences were also seen after 1 month and 1 year. It was also noted that in patients with a history of angina pectoris, the highest levels of fT4 were found in patients classified with unstable angina pectoris. Jung et al. [51] examined the association of thyroid function with CAD in euthyroid angina pectoris patients and showed that fT4 levels were associated with the presence and the severity of CAD. Jung et al. [51] study also suggests that elevated serum fT4 levels, even within normal range, could be a risk factor for CAD. Our study extends the data of Jung et al. [51] by showing that elevated fT4 levels during rehabilitation are related with long-term mortality in CAD patients.

Kozdag et al. [45] studied a group of 111 patients with ischemic and non-ischemic dilated cardiomyopathy and advanced NYHA class (III-IV), and showed that patients with lower fT3/fT4 ratio had a significantly less favorable outcome, as compared with those having higher fT3/fT4 ratio during 12 months of follow-up. Studies also find that NT-pro-BNP levels predict cardiac-related mortality in HF patients and patients with congenital heart disease [9–11, 52]. Recent review suggests that NT-pro-BNP assessment alone could be a useful tool predicting all-cause mortality in stable CAD patients [53]. However, we found that not only higher levels of NT-pro-BNP but also fT4 and lower fT3/fT4 ratio during cardiac rehabilitation were associated with long-term mortality in patients after ACS. Thus, in practical terms, the determination of fT4 level and fT3/fT4 ratio together with NT-pro-BNP, are valuable and simple predictors for the identification of CAD patients that are more likely to experience negative long-term outcomes after cardiac rehabilitation.

However, despite this relationship, using fT4 levels as a prognostic indicator in clinical settings will require more research to establish its validity. For example, future research could look at the influence of NT-pro-BNP and inflammatory markers concentration changes on fT4 levels in order to establish possible mediation/moderation effects on mortality. In the present form our findings may not be clinically relevant, but should be used to create multifactorial risk for mortality models.

Despite our consistent results, there were some limitations of the study that should be noted. Particularly, in terms of generalizability, as the majority of study participants had mild to moderate HF and all study patients attended a single-center in-patient cardiac rehabilitation program after being treated for ACS. Thus, the results may not apply to patients with more advanced HF and those who do not attend cardiac rehabilitation programs. Another limitation of our study was that we did not measure the fT3 level and other thyroid hormones in acute stage of coronary syndromes and therefore did not established variations of the fT3 before cardiac rehabilitation.

Conclusions

This study demonstrated that thyroid hormones characteristics such as fT4 level and fT3/fT4 ratio together with NT-pro-BNP level may be valuable predictors of long-term outcomes of CAD patients after experiencing ACS. Additional research is needed to determine how and when these prognostic indicators should be operationalized in a clinical setting and how treatment should be prioritized in higher-risk cardiac rehabilitation patients.

Abbreviations

ACS: acute coronary syndrome; CAD: coronary artery disease; CRP: C-reactive protein; fT3: free T3; fT4: free T4; HF: heart failure; HR: hazard ratio; hs-CRP: high-sensitivity CRP; IL-6: interleukin-6; ln: natural-log transformed; LVEF: left ventricular ejection fraction; MI: myocardial infarction; NT-pro-BNP: N-terminal pro-B-type natriuretic peptides; NYHA: New York Heart Association; rT3: reverse T3; SD: standard deviation; T3: total triiodothyronine; T4: total thyroxine; TSH: thyroid-stimulating hormone.

Competing interests

The authors declare that they have no competing interests.

Authors' contributions

JB wrote the manuscript and served as an expert on cardiology. NM served as an expert in endocrinology providing substantive feedback on the analysis and made major contributions to the writing of the manuscript. AP was involved with the statistical analysis and assisted with final solutions and presentation of the data. JB§ contributed substantially to the improvements of the analysis of the written manuscript. RB was guarantor of this work and, as such, made leading contributions to conception and design of the study. All authors read and approved the final manuscript, except RB, who very sadly passed away while the manuscript was still under construction.

Acknowledgements

This research was funded by the European Social Fund under the Global Grant measure, Grant VP1-3.1-SMM-07-K-02-060.

References

1. Klein I, Ojamaa K. Thyroid hormone and the cardiovascular system. N Engl J Med. 2001;344(7):501–9.
2. Yin WH, Chen JW, Feng AN, Lin SJ, Young S. Multimarker approach to risk stratification among patients with advanced chronic heart failure. Clin Cardiol. 2007;30(8):397–402.
3. Damman P, Beijk MA, Kuijt WJ, Verouden NJ, van Geloven N, Henriques JP, et al. Multiple biomarkers at admission significantly improve the prediction of mortality in patients undergoing primary percutaneous coronary intervention for acute ST-segment elevation myocardial infarction. J Am Coll Cardiol. 2011;57(1):29–36.
4. Klein I, Danzi S. Thyroid disease and the heart. Circulation. 2007;116(15):1725–35.
5. Mair J, Hammerer-Lercher A, Puschendorf B. The impact of cardiac natriuretic peptide determination on the diagnosis and management of heart failure. Clin Chem Lab Med. 2001;39(7):571–88.
6. de Lemos JA, Morrow DA, Bentley JH, Omland T, Sabatine MS, McCabe CH, et al. The prognostic value of B-type natriuretic peptide in patients with acute coronary syndromes. N Engl J Med. 2001;345(14):1014–21.
7. Pfister R, Tan D, Thekkanal J, Hellmich M, Schneider CA. NT-pro-BNP is associated with long-term outcome in a heterogeneous sample of cardiac inpatients. Eur J Intern Med. 2007;18(3):215–20.
8. Grabowski M, Filipiak KJ, Malek LA, Karpinski G, Huczek Z, Stolarz P, et al. Admission B-type natriuretic peptide assessment improves early risk stratification by Killip classes and TIMI risk score in patients with acute ST elevation myocardial infarction treated with primary angioplasty. Int J Cardiol. 2007;115(3):386–90.
9. Gegenhuber A, Mueller T, Dieplinger B, Poelz W, Pacher R, Haltmayer M. B-type natriuretic peptide and amino terminal proBNP predict one-year mortality in short of breath patients independently of the baseline diagnosis of acute destabilized heart failure. Clin Chim Acta. 2006;370(1–2):174–9.
10. Hammerer-Lercher A, Neubauer E, Muller S, Pachinger O, Puschendorf B, Mair J. Head-to-head comparison of N-terminal pro-brain natriuretic peptide, brain natriuretic peptide and N-terminal pro-atrial natriuretic peptide in diagnosing left ventricular dysfunction. Clin Chim Acta. 2001;310(2):193–7.
11. Koglin J, Pehlivanli S, Schwaiblmair M, Vogeser M, Cremer P, von Scheidt W. Role of brain natriuretic peptide in risk stratification of patients with congestive heart failure. J Am Coll Cardiol. 2001;38(7):1934–41.
12. Biondi B. Mechanisms in endocrinology: heart failure and thyroid dysfunction. Eur J Endocrinol. 2012;167(5):609–18.
13. Iervasi G, Molinaro S, Landi P, Taddei MC, Galli E, Mariani F, et al. Association between increased mortality and mild thyroid dysfunction in cardiac patients. Arch Intern Med. 2007;167(14):1526–32.
14. Ascheim DD, Hryniewicz K. Thyroid hormone metabolism in patients with congestive heart failure: the low triiodothyronine state. Thyroid. 2002;12(6):511–5.
15. Zhang B, Peng W, Wang C, Li W, Xu Y. A low fT3 level as a prognostic marker in patients with acute myocardial infarctions. Internal Med (Tokyo, Japan). 2012;51(21):3009–15.
16. Kimura T, Kanda T, Kotajima N, Kuwabara A, Fukumura Y, Kobayashi I. Involvement of circulating interleukin-6 and its receptor in the development of euthyroid sick syndrome in patients with acute myocardial infarction. Eur J Endocrinol. 2000;143(2):179–84.
17. Friberg L, Werner S, Eggertsen G, Ahnve S. Rapid down-regulation of thyroid hormones in acute myocardial infarction: is it cardioprotective in patients with angina? Arch Intern Med. 2002;162(12):1388–94.
18. Pingitore A, Landi P, Taddei MC, Ripoli A, L'Abbate A, Iervasi G. Triiodothyronine levels for risk stratification of patients with chronic heart failure. Am J Med. 2005;118(2):132–6.
19. Shanoudy H, Soliman A, Moe S, Hadian D, Veldhuis JD, Iranmanesh A, et al. Early manifestations of "sick euthyroid" syndrome in patients with compensated chronic heart failure. J Card Fail. 2001;7(2):146–52.
20. Passino C, Pingitore A, Landi P, Fontana M, Zyw L, Clerico A, et al. Prognostic value of combined measurement of brain natriuretic peptide and triiodothyronine in heart failure. J Card Fail. 2009;15(1):35–40.
21. Nessler J, Nessler B, Golebiowska-Wiatrak R, Palka I, Gackowski A, Kitlinski M, et al. Serum biomarkers and clinical outcomes in heart failure patients treated de novo with carvedilol. Cardiol J. 2013;20(2):144–51.
22. Cesari M, Penninx BW, Newman AB, Kritchevsky SB, Nicklas BJ, Sutton-Tyrrell K, et al. Inflammatory markers and onset of cardiovascular events: results from the Health ABC study. Circulation. 2003;108(19):2317–22.
23. Pannitteri G, Marino B, Campa PP, Martucci R, Testa U, Peschle C. Interleukins 6 and 8 as mediators of acute phase response in acute myocardial infarction. Am J Cardiol. 1997;80(5):622–5.
24. Smith DA, Irving SD, Sheldon J, Cole D, Kaski JC. Serum levels of the antiinflammatory cytokine interleukin-10 are decreased in patients with unstable angina. Circulation. 2001;104(7):746–9.
25. Nian M, Lee P, Khaper N, Liu P. Inflammatory cytokines and postmyocardial infarction remodeling. Circ Res. 2004;94(12):1543–53.
26. Boelen A, Platvoet-Ter Schiphorst MC, Wiersinga WM. Association between serum interleukin-6 and serum 3,5,3'-triiodothyronine in nonthyroidal illness. J Clin Endocrinol Metab. 1993;77(6):1695–9.

27. Stouthard JM, van der Poll T, Endert E, Bakker PJ, Veenhof CH, Sauerwein HP, et al. Effects of acute and chronic interleukin-6 administration on thyroid hormone metabolism in humans. J Clin Endocrinol Metab. 1994;79(5):1342–6.
28. Bartalena L, Bogazzi F, Brogioni S, Grasso L, Martino E. Role of cytokines in the pathogenesis of the euthyroid sick syndrome. Eur J Endocrinol. 1998;138(6):603–14.
29. Lubrano V, Pingitore A, Carpi A, Iervasi G. Relationship between triiodothyronine and proinflammatory cytokines in chronic heart failure. Biomed Pharmacother. 2010;64(3):165–9.
30. Osman R, L'Allier PL, Elgharib N, Tardif JC. Critical appraisal of C-reactive protein throughout the spectrum of cardiovascular disease. Vasc Health Risk Manag. 2006;2(3):221–37.
31. Steg PG, James SK, Atar D, Badano LP, Blomstrom-Lundqvist C, Borger MA, et al. ESC Guidelines for the management of acute myocardial infarction in patients presenting with ST-segment elevation. Eur Heart J. 2012;33(20):2569–619.
32. Piepoli MF, Corra U, Benzer W, Bjarnason-Wehrens B, Dendale P, Gaita D, et al. Secondary prevention through cardiac rehabilitation: from knowledge to implementation. A position paper from the Cardiac Rehabilitation Section of the European Association of Cardiovascular Prevention and Rehabilitation. Eur J Cardiovasc Prev Rehabil. 2010;17(1):1–17.
33. Montalescot G, Sechtem U, Achenbach S, Andreotti F, Arden C, Budaj A, et al. 2013 ESC guidelines on the management of stable coronary artery disease: the Task Force on the management of stable coronary artery disease of the European Society of Cardiology. Eur Heart J. 2013;34(38):2949–3003.
34. Burkauskas J, Mickuviene N, Brozaitiene J, Staniute M, Podlipskyte A, Rastenyte D, et al. Gene-environment interactions connecting Low triiodothyronine syndrome and outcomes of cardiovascular disease (GET-VASC): study protocol. Biological Psychiatry and Psychopharmacology. 2014; 16(2):66–73.
35. Staniute M, Brozaitiene J, Burkauskas J, Kazukauskiene N, Mickuviene N, Bunevicius R. Type D personality, mental distress, social support and health-related quality of life in coronary artery disease patients with heart failure: a longitudinal observational study. Health Qual Life Outcomes. 2015;13:1.
36. DeLong ER, DeLong DM, Clarke-Pearson DL. Comparing the areas under two or more correlated receiver operating characteristic curves: a nonparametric approach. Biometrics. 1988;44(3):837–45.
37. Pfister R, Strack N, Wielckens K, Malchau G, Erdmann E, Schneider CA. The relationship and prognostic impact of low-T3 syndrome and NT-pro-BNP in cardiovascular patients. Int J Cardiol. 2010;144(2):187–90.
38. Mayer Jr O, Simon J, Cech J, Rosolova H, Hrbkova J, Pikner R, et al. Even mild changes in free thyroxine could influence the degree of heart failure measured by its biological surrogates. Physiol Res. 2008;57(4):525–9.
39. Iervasi G, Pingitore A, Landi P, Raciti M, Ripoli A, Scarlattini M, et al. Low-T3 syndrome: a strong prognostic predictor of death in patients with heart disease. Circulation. 2003;107(5):708–13.
40. Friberg L, Drvota V, Bjelak AH, Eggertsen G, Ahnve S. Association between increased levels of reverse triiodothyronine and mortality after acute myocardial infarction. Am J Med. 2001;111(9):699–703.
41. Chuang CP, Jong YS, Wu CY, Lo HM. Impact of triiodothyronine and N-terminal pro-B-type natriuretic peptide on the long-term survival of critically ill patients with acute heart failure. Am J Cardiol. 2014;113(5):845–50.
42. Selvaraj S, Klein I, Danzi S, Akhter N, Bonow RO, Shah SJ. Association of serum triiodothyronine with B-type natriuretic peptide and severe left ventricular diastolic dysfunction in heart failure with preserved ejection fraction. Am J Cardiol. 2012;110(2):234–9.
43. Opasich C, Pacini F, Ambrosino N, Riccardi PG, Febo O, Ferrari R, et al. Sick euthyroid syndrome in patients with moderate-to-severe chronic heart failure. Eur Heart J. 1996;17(12):1860–6.
44. Coceani M, Iervasi G, Pingitore A, Carpeggiani C, L'Abbate A. Thyroid hormone and coronary artery disease: from clinical correlations to prognostic implications. Clin Cardiol. 2009;32(7):380–5.
45. Kozdag G, Ural D, Vural A, Agacdiken A, Kahraman G, Sahin T, et al. Relation between free triiodothyronine/free thyroxine ratio, echocardiographic parameters and mortality in dilated cardiomyopathy. Eur J Heart Fail. 2005;7(1):113–8.
46. Peeters RP, Wouters PJ, van Toor H, Kaptein E, Visser TJ, Van den Berghe G. Serum 3,3′,5′-triiodothyronine (rT3) and 3,5,3′-triiodothyronine/rT3 are prognostic markers in critically ill patients and are associated with postmortem tissue deiodinase activities. J Clin Endocrinol Metab. 2005;90(8):4559–65.
47. Pingitore A, Iervasi G, Barison A, Prontera C, Pratali L, Emdin M, et al. Early activation of an altered thyroid hormone profile in asymptomatic or mildly symptomatic idiopathic left ventricular dysfunction. J Card Fail. 2006;12(7):520–6.
48. Li X, Chen C, Gan F, Wang Y, Ding L, Hua W. Plasma NT pro-BNP, hs-CRP and big-ET levels at admission as prognostic markers of survival in hospitalized patients with dilated cardiomyopathy: a single-center cohort study. BMC Cardiovasc Disord. 2014;14:67.
49. Hawkes AL, Patrao TA, Ware R, Atherton JJ, Taylor CB, Oldenburg BF. Predictors of physical and mental health-related quality of life outcomes among myocardial infarction patients. BMC Cardiovasc Disord. 2013;13:69.
50. Leon de la Fuente R, Naesgaard PA, Nilsen ST, Woie L, Aarsland T, Gallo P, et al. B-type natriuretic peptide and high sensitive C-reactive protein predict 2-year all cause mortality in chest pain patients: a prospective observational study from Salta, Argentina. BMC Cardiovasc Disord. 2011;11:57.
51. Jung CH, Rhee EJ, Shin HS, Jo SK, Won JC, Park CY, et al. Higher serum free thyroxine levels are associated with coronary artery disease. Endocr J. 2008;55(5):819–26.
52. Popelova JR, Kotaska K, Tomkova M, Tomek J. Usefulness of N-terminal Pro-brain natriuretic peptide to predict mortality in adults with congenital heart disease. Am J Cardiol. 2015;116(9):1425–30.
53. Wei G, Yaqi R, Ningfu W, Xuwei H. N-terminal prohormone B-type natriuretic peptide and cardiovascular risk in stable coronary artery disease: a meta-analysis of nine prospective studies. Rev Cardiovasc Med. 2013;14(2–4):e92–8.

6

Acute coronary syndrome in young Sub-Saharan Africans

Moustapha Sarr[1], Djibril Mari Ba[1], Mouhamadou Bamba Ndiaye[1*], Malick Bodian[1], Modou Jobe[1], Adama Kane[1], Maboury Diao[1], Alassane Mbaye[2], Mouhamadoul Mounir Dia[1], Soulemane Pessinaba[1], Abdoul Kane[2] and Serigne Abdou Ba[1]

Abstract

Background: Coronary heart disease remains the leading cause of death in developed countries. In Africa, the disease continues to rise with varying rates of progression in different countries. At present, there is little available work on its juvenile forms. The objective of this work was to study the epidemiological, clinical and evolutionary aspects of acute coronary syndrome in young Sub-Saharan Africans.

Methods: This was a prospective multicenter study done at the different departments of cardiology in Dakar. We included all patients of age 40 years and below, and who were admitted for acute coronary syndrome between January 1st, 2005 and July 31st, 2007. We collected and analyzed the epidemiological, clinical, paraclinical and evolutionary data of the patients.

Results: Hospital prevalence of acute coronary syndrome in young people was 0.45% (21/4627) which represented 6.8% of all cases of acute coronary syndrome admitted during the same period. There was a strong male predominance with a sex-ratio (M:F) of 6. The mean age of patients was 34 ± 1.9 years (range of 24 and 40 years). The main risk factor was smoking, found in 52.4% of cases and the most common presenting symptom was chest pain found in 95.2% of patients. The average time delay before medical care was 14.5 hours. Diagnosis of ST- elevation myocardial infarction in 85.7% of patients and non-ST-elevation myocardial infarction in 14.3% was made by the combination electrocardiographic features and troponin assay. Echocardiography found a decreased left ventricular systolic function in 37.5% of the patients and intraventricular thrombus in 20% of them. Thrombolysis using streptokinase was done in 44.4% of the patients with ST- elevation myocardial infarction. Hospital mortality was 14.3%.

Conclusion: Acute coronary syndrome is present in young Sub-Saharan Africans. The main risk factor found was smoking.

Keywords: Acute coronary syndrome, Young Sub-Saharan African, Dakar

Background

Coronary heart disease remains the leading cause of death in developed countries. It is usually seen from the fifth to the seventh decades of life, but some cases in young people have been reported [1,2]. In Africa, while the work of the first European doctors that arrived on the continent claimed the low occurrence or even absence of atherosclerosis and its clinical manifestations, different schools of cardiology have shown not only their emergence, but especially their increase although at different rates in different countries [3,4]. On the other hand, few studies have been published on young people (5).

The objective of this work was to study the epidemiological, as well as the clinical and evolutionary peculiarities of acute coronary syndrome (ACS) in the young Sub-Saharan Africans of age 40 years and below.

Methods

This was a prospective multicenter study conducted at the respective cardiology departments of Aristide Le Dantec

* Correspondence: bambandiaye75@yahoo.fr
[1]Service de Cardiologie, CHU Aristide Le Dantec University Hospital, PO Box 6633, Dakar étoile, Avenue Pasteur, Dakar, Senegal
Full list of author information is available at the end of the article

University Hospital, Grand Yoff General Hospital and Principal Hospital of Dakar over a period of 31 months (January 1st 2005 to July 31st 2007), in Dakar, Senegal.

All patients with an age of 40 years and below, admitted for acute coronary syndrome on the basis of anginal pain at rest, suggestive electrocardiographic changes and elevated troponin I levels, were included. Patients with more than 40 years of age, those with stable angina, and those with semi-recent or sequel of coronary syndrome were excluded from the study.

We studied data on age, gender, past history including history of diabetes, hypertension, smoking, alcoholism, sedentarism (less than 30 minutes or more of moderate-intensity physical activity on most days of the week), obesity; family history of coronary heart disease at a young age (before 55 years in men and 65 years in women), use of estrogen-progestin contraceptives, stable angina and stress.

We sought the presence of chest pain, dyspnea and gastrointestinal symptoms.

We also noted the time delay before admission, the management given, and the vital parameters (blood pressure, heart rate, respiratory rate, temperature, body mass index).

All patients had a complete physical examination and a laboratory assessment. Troponin I assay was done using Architect STAT chemiluminescent microparticle immunoassay (Abbot). The other tests included blood glucose level on admission, total cholesterol and its fractions, and triglycerides. On the ECG, we looked for subepicardial or subendocardial lesion, subepicardial or subendocardial ischemia, abnormal Q waves, rhythm and conduction abnormalities. We have also looked for signs of venous stasis on the chest x-ray and evaluated using Doppler echocardiography (which was performed during the first 24 hours of admission), the left ventricle wall motion, left ventricular ejection fraction using Simpson's biplanar method, and the presence of intracavitary thrombus. Treatment modalities were evaluated as well as evolution during hospitalization.

The study protocol was approved by the Ethics Committee of the Ministry of Health and Social Welfare, Senegal (Comité d'éthique du Ministère de la Santé et l'Action Sociale). A signed consent form was obtained from each of the study participants.

The studied parameters were entered into an electronic questionnaire using Epi Info version 6.0 of the World Health Organization. Data analysis was performed using SPSS 15.0 (Statistical Package for Social Sciences). Quantitative data were expressed as mean ± standard deviation.

Results

Hospital prevalence of acute coronary syndrome in young patients was 0.45% (21/4627), meaning 6.8% (21/309) of patients admitted for acute coronary syndrome during the same period. Eighteen patients (85.7%) were males and three patients (14.3%) were females, giving a ratio of 6:1. The mean age of patients was 34 ± 1.9 years with a range of 24 and 40 years. In women, the mean age was 37 years and among men it was 34 years.

The risk factors in our patients (Table 1) were dominated by active smoking found in 11 patients (52.4%). The average number of pack-years was 8.10 ± 2.3 and ranged from 1 to 17 pack-years.

Five patients (23.8%) had no risk factors, seven patients (33.3%) had one risk factor and the remaining patients (42.9%) had more than one.

Chest pain was present in 20 patients (95.2%). In 65% of cases, it was typical anginal pain and inaugural in 70% of cases. The average time delay before medical care was given was 14.5 hours, with extremes of 03 and 48 hours.

On admission, blood pressure was greater than or equal to 140 and/or 90 mmHg in three patients (14.3%). Average body mass index was 23.5 ± 1.5 kg / m^2. No patient was found to be obese.

Systemic examination was strictly normal in 18 patients (95.2%). Three patients however showed signs of left ventricular failure (Killip II).

Mean troponin I level found was 29 ± 40.9 ng/ml (0.01 to 401.6 ng/ ml). Two patients had levels below 0.05 ng/ml. Average blood glucose level was 1.2 ± 0.4 g/l (0.6 to 3.83 g/l). It was found to be 1.24 g/l in 4 patients (21%). Mean total cholesterol was 1.4 ± 0.2 g/l (0.85 to 2.58 g/l). Hypercholesterolaemia was present in two patients, LDL cholesterol greater than 1.6 g/l in one patient and HDL cholesterol less than 0.4 g/l in seven patients (41.2%). Two patients had a triglyceride level greater than 1.5 g/l.

Electrocardiogram revealed an acute coronary syndrome with persistent ST-elevation in 18 patients (85.7%) and non ST-elevation acute coronary syndrome in three patients (14.3%).

Topographically, the anterior and inferior territories were the most represented and found respectively in 14

Table 1 Risk factors found in the study population

Risk factors	Number	%
Tobacco smoking	11	52.4
Stress	9	42.9
Sedentarism	3	14.3
Hypertension	3	14.3
Hypercholesterolemia	2	9.5
Heredity	2	9.5
Diabetes	1	4.8

(66, 7%) and 7 patients (33.3%). An extension to the right ventricle was observed in one patient. We also noted two cases of ventricular tachycardia and complete atrioventricular block in one patient.

Chest radiography showed a cardiomegaly in four patients (21%). Doppler echocardiography revealed impaired segmental kinetics in 12 patients (60%). The mean ventricular ejection fraction was 52.2 ± 8.5% (20-80%). Systolic dysfunction was found in six patients and left ventricular thrombus in four.

Concerning treatment, thrombolysis using streptokinase was performed in eight patients, accounting for 44.4% of patients with ST-elevation.

Low molecular weight heparin was used in 19 patients (90.5%), aspirin in 20 patients (95.2%), clopidogrel in 7 patients (33.3%) beta blockers in 17 patients (81%), angiotensin converting enzyme inhibitors in 17 patients (81%), statins in 14 patients (66.7%) and analgesics in 13 patients (62%).

The evolution during hospitalization after a mean hospital stay of 18.7 ± 4.5 days (1–37 days) was favorable in 18 patients (85.7%). Three deaths (14.3%) were recorded, two of which were due to sudden death from ventricular fibrillation and one due to cardiogenic shock.

Discussion

In our study, the prevalence of acute coronary syndrome before age 40 was 0.45% with an incidence of 6.8% on all patients with coronary heart disease hospitalized during the same period.

Data on the incidence of acute coronary syndrome in young people are rare in Africa [5,6]. However, Wade found a prevalence of 0.03% and an incidence of 5.7% [7].

This incidence of 6.8% is bringing our numbers in the range of the European and American literature (4-10%) [8-12] and could be an evidence of a real epidemiological transition.

The mean age of our patients was 34 years. Tricot [13], and Dolder [8] found, respectively, a mean age of 36 years and 35.4 years. However in India the youngest age reported for acute coronary syndrome was in a 14 year-old [14].

Our study confirms male predominance as has been emphasized in previous works [2,7,9,10,14].

Smoking was found to be the main risk factor and is often found in the occurrence of coronary events in young patients [15]. Indeed, most works on the occurrence of coronary syndrome in young patients have a disease pattern dominated by monotonous smoking [9,16,17].

This is reflected in our work where smoking is found in 52.4% of cases. This rate seems more important in European series, where it has been reported to be up to 93% [13]. The use of hard drugs, as was the case with one of our patients, may be associated with the occurrence of a coronary event [18,19].

The delay in our work (14.5 hours) is close to what is found in some Africans like in Tunisia [20].This period is shorter in the European series [21,22].

Clinically, acute coronary syndrome in young patients does not appear much different from that of the elderly. This has been emphasized by several authors [9,14,23,24]. The picture of acute coronary syndrome is dominated by pain in both the young as well as in the elderly.

Elevation of troponin levels form part of the definition of acute coronary syndrome [25]. This high rate of troponin assay in our work translates into a better integration of this biological parameter in the management of acute coronary syndrome. Concerning cardiomegaly found in 4 patients on chest X-ray at admission, no conclusion could be drawn as data on the existence cardiomyopathies or other heart disease could be established.

In our study we found using Doppler echocardiography an impaired left ventricular systolic function in 37.5% of cases versus 63.3% found by Renambot J et al. However, the mean age of patients in this series was 47.1 years ± 4 [26]. Left intraventricular thrombus in the apical region was found in 20% of our patients. These results confirm data from the literature [27,28]. Segmental abnormality observed in only 60% of the cases might be primarily the effect of thrombolytic therapy. Also the degree of myocardial damage may not have been severe enough to lead segmental abnormality.

The impact of thrombolytic therapy on mortality with a time-dependent effect has been reported by several studies [29-31]. It is now clear that thrombolysis can significantly reduce mortality of patients with acute coronary syndrome. In our work, steptokinase being the only available thrombolytic in our hospitals, was used in 44.4% of patients admitted with an ST-elevation acute coronary syndrome. The reasons for the low use of thrombolytics in this study were due to many factors including low awareness level of the population about acute coronary syndrome, poor transport and communication network to reach referral centers, lack of available electrocardiography in health centers which are located close to patients, delayed referral from health centers of suspected cases and inability to meet the high cost of thrombolytic treatment. The favorable outcome in young adults, as seen in our work (85.7%) seems higher than that observed in the elderly.

Heart failure is a common and serious complication of acute myocardial infarction. It was present in our work in 14.3% of patients. This was found in 18.2% and 9.2% respectively in the series of Al-Khadra and Kanitz [14,24]. A relationship between age and heart failure has been reported by Magid with a greater frequency of occurrence in the elderly compared to young subjects [32].

The ventricular arrhythmias are responsible for 30-40% of deaths occurring during the first 12 hours of a myocardial infarction. In our work, ventricular fibrillation was responsible for two deaths during the acute phase.

Conclusion

The occurrence of acute coronary syndrome is a reality in young Sub-Saharan Africans. The main risk factor is smoking. Complications are not rare and the mortality remains high.

Competing interests
The authors declare that they have no competing interests

Authors' contributions
MS, DMB, MBN and SAB designed the study protocol, participated in the data collection and contributed in analyzing the data and writing of the draft manuscript. MB, MJ, AdK and MD participated in data analysis and critically revising the manuscript for important intellectual content. AM, MMD, SP and AK participated in study design and in data analysis. All authors have read and approved the final version of the manuscript.

Author details
[1]Service de Cardiologie, CHU Aristide Le Dantec University Hospital, PO Box 6633, Dakar étoile, Avenue Pasteur, Dakar, Senegal. [2]Service de Cardiologie, Hôpital Général de Grand Yoff, Dakar, Senegal.

References
1. Benomar M, Berrada M: **Fréquence et aspects épidémiologiques de l'infarctus du myocarde de l'adulte jeune marocain.** *Cœur et Med Inter* 1973, **XII**(3):409–415.
2. Bensaid J: **L'infarctus du myocarde de 20 à 40 ans.** *La revue du praticien* 1979, **53:**4091–4094.
3. Shavadia J, Yonga G, Otieno H: **A prospective review of acute coronary syndromes in an urban hospital in sub-Saharan Africa.** *Cardiovasc J Afr* 2012, **23:**318–321.
4. Shaper A: **Cardiovascular studies in the Samburu tribe of northern Kenya.** *Am Heart J* 1962, **63:**437.
5. Wyndham CH, Seftel HC, Pilcher GJ, Baker SG: **Prevalence of hypercholesterolemia in young Afrikaners with myocardial infarction. Ischemic heart disease risk factors.** *S Afr Med J* 1978, **71**(3):139–142.
6. Charles D, Barabe P, Talbi D: **Infarctus du myocarde en Algérie. A propos de 30 observations.** *Cardiol Trop* 1982, **8**(29):13–19.
7. Wade B, Djimadoum N, Charles D: **L'infarctus du myocarde chez le jeune Sénégalais. Etude étiologique et clinique de 14 cas.** *Cardiologie Tropicale* 1996, **22:**39–44.
8. Dolder MA, Olivier MF: **Myocardial infarction in young men: study of risk factors in nine countries.** *Br Heart J* 1975, **37:**493–503.
9. Joussein-Remacle S, Delarche N, Bader H, Bader H, Lasserre R, Estrade G: **Facteurs de risque de l'infarctus du myocarde du sujet jeune: registre prospectif sur un an.** *Ann Cardiol Angeiol* 2006, **55:**204–209.
10. Kannel WB, Abbott RD: **Incidence and prognosis of unrecognized myocardial infarction.** *N Engl J Med* 1984, **311:**1144–1147.
11. Migliaresi P, Celentano P, Palmieri V, Pezzullo S, Martino S, Bonito M, Guillaro B, *et al*: **Knowledge of cardiovascular risk factors and awareness of non-pharmacological approach for risk prevention in young: the cardiovascular risk prevention project "help your heart stay young".** *Nutr Metab Cardiovasc Dis* 2007, **17:**468–472.
12. Ruiz-Bailen M, Dehayos EA, Ramos-Cadra JA, Díaz-Castellanos MA, Issa-Khozouz Z, Reina-Toral A, López-Martínez A, *et al*: **Influence of age on clinical course, management and mortality of acute myocardial infarction in the spanish population.** *Int J Cardiol* 2002, **85:**285–296.
13. Tricot R, Laffay N, Fillatre D: **L'infarctus du sujet jeune.** In *Entretiens de Bichat, (Médecine).* Paris: Expansions scient.fr.ed; 1974:93–98.
14. Al-khadra AH: **Clinical profile of young patients with acute myocardial infarction in Saudi Arabia.** *Int J Cardiol* 2003, **91:**9–13.
15. Thomas D: **Athérosclérose.** In *Cardiologie.* Paris: Ellipses; 1994:135–151.
16. Bauters C: **De la plaque d'athérome à la plaque instable.** In *ANGOR De la douleur thoracique à la plaque vulnérable.* Edited by François D. Paris: EDITIONS scientifiques & LC; 2003:41–52.
17. Collet JP, Ripoli L, Choussat R, Lison L, Montalescot G: **La maladie athérothrombotique coronaire du sujet jeune: état des lieux.** *Sang. Thrombose Vaisseaux* 2000, **12:**218–225. N°24.
18. Hollander JE, Hoffman RS, Gennis P, Fairweather P, Feldman JA, Fish SS, DiSano MJ, *et al*: **Cocaine-associated chest pain: one-year follow-up.** *Acad Emerg Med* 1995, **2:**179–184.
19. Kloner RA, Rezkalla SH: **Cocaine and the heart.** *N Engl J Med* 2003, **348:**487–517.
20. Mahdhaoui A, Bouraoui H, Majdoub MA, Ben Abdelaziz A, Trimeche B, Zaaraoui J, Jeridi G, *et al*: **Délais de prise en charge de l'IDM en phase aiguë : résultats d'une enquête dans la région de Sousse (Tunisie).** *Ann Cardiol Angeiol* 2003, **52:**15–19.
21. De Lopagno SM: **Syndrome coronarien aigu: analyse des délais de la prise en charge.** *Thèse Med, Genève* 2004:. No 10397.
22. Pistavos C, Panagiotakos DB, Antonoulas A, Zombolos S, Kogias Y, Mantas Y, Stravopodis P, *et al*: **Epidemiology of acute coronary syndromes in a Mediterranean country; aims, design and baseline characteristics of the Greek study of acute coronary syndrome (GREECS).** *BMC Public Health* 2005, **5:**23.
23. Benacerraf A, Castilloy-Fennoy A, Goffinet D, Krantz D: **L'infarctus du myocarde avant 36 ans: à propos de 20 cas.** *Arch Mal Cœur* 1978, **77**(7):756–764.
24. Kanitz MG, Giovannucci SJ, Jones JS, Mott M: **Myocardial infarction in young adults: Risk factors and clinical features.** *Emerg Med J* 1996, **14:**139–145.
25. Capolaghi B, Charbonnier B, Dumonet M, Hennache B, Henninot J, Laperche T, *et al*: **Recommandations sur la prescription, le dosage et l'interprétation des troponines cardiaques.** *Ann Biol Clin* 2005, **63:**245–261.
26. Renambot J, Traore I, Chauvet J, *et al*: **Relative rareté des indications opératoires dans la maladie coronaire chez les noirs africains: etude de 90 cas.** *Cardiol Trop* 1991, **17:**89–95.
27. Ba A: **Les cardiopathies ischémiques: étude prospective à propos de 69 cas colligés à la clinique cardiologique du CHU de Dakar.** *Thèse Med Dakar* 2002. No. 11.
28. Mboup MC: **Les syndromes coronariens aigus: etude prospective à propos de 59 cas colligés en milieu hospitalier dakarois.** *Thèse Med Dakar* 2006. No. 71.
29. EMERAS (Estudio Multicentrico Estreptoquinasa Republicas de America del Sur) Collaborative Group: **Randomized trial of the late thrombolysis in acute myocardial infarction.** *Lancet* 1993, **342:**767.
30. LATE (Late Assessment of Thrombolytic Efficacity) Study Group: **Late Assessment of Thrombolytic Efficacity (LATE) Study with alteplase 6–24 hours after onset of acute myocardial infarction.** *Lancet* 1993, **342:**759–766.
31. Weaver WD: **Time to thrombolytic treatment: factors affecting delay and their influences on outcome.** *J Am Coll Cardiol* 1995, **25:**3S–9S.
32. Magid DJ: **Older emergency departement patients with acute myocardial infarction receive lower quality of care than younger patients.** *Ann Emerg Med* 2005, **46:**14–21.

SMARTphone-based, early cardiac REHABilitation in patients with acute coronary syndromes [SMART-REHAB Trial]

Matias B. Yudi[1,2*], David J. Clark[1,2], David Tsang[3], Michael Jelinek[2,4,5], Katie Kalten[1], Subodh Joshi[6], Khoa Phan[6], Arthur Nasis[7], John Amerena[8], Sandeep Arunothayaraj[4], Chris Reid[9] and Omar Farouque[1,2]

Abstract

Background: There are well-documented treatment gaps in secondary prevention of coronary heart disease and no clear guidelines to assist early physical activity after acute coronary syndromes (ACS). Smartphone technology may provide an innovative platform to close these gaps. This paper describes the study design of a randomized controlled trial assessing whether a smartphone-based secondary prevention program can facilitate early physical activity and improve cardiovascular health in patients with ACS.

Methods: We have developed a multi-faceted, patient-centred smartphone-based secondary prevention program emphasizing early physical activity with a graduated walking program initiated on discharge from ACS admission. The program incorporates; physical activity tracking through the smartphone's accelerometer with interactive feedback and goal setting; a dynamic dashboard to review and optimize cardiovascular risk factors; educational messages delivered twice weekly; a photographic food diary; pharmacotherapy review; and support through a short message service. The primary endpoint of the trial is change in exercise capacity, as measured by the change in six-minute walk test distance at 8-weeks when compared to baseline. Secondary endpoints include improvements in cardiovascular risk factor status, psychological well-being and quality of life, medication adherence, uptake of cardiac rehabilitation and re-hospitalizations.

Discussion: This randomized controlled trial will use a smartphone-phone based secondary prevention program to emphasize early physical activity post-ACS. It will provide evidence regarding the feasibility and utility of this innovative platform in closing the treatment gaps in secondary prevention.

Keywords: Cardiac rehabilitation, Secondary prevention, Acute coronary syndromes, mhealth, Smartphone application

Background

Coronary heart disease (CHD) is the leading cause of mortality and morbidity in the world [1]. In 2012 CHD accounted for approximately 7.4 million lives, an increase of 23 % (1.4 million) from CHD deaths in 2000 [1]. Patients at highest risk of premature death, myocardial infarction and re-hospitalization are those with known CHD [2]. Consequently international guidelines strongly advocate proven secondary prevention strategies such evidence-based pharmacological therapy, cardiovascular risk factor optimization, cardiac rehabilitation and adherence to diet and physical activity recommendations [3].

Cardiac rehabilitation provides a comprehensive secondary prevention framework based on extensive scientific evidence. A recent Cochrane review revealed cardiac rehabilitation was associated with a 13 % decrease in

* Correspondence: matiasyudi@gmail.com
[1]Department of Cardiology, Austin Health, Melbourne, Australia
[2]Department of Medicine, University of Melbourne, Melbourne, Australia
Full list of author information is available at the end of the article

all-cause mortality and a 26 % decrease in cardiovascular mortality [4]. This result is consistent with several other meta-analyses [5–7].

However, there is poor translation of scientific evidence into clinical practice. Cardiac rehabilitation services are underutilized as highlighted by low referral rates and even lower completion rates [8–12]. In addition, utilization of recommended pharmacological therapy and compliance with dietary and physical activity guidelines is suboptimal [13–16]. Lastly, outpatient cardiac rehabilitation often starts weeks to months after the index event, even with the utilization of new technology [17]. This delay creates a missed opportunity to immediately reinforce the importance of physical activity and lifestyle changes. Furthermore, the delay in cardiac rehabilitation has been associated with delayed resumption of work [18].

The drawbacks of conventional cardiac rehabilitation have resulted in the development of innovative models of care. In the seminal paper by Vale et al, regular personal coaching via telephone has been shown to be effective in reducing total cholesterol levels and other cardiovascular risk factors [19]. Systematic reviews and meta-analyses have shown telehealth interventions for secondary prevention, limited to telephone calls, internet and videoconferencing technologies, offer an effective alternative model of secondary prevention care [20, 21].

Most recently, the Tobacco, Exercise and Diet Messages (TEXT ME) study showed a lifestyle-focused text-messaging service lowered LDL-cholesterol level, and blood pressure while increasing smoking cessation rates and physical activity in patients with known CHD [22].

Smartphone technology is an advance on previous telehealth and text-message based technologies. It has the potential to revolutionize the landscape of secondary prevention as it can provide a platform for a patient-centred program with the capacity to incorporate education, real-time feedback, motivation, reminders and support. Furthermore, it is a tool that can be used to monitor diet, physical activity, medications and cardiovascular risk factor parameters. Lastly and most importantly, a smartphone-based program can be started immediately, delivered from anywhere at any time and for extended periods of time.

Four studies have been published incorporating smartphone technology for the delivery of cardiac rehabilitation. Worringham et al. assessed a walking-based cardiac rehabilitation program with single-lead ECG, heart rate and GPS-based speed and location transmitted via smartphone for real-time monitoring by a qualified exercise scientist. [23] Six patients were evaluated in 134 exercise sessions with improvements in exercise capacity (improvement in 6-minute walk test from 524 m to 637 m, $p < 0.01$) and health status measured by SF-36 form. Korzeniowska-Kubacka et al. assessed a mobile device with preprogrammed exercise training sessions with audio and visual clues and a 3-lead ECG monitor [24]. In this non-randomized trial, 30 patients were assigned to the mobile device intervention with 10 supervised exercise sessions and 14 sessions with the mobile device at home. The control group of 32 patients had 24 supervised exercise sessions. There was in improvement in exercise capacity in the mobile arm ($p < 0.05$) but no difference in blood pressure. Blasco et al. assessed a web-based telemonitoring system that provided patients with self-measurement devices and connected them to a cardiologist who accessed the data and sent recommendations via short message service (SMS) [25]. In this single-blinded, randomized controlled trial of 203 acute coronary syndrome survivors, patients in the telemonitoring group were more likely to improve at least one risk factor (RR 1.4, 95 % CI 1.1–1.7) and achieve targets for BP (62.1 % vs 42.9 %, $p = 0.01$) and HbA1c (86.4 % vs 54.2 %, $p = 0.02$). Varnfield et al. compared the effectiveness of smartphone-based cardiac rehabilitation versus traditional care on cardiac rehabilitation uptake, adherence and completion in a randomized controlled trial [17]. 120 patients were randomized to the two groups for a 6-week cardiac rehabilitation program followed by a 6-month self-maintenance period. The smartphone based model included health and exercise monitoring, motivational and educational material delivery and weekly mentoring consultations. The trial met its primary end point with the smartphone based rehabilitation program showing significantly higher uptake (94 % vs. 68 %, $P < 0.05$) and completion (80 % vs. 47 %, $p < 0.05$).

The exponential growth and availability of smartphone technology provides a novel opportunity to optimize secondary prevention of coronary heart disease [26]. However, further studies are needed to examine the value of this approach and to demonstrate improvements in objective outcomes.

AIM

The aim of this study is to assess the impact of a smartphone-based secondary prevention program (SSPP), initiated on discharge in patients with acute coronary syndromes, on exercise capacity, cardiovascular risk factors, quality of life and mood.

Hypothesis

The primary hypothesis is that a SSPP would improve exercise capacity, as measured by a 6-minute walk test, compared to standard care. Secondary hypotheses are: A SSPP will result in improvement in cardiac depression and quality of life scores as well as in cardiovascular risk factors (lipid profile, blood pressure, HbA1C, anthropometry) and secondary prevention pharmacotherapy use between the groups.

Methods/design

The study design is single-blinded, two-arm, parallel, randomized control trial. The study design is displayed in Fig. 1. The protocol conforms to the SPIRIT 2013 statement and the intervention is described in accordance with the CONSORT-EHEALTH checklist. [27–30]

Eligibility and recruitment

Patient over the age of 18 with a diagnosis of an acute coronary syndrome and documented coronary artery disease on coronary angiography (coronary artery stenosis >50 %), who are treated either medically or with percutaneous coronary intervention will be eligible for inclusion. The other major inclusion criteria will be personal ownership of a smartphone.

Exclusion criteria include untreated ventricular tachycardia, severe heart failure, significant residual coronary artery disease requiring revascularization, treatment with coronary artery bypass surgery, coexisting disease with a life expectancy less than 1 year and/or significant exercise limitations for reasons other than CHD.

Recruitment will occur during hospital admission at six major university affiliated teaching hospitals in Victoria, Australia. All patients admitted with acute coronary syndromes will be screened and those meeting the entry criteria will be selected. Potential participants will receive study information and informed consent will be obtained.

Sample size calculation

A sample size of 152 participants (76 per group) will be required to detect a minimal clinically important difference of 25 m for the six-minute walk test with 80 % power at 5 % level of significance [31, 32]. To account for an estimated 20 % loss to follow-up, 100 patients in each arm will be recruited.

Ethics approval

The Austin Health Human Research Ethics Committee granted approval for the trial (HREC/14/AUSTIN/128).

Randomization and blinding

Eligible patients will be randomized in a 1:1 fashion to smartphone-based secondary prevention program or usual care through a computerized randomization program. Randomization will be stratified by study site and be overseen by the Centre of Cardiovascular Research and Education in Therapeutics at Monash University; an independent research body within the School of Public Health and Preventive Medicine at Monash University, Melbourne, Australia. Baseline assessment, including the 6-minute walk test, will occur prior to randomization. Assessors of the primary outcome are blind to treatment allocation; however participants are not blinded.

Intervention

The smartphone-based secondary prevention program will be delivered over 8 weeks starting at time of discharge from hospital through a smartphone application (app). Participants in the smartphone intervention cohort will download the intervention application ("app") into their smartphone. They will then receive education on how to use the app. The SSPP is a multi-faceted intervention with particular emphasis on early physical activity. The app provides a platform to deliver a comprehensive secondary prevention program (Fig. 2). Participants can

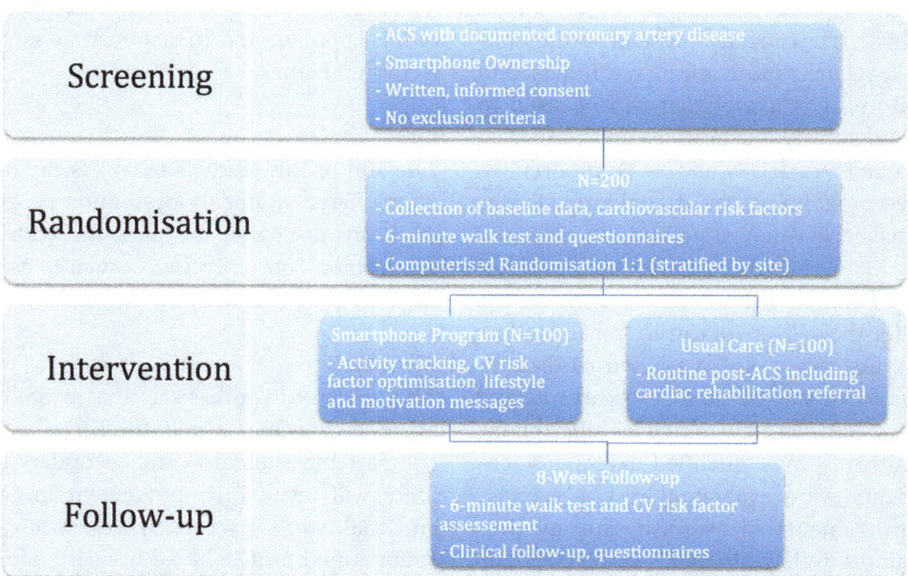

Fig. 1 Randomized Control Trial Design and Flow

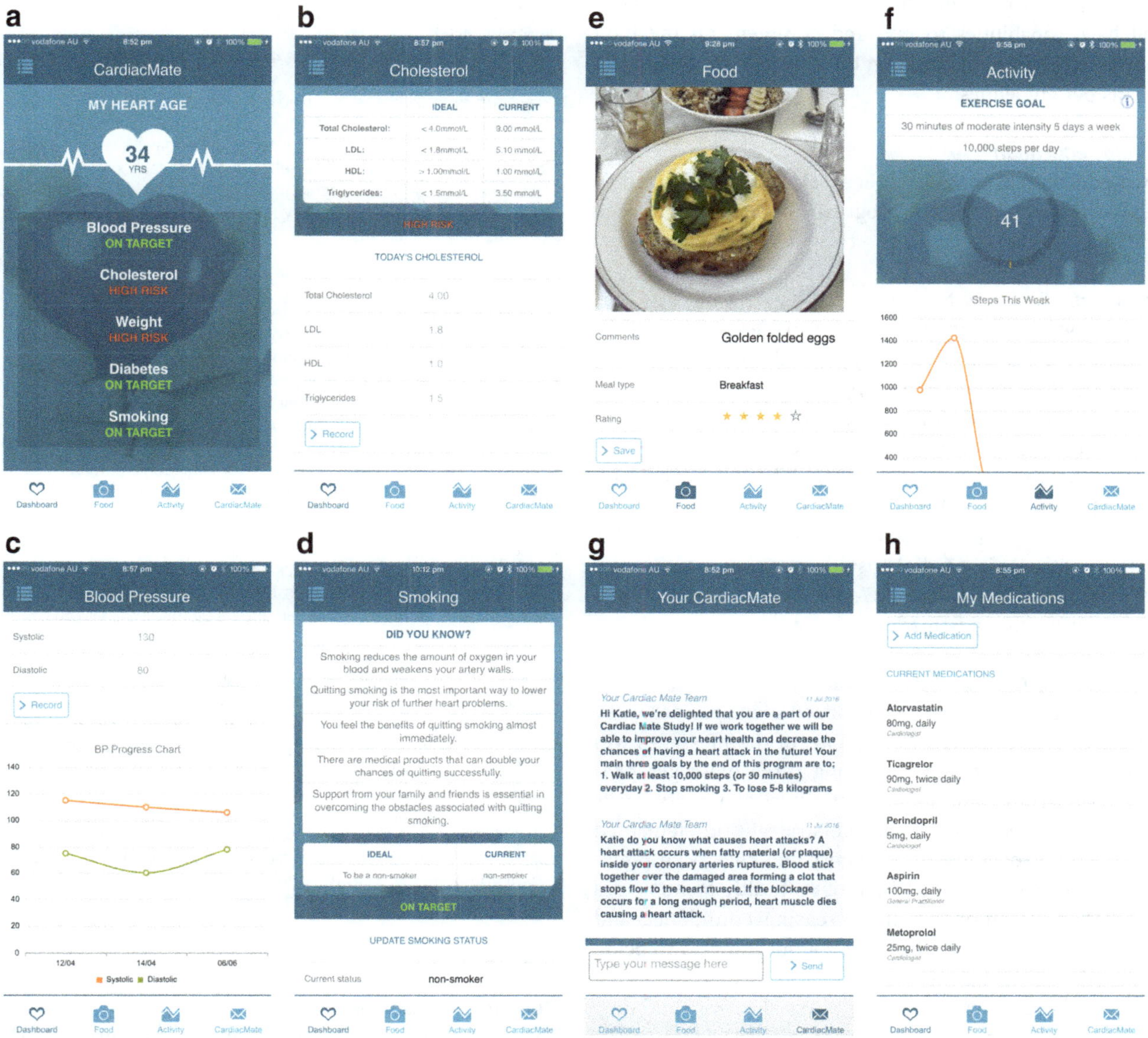

Fig. 2 Smartphone application interface depicting interactive dashboard (**a**), cholesterol page (**b**), blood pressure progress chart (**c**), smoking education page (**d**), photographic food diary (**e**), activity tracking page (**f**), individualized messaging service (**g**) and medication page (**h**)

log off the app at any time effectively not undertaking the SSPP. The different components of the SSPP are discussed in detail below.

Exercise prescription

Patients will have access to real-time feedback of their activity levels through the app's activity tracker which links to the smartphone's accelerometer feature. Patients will be able to monitor the number of steps taken and the distance walked. Patients will undertake a graded walking program increasing in time and intensity over the 8 weeks. Their aim will be to achieve 30 min of walking a day for at least 5 days every week, in accordance with guideline recommendations [3]. Patients will be encouraged to progress to moderate intensity activity, defined as a noticeable increase in depth and rate of breathing while still being able to talk comfortably, within 2 weeks.

Dynamic tracking of cardiovascular risk factors

Patients will have an interactive personal dashboard highlighting the status of their cardiovascular risk factors. Blood pressure, cholesterol levels, glucose levels, weight, smoking status will be graded depending whether they are at recommended target levels [3]. Patients will record this information in the app prior to discharge and will be able to update this at anytime.

Dietary habits

Dietary habits will be tracked through the app via access to the phone's inbuilt camera. Patients will be encouraged to photograph the food they consume. They will have capabilities to rate and comment on the food they are communing based on their perception of an ideal diet as per guidelines.

Cardiac education

Two educational messages per week will be delivered to the participants as they progress through the 8-week SSPP.

Cardiac medication list

Patients will input their discharge medications into the app prior to leaving hospital. The medication list will be reviewed to ensure that appropriate evidence-based pharmacotherapy (dual antiplatelet therapy, statin, angiotensin converting enzyme inhibitor/angiotensin receptor blocker, beta-blocker) has been prescribed. If a particular class of drug has not been prescribed, the patient will be notified through the app and encouraged to discuss this further with their cardiologist or general practitioner. Participants will be able to edit their medication list whenever a change is made.

Interactive and personalized feedback

Patients will receive five personalized messages per week via the app messaging service. Two of the messages will be educational and the remaining three messages provide goal setting and feedback on physical activity levels and diet. The behavioural change strategies implemented are based on social cognitive theory and have been previously successfully applied in mobile health technologies [33]. There is emphasis on increasing confidence and motivation to exercise while overcoming barriers to being physically active. Furthermore, there is clear goal setting prescribed every week regarding physical activity and diet. Feedback is given based on exercise levels (automated) and diet (personalized). The app allows the patient to analyze their own physical activity and assess their progress towards their individualized goal. Table 1 shows sample messages.

Support

The messaging service also allows the patient to initiate contact if they have any questions regarding their cardiac condition or rehabilitation process. Replies will be made within one business day.

Standard care

Regardless of the treatment arm, all patients will receive standard of care treatment post-ACS. This includes in-patient cardiology review, pre-discharge planning, formal communication with general practitioner through a discharge summary letter, referral to cardiac rehabilitation, promotion of self care and a chest pain action plan.

Table 1 Sample Messages

Physical Activity
- Hi [name], walking is a great type of exercise for people with coronary heart disease – I see you did xxxx steps yesterday. Over the next few days, aim to walk at least 500 steps more a day!
- Hi [name], well done on your activity over the past week! For this week, your goal is to walk for at least 20 min a day. Given your best last week was xxxx steps, this week you should reach xxxx steps a day!
- Hi [name], well done on reaching xxxx steps last week! This week, your aim is to walk 30 min a day everyday. Make it a routine as they benefits will last a lifetime!

Dietary Habits
- Hi [name], diet is very important in reducing the risk of future heart attacks. Your aim for the week is to try and eat 5 serving of vegetables everyday. Make sure you take photos of your meals so you are accountable for what you are eating!
- Hi [name], making small, healthy changes in the food and drinks that you have can make a big difference. Over the next week can you try and eliminate all soft drinks and junk food. Keep us posted with your electronic food diary!
- Hi [name], did you know that oily fish contains polyunsaturated fat that helps to lower your cholesterol? You should try and have 2–3 serves of fish each week.

Educational
- [Name], do you know what causes heart attacks? A heart attack occurs when fatty material (or plaque) inside your coronary arteries ruptures. Blood sticks together over the damaged area forming a clot that stops flow to the heart muscle. If the blockage occurs for a long enough period, heart muscle dies causing a heart attack.
- [Name], did you know it is essential to take your prescribed medications? They will reduce your risk of further heart attacks, strokes and premature death. You should be taking 5 medications for your heart. Check with your doctor if you have any questions about them or if need a new script – suddenly stopping your medications can place you at high risk of further heart attacks.
- [Name], did you know most people can have sex soon after a heart attack? If you can walk up two flights of stairs without getting breathless or having chest pain, you are probably well enough to have sex. If you have any concerns, don't hesitate to contact your doctor.

Outcome assessment

Participants will be evaluated at baseline, prior to discharge from hospital, and at 8 weeks, as an outpatient. The initial assessment will include explanation of study protocol and signing of consent forms. Patients assigned to SSPP will undertake app training to ensure they can maximize their experience. Baseline evaluation will include measurement and assessment of height, weight, waist circumference, resting heart rate and blood pressure, smoking status, fasting cholesterol and glucose levels and exercise capacity measured by a six-minute walk test.

Primary outcome

The primary outcome is change in six-minute walk distance that will be measured in standardized fashion [34]. The initial test will be undertaken prior to hospital discharge and this will be repeated at 8 weeks as an outpatient, without monitoring.

Secondary outcomes

In general, all secondary outcomes will be measured at baseline and at 8-week follow-up. Table 2 summarises the secondary outcomes of our study.

Body mass index will be derived from the weight (kg) divided by height (m) squared. Waist circumference will be measured using an anthropometric tape placed around the participant's waist at the level of the umbilicus. An electronic sphygmomanometer with pulse oximetry will be used to assess the systolic and diastolic blood pressure as well as resting heart rate.

Fasting glucose and cholesterol levels will be measured after 12 h of fasting. It will be analyzed at the pathology department of the corresponding hospital in standard fashion.

Smoking status, medication compliance and current medication list will be assessed via self-reporting at the 8-week assessment. The date the participant returns to work, if applicable, will also be collected to assess the time to resumption of work after acute coronary syndromes.

Uptake, adherence and completion of a cardiac rehabilitation program will be assessed. Uptake is defined as attending at least one exercise session for traditional cardiac rehabilitation or uploading 1 day's physical activity in the SSPP. Adherence is defined as attending 4 weeks' or uploading 12-days of activity over 4 weeks of physical activity. Completion is defined as showing adherence to cardiac rehabilitation and attending the 8-week assessment session.

Major adverse cardiovascular events (MACE) will be recorded. MACE is defined as the composite of death, myocardial infarction, stroke and unplanned revascularization.

Assessment for depression will be undertaken with the Cardiac Depression Scale (CDS) and Depression Scale – Short Form (DS-SF) [35]. Assessment of anxiety will be undertaken with the use of the Hospital Anxiety and Depression Scale (HADS). Change in quality of life will be assessed by the SF-36 questionnaire [36].

The EQ5D will be used to obtain a single preference index for calculation of Quality Adjusted Life Years (QALY) to assess cost per QALY for comparison to standard care. Health care utilization will be recorded for adverse events including presentation to hospital and/or general practitioner for symptoms of coronary heart disease or heart failure.

Table 2 Primary and secondary endpoints

Primary Outcome
• Change in six-minute walk test distance
Secondary Outcomes
• Fasting lipid levels (TC, LDL-C, HDL-C, TG)
• Fasting glucose
• Resting blood pressure
• Weight and body mass index
• Waist circumference
• Smoking status (self-reported)
• Uptake, Adherence and Completion of cardiac rehabilitation
• Major adverse cardiovascular events
• Cardiovascular hospital re-admissions
• Depression assessment (CDS and DS-SF questionnaires)
• Anxiety assessment (HADS questionnaire)
• Quality of life assessment (SF-36 questionnaire)
• Health outcome assessment (EQ-5D questionnaire)
• Time to return to work
• Secondary prevention pharmacotherapy use (self-reported)
• Six minute walk test distance at 8-weeks

Statistical analysis

Statistical analyses will be performed using SPSS (IBM, USA). Baseline characteristics will be summarized using descriptive statistics. Continuous variables will be described as mean and standard deviation and be compared using Student's t test. Categorical variables will be described as frequencies and percentages and compared using Fisher's exact or chi-square tests as appropriate. Treatment evaluation will be performed on an intention to treat (ITT) analysis.

Discussion

This novel study aims to evaluate the impact of a smartphone based secondary prevention program on functional capacity of patients with acute coronary syndromes. The benefit of comprehensive secondary prevention programs incorporating physical activity is well recognised. Smartphone technology could hold the key to bridging the well documented gap between scientific evidence and clinical practice.

This randomised clinical trial also aims to build the scientific base supporting alternative models of secondary prevention care in patients post acute myocardial infarction. Of particular note, is the initiation of this program as soon as the patient is discharged from hospital post their index event. This is a crucial period of recovery and immediate initiation of smartphone based secondary prevention program may facilitate early physical activity and return to normal daily function, including resumption of work.

The primary endpoint aims to objectively assess improvement in physical activity through the use of the six-minute walk test. Near maximal exercise testing is safe in patients with uncomplicated myocardial infarction prior to discharge and thus early mobilisation should be encouraged [37, 38]. The superiority trial design is suitable to detect a minimal clinically important difference in 6-minute walk distance [31]. It is postulated the improvement will be due to earlier initiation of an exercise program and increase in uptake and adherence with cardiac rehabiliation.

Acknowledgements

Dr Matias Yudi is supported by a National Health and Medical Research Council of Australia Postgraduate Scholarship and a National Heart Foundation of Australia Health Professional Scholarship.

Funding
The Victorian Cardiac Clinical Network and the National Heart Foundation of Australia, through a Vanguard Grant, have funded this study. They did not have any role in the design of this study protocol.

Authors' contributions
MY, MJ, DC, OF developed the concept, obtained funding, and designed the trial protocol. DT, KK, SJ, KP, AN, JA, SA contributed to the study design. CR provided statistical analysis support. All authors read and approved the final document.

Competing interests
The authors declare that they have no competing interests.

Author details
[1]Department of Cardiology, Austin Health, Melbourne, Australia. [2]Department of Medicine, University of Melbourne, Melbourne, Australia. [3]Department of Cardiology, Western Health, Melbourne, Australia. [4]Department of Cardiology, St Vincent's Hospital, Melbourne, Australia. [5]Department of Heart and Mind, Australian Catholic University, Melbourne, Australia. [6]Monash Heart, Monash Health, Melbourne, Australia. [7]Department of Cardiology, Royal Melbourne Hospital, Melbourne, Australia. [8]Department of Cardiology, Barwon Health, Geelong, Australia. [9]School of Public Health, Curtin University, Perth, Western Australia, Australia.

References

1. The Top 10 Causes of Death. Fact Sheet Number 310. [http://www.who.int/mediacentre/factsheets/fs310/en/index.html]. Accessed 31 Aug 2016.
2. Briffa TG, Hobbs MS, Tonkin A, Sanfilippo FM, Hickling S, Ridout SC, Knuiman M. Population trends of recurrent coronary heart disease event rates remain high. Circ Cardiovasc Qual Outcomes. 2011;4(1):107–13.
3. Smith Jr SC, Benjamin EJ, Bonow RO, Braun LT, Creager MA, Franklin BA, Gibbons RJ, Grundy SM, Hiratzka LF, Jones DW, et al. AHA/ACCF secondary prevention and risk reduction therapy for patients with coronary and other atherosclerotic vascular disease: 2011 update: a guideline from the American heart association and American college of cardiology foundation endorsed by the world heart federation and the preventive cardiovascular nurses association. J Am Coll Cardiol. 2011;58(23):2432–46.
4. Heran BS, Chen JM, Ebrahim S, Moxham T, Oldridge N, Rees K, Thompson DR, Taylor RS. Exercise-based cardiac rehabilitation for coronary heart disease. Cochrane Database Syst Rev. 2011;7:CD001800.
5. Clark AM, Hartling L, Vandermeer B, McAlister FA. Meta-analysis: secondary prevention programs for patients with coronary artery disease. Ann Intern Med. 2005;143(9):659–72.
6. Lawler PR, Filion KB, Eisenberg MJ. Efficacy of exercise-based cardiac rehabilitation post-myocardial infarction: a systematic review and meta-analysis of randomized controlled trials. Am Heart J. 2011;162(4):571–84. e572.
7. Taylor RS, Brown A, Ebrahim S, Jolliffe J, Noorani H, Rees K, Skidmore B, Stone JA, Thompson DR, Oldridge N. Exercise-based rehabilitation for patients with coronary heart disease: systematic review and meta-analysis of randomized controlled trials. Am J Med. 2004;116(10):682–92.
8. Suaya JA, Shepard DS, Normand SL, Ades PA, Prottas J, Stason WB. Use of cardiac rehabilitation by Medicare beneficiaries after myocardial infarction or coronary bypass surgery. Circulation. 2007;116(15):1653–62.
9. Johnson N, Fisher J, Nagle A, Inder K, Wiggers J. Factors associated with referral to outpatient cardiac rehabilitation services. J Cardpulm Rehabil. 2004;24(3):165–70.
10. Chew DP, French J, Briffa TG, Hammett CJ, Ellis CJ, Ranasinghe I, Aliprandi-Costa BJ, Astley CM, Turnbull FM, Lefkovits J, et al. Acute coronary syndrome care across Australia and New Zealand: the SNAPSHOT ACS study. Med J Aust. 2013;199(3):185–91.
11. Bunker S, McBurney H, Cox H, Jelinek M. Identifying participation rates at outpatient cardiac rehabilitation programs in Victoria, Australia. J Cardpulm Rehabil. 1999;19(6):334–8.
12. Scott IA, Lindsay KA, Harden HE. Utilisation of outpatient cardiac rehabilitation in Queensland. Med J Aust. 2003;179(7):341–5.
13. Chow CK, Jolly S, Rao-Melacini P, Fox KA, Anand SS, Yusuf S. Association of diet, exercise, and smoking modification with risk of early cardiovascular events after acute coronary syndromes. Circulation. 2010;121(6):750–8.
14. Briffa TG, Kinsman L, Maiorana AJ, Zecchin R, Redfern J, Davidson PM, Paull G, Nagle A, Denniss AR. An integrated and coordinated approach to preventing recurrent coronary heart disease events in Australia. Med J Aust. 2009;190(12):683–6.
15. Heeley EL, Peiris DP, Patel AA, Cass A, Weekes A, Morgan C, Anderson CS, Chalmers JP. Cardiovascular risk perception and evidence–practice gaps in Australian general practice (the AusHEART study). Med J Aust. 2010;192(5):254–9.
16. Kotseva K, Wood D, De Bacquer D, De Backer G, Ryden L, Jennings C, Gyberg V, Amouyel P, Bruthans J, Castro Conde A, et al. EUROASPIRE IV: a European society of cardiology survey on the lifestyle, risk factor and therapeutic management of coronary patients from 24 European countries. Eur J Prev Cardiol. 2016;23(6):636–48.
17. Varnfield M, Karunanithi M, Lee CK, Honeyman E, Arnold D, Ding H, Smith C, Walters DL. Smartphone-based home care model improved use of cardiac rehabilitation in postmyocardial infarction patients: results from a randomised controlled trial. Heart. 2014;100(22):1770–9.
18. Worcester MU, Elliott PC, Turner A, Pereira JJ, Murphy BM, Le Grande MR, Middleton KL, Navaratnam HS, Nguyen JK, Newman RW, et al. Resumption of work after acute coronary syndrome or coronary artery bypass graft surgery. Heart Lung Circ. 2014;23(5):444–53.
19. Vale MJ, Jelinek MV, Best JD, Dart AM, Grigg LE, Hare DL, Ho BP, Newman RW, McNeil JJ, Group CS. Coaching patients on achieving cardiovascular health (COACH): a multicenter randomized trial in patients with coronary heart disease. Arch Intern Med. 2003;163(22):2775–83.
20. Neubeck L, Redfern J, Fernandez R, Briffa T, Bauman A, Freedman SB. Telehealth interventions for the secondary prevention of coronary heart disease: a systematic review. Eur J Cardiovasc Prev Rehabil. 2009;16(3):281–9.
21. Huang K, Liu W, He D, Huang B, Xiao D, Peng Y, He Y, Hu H, Chen M, Huang D. Telehealth interventions versus center-based cardiac rehabilitation of coronary artery disease: a systematic review and meta-analysis. Eur J Prev Cardiol. 2015;22(8):959–71.
22. Chow CK, Redfern J, Hillis GS, Thakkar J, Santo K, Hackett ML, Jan S, Graves N, de Keizer L, Barry T, et al. Effect of lifestyle-focused text messaging on risk factor modification in patients with coronary heart disease: a randomized clinical trial. JAMA. 2015;314(12):1255–63.
23. Worringham C, Rojek A, Stewart I. Development and feasibility of a smartphone, ECG and GPS based system for remotely monitoring exercise in cardiac rehabilitation. PLoS One. 2011;6(2):e14669.
24. Korzeniowska-Kubacka I, Dobraszkiewicz-Wasilewska B, Bilinska M, Rydzewska E, Piotrowicz R. Two models of early cardiac rehabilitation in male patients after myocardial infarction with preserved left ventricular function: comparison of standard out-patient versus hybrid training programmes. Kardiol Pol. 2011;69(3):220–6.
25. Blasco A, Carmona M, Fernandez-Lozano I, Salvador CH, Pascual M, Sagredo PG, Somolinos R, Munoz A, Garcia-Lopez F, Escudier JM, et al. Evaluation of a telemedicine service for the secondary prevention of coronary artery disease. J Cardiopulm Rehabil Prev. 2012;32(1):25–31.
26. Neubeck L, Lowres N, Benjamin EJ, Freedman SB, Coorey G, Redfern J. The mobile revolution–using smartphone apps to prevent cardiovascular disease. Nat Rev Cardiol. 2015;12(6):350–60.
27. Chan AW, Tetzlaff JM, Gotzsche PC, Altman DG, Mann H, Berlin JA, Dickersin K, Hrobjartsson A, Schulz KF, Parulekar WR, et al. SPIRIT 2013 explanation and elaboration: guidance for protocols of clinical trials. BMJ. 2013;346:e7586.
28. Chan AW, Tetzlaff JM, Altman DG, Laupacis A, Gotzsche PC, Krleza-Jeric K, Hrobjartsson A, Mann H, Dickersin K, Berlin JA, et al. SPIRIT 2013 statement: defining standard protocol items for clinical trials. Ann Intern Med. 2013;158(3):200–7.
29. Chan AW, Tetzlaff JM, Altman DG, Dickersin K, Moher D. SPIRIT 2013: new guidance for content of clinical trial protocols. Lancet. 2013;381(9861):91–2.
30. Eysenbach G, Group C-E. CONSORT-EHEALTH: improving and standardizing evaluation reports of Web-based and mobile health interventions. J Med Internet Res. 2011;13(4):e126.
31. Gremeaux V, Troisgros O, Benaim S, Hannequin A, Laurent Y, Casillas JM, Benaim C. Determining the minimal clinically important difference for the six-minute walk test and the 200-meter fast-walk test during cardiac

rehabilitation program in coronary artery disease patients after acute coronary syndrome. Arch Phys Med Rehabil. 2011;92(4):611–9.
32. Beatty AL, Schiller NB, Whooley MA. Six-minute walk test as a prognostic tool in stable coronary heart disease: data from the heart and soul study. Arch Intern Med. 2012;172(14):1096–102.
33. Winter SJ, Sheats JL, King AC. The use of behavior change techniques and theory in technologies for cardiovascular disease prevention and treatment in adults: a comprehensive review. Prog Cardiovasc Dis. 2016;58(6):605–12.
34. Laboratories ATSCoPSfCPF. ATS statement: guidelines for the six-minute walk test. Am J Respir Crit Care Med. 2002;166:111–7.
35. Hare DL, Davis CR. Cardiac depression scale: validation of a new depression scale for cardiac patients. J Psychosom Res. 1996;40(4):379–86.
36. Brown N, Melville M, Gray D, Young T, Munro J, Skene AM, Hampton JR. Quality of life four years after acute myocardial infarction: short form 36 scores compared with a normal population. Heart. 1999;81(4):352–8.
37. Topol EJ, Juni JE, O'Neill WW, Nicklas JM, Shea MJ, Burek K, Pitt B. Exercise testing three days after onset of acute myocardial infarction. Am J Cardiol. 1987;60(13):958–62.
38. Jelinek VM, Ziffer RW, McDonald IG, Wasir H, Hale GS. Early exercise testing and mobilization after myocardial infarction. Med J Aust. 1977;2(18):589–93.

8

In-hospital free fatty acids levels predict the severity of myocardial ischemia of acute coronary syndrome

Pei Ma, Lu Han, Zhihua Lv, Wei Chen, Hanning Hu, Jiancheng Tu, Xin Zhou* and Song-Mei Liu*

Abstract

Background: We aimed to assess whether the levels of FFAs (free fatty acids) in ACS (acute coronary syndrome) patients depend on the extent of myocardial ischemia during the subacute phase of ACS attack.

Methods: A total of 892 consecutive CAD (coronary artery disease) subjects undergoing coronary angiography were enrolled. The FFAs contents were measured based on enzymatic assay. The relationship between FFAs and Gensini score and ACS susceptibility was assessed.

Results: In the overall population, the upper FFAs quartile was accompanied with higher ischemia parameters and increased occurrence of ACS and STEMI (ST-segment elevation myocardial infarction) ($P < 0.05$). The FFAs concentrations were approximately 1.5-fold higher in ACS than in stable CAD patients, roughly 1.3-fold higher in STEMI than non-STEMI ACS patients and probably 1.3-fold higher in non-STEMI ACS than in stable CAD patients. After adjusted for traditional cardiovascular risk factors, the FFAs level remained a risk factor for a higher Gensini score with more than 40 ($P < 0.001$) and prevalent ACS ($P < 0.001$). After adjusted for traditional risk factors, FFAs levels after natural logarithm transformation were associated with hs-CRP and WBC counts in ACS patients. A multiplicative interaction was found between hs-CRP, WBC counts and FFAs in incident ACS and higher Gensini score ($P < 0.001$).

Conclusions: Higher in-hospital levels of FFAs persist and may reflect the severity of ischemia and necrosis during the subacute phase of ACS attack.

Keywords: Acute coronary syndrome, Free fatty acids, Gensini score

Background

Plasma free fatty acids (FFAs) levels are elevated within 12 h after the onset of acute myocardial infarction (AMI) [1], moreover, elevated FFAs are associated with worse outcomes including increased risk of arrhythmia [2], sudden cardiac death and total mortality [3]. Although most FFAs are bound to albumin, a small fraction is unbound FFA (FFAu); FFAu increases in the ischemic, under-perfused myocardium rapidly within 30 min, which is considered to be more sensitive in physiologic changes than bound FFAs.

Inflammation plays a critical role throughout the atherosclerotic stage in various vessels, ranging from fatty streak formation to cardiovascular events [4, 5]. Among the potential inflammation biomarkers, C-reactive protein, the classical acute-phase protein, functions as a highly sensitive systemic marker of inflammation and tissue damage and can be measured by high-sensitivity assay (hs-CRP). Numerous epidemiological studies have demonstrated that hs-CRP had a clear prognostic value for predicting major cardiovascular events and mortality [6, 7].

Increased FFAu is an early predictor of ischemia in ACS (acute coronary syndrome) [8]. Our previous study found that plasma FFA compositions were dysregulated in CAD (coronary artery disease) patients, partly influenced by age and gene polymorphisms [9, 10]. Therefore the objective of our study was to explore the association between total FFAs and the severity of myocardial

* Correspondence: zhouxjyk@163.com; smliu@whu.edu.cn
Center for Gene Diagnosis, Zhongnan Hospital of Wuhan University, Donghu Road 169#, Wuhan 430071, Hubei, PR China

ischemia of ACS during subacute phase, and further investigated whether this was influenced by hs-CRP.

Methods

Subjects

The study was approved by the medical ethical committee of Zhongnan Hospital of Wuhan University. All participants were Han population from China, who gave their informed, written consent. From 2012 to 2014, we consecutively recruited patients who underwent selective coronary angiography for suspected coronary atherosclerosis and who were admitted within 24 h from chest pain at cardiovascular department. The diagnosis of CAD was defined as the presence of coronary lesions ≥50 % in at least one major artery segment assessed by two independent cardiologists who had no information of the patients' clinical characteristics and biochemical results. We excluded all patients with additional complications including viral hepatitis, tumor, autoimmune disease, serious liver or renal dysfunction, myocardiopathy or valvular heart disease and patients received with heparin treatment.

Serial blood samples were taken after admission for routine laboratory parameter tests, including liver function, kidney function, lipids and lipoproteins and myocardial enzymes. Estimated glomerular filtration rate (eGFR) was calculated using the Modification of Diet in Renal Disease (MDRD) study equation: eGFR = 186 × ((serumcreatinine)^(- 1.154)) × ((age)^(-0.203)) × [0.742 if female]. AMI was defined by typical clinical symptoms, electrocardiograph changes and positive serum biomarkers [11, 12]. Unstable angina (UA) was established based on the criteria of Brawmwald using clinical symptoms, non-ST segment elevation and negative serum biomarkers [13].

Assay of FFAs content

Serum samples were collected, separated and stored at −80 °C within 24 h of admission. Samples were incubated for 15 min at room temperature and then a single determination of FFAs content was tested by enzymatic assay (Clinimate NEFA, Tokyo, Japan).

Angiographic analysis

Catheterization and multiple views were imaged and maximal stenosis in each coronary artery segment was evaluated by a cardiologist according to the segmental classification system of the Coronary Artery Surgery Study. The extent of angiographically documented CAD was quantified in the left anterior descending artery, the left circumflex artery, and the right coronary artery, the criteria were as follows: normal coronary arteries (smooth, with either no stenosis or stenosis of <10 % of the luminal diameter), mild coronary arteries (stenosis of 10 % to 50 % of the luminal diameter in ≥ 1 coronary artery), or 1, 2 or 3-vessel disease, defined as stenosis of more than 50 % of the luminal diameter.

Gensini score

To assess coronary artery disease burden based on coronary angiogram, the Gensini score was calculated according to Gensini scoring system [14]. The Gensini score equaled the sum of all segment scores (where each segment score equaled the segment weighting factor multiplied by the severity score). Severity scores assigned to the specific percentages of luminal diameter reduction of the coronary artery segment were 32 for 100 %, 16 for 99 %, 8 for 90 %, 4 for 75 %, 2 for 50 %, and 1 for 5 %.

Statistical analysis

Variables were expressed as the mean ± SD, median (25th–75th percentile) or proportions and compared using Mann–Whitney *U*-test, Kruskal-Wallis H-test or the χ^2 test in univariable analysis. Binary logistic regression analysis was used to identify correlated risk factors. All analyses were performed using PASW Statistics, version 13.0 (SPSS, Chicago, IL, USA).

Results

Clinical characteristic

The study population consisted of 404 SCAD (stable coronary artery disease) patients, including 294 chronic stable angina patients (male 56.1 %, aged 68 ± 11),110 old myocardial infarction patients (male 76.4 %, aged 66 ± 12) and 488 ACS patients, including 108 UA patients (male 56.6 %, aged 68 ± 11), 191 NSTEMI (non-ST segment elevation myocardial infarction) patients (male 76.2 %, aged 67 ± 13) and 189 STEMI (ST segment elevation myocardial infarction) patients (male 82.4 %, aged 62 ± 13).

The baseline demographic, clinical characteristics and laboratory parameters according to the quartiles of the FFAs levels (Q1 0.12–0.37, $n = 223$; Q2 0.38–0.54, $n = 218$; Q3 0.55–0.78, $n = 228$; Q4 0.79–4.57, $n = 223$) for the study population were summarized in Table 1. The distribution of FFAs quartiles were slightly unbalanced with traditional cardiovascular risk factors such as age, smoking, fasting blood glucose, hs-CRP and the atherogenic lipid parameters including TC, LDL-C, TG ($P < 0.05$). In addition, the necrosis and ischemia parameters dramatically increased according to FFAs quartiles such as cTnT, CK-MB, maximal stenosis and Gensini score ($P < 0.05$).

Association of FFAs with severity of ischemia and necrosis

The FFAs levels in ACS patients were higher than in SCAD patients ((0.68 mmol/l (0.45, 0.911) vs. 0.44 mmol/l (0.3, 0.63), $P < 0.001$, respectively)) (Fig. 1a), which remained a significant correlation after adjustment for age and gender ($P < 0.001$). Among patients with ACS, the

Table 1 Clinical characteristic of study population

	Q1 ($n = 223$)	Q2 ($n = 218$)	Q3 ($n = 228$)	Q4 ($n = 223$)	*P*
FFAs (mmol/l)	0.27 (0.21, 0.32)	0.46 (0.42, 0.49)	0.65 (0.59, 0.72)	1.01 (0.88, 1.28)	-
Demographics					
Age (y)	63 ± 13	60 ± 10.4	60 ± 10.4	62 ± 12	0.021
Male (%)	65.5	67.9	70.6	66.8	NS
Risk factors					
SBP (mmHg)	141 ± 24	133 ± 16	134 ± 21	124 ± 20	NS
DBP (mmHg)	82 ± 11	79 ± 11	82 ± 15	75 ± 11	NS
HR (bpm)	72 ± 7	74 ± 15	75 ± 8	74 ± 14	0.01
Smoking (%)	33.8	51.9	51.3	49.7	0.005
Hypertension (%)	67.7	69.3	65.4	57.4	0.043
Diabetes mellitus (%)	26.9	30.3	31.3	29.6	NS
Hyperlipidemia (%)	58.7	62.4	70.2	66.4	0.048
Laboratory parameter					
TC (mmol/l)	4.04 ± 0.86	4.28 ± 1.04	4.78 ± 1.56	4.3 ± 0.88	<0.001
HDL-C (mmol/l)	1 ± 0.2	1.05 ± 0.2	0.99 ± 0.21	1 ± 0.2	NS
LDL-C (mmol/l)	2.5 ± 0.92	2.73 ± 0.83	2.93 ± 0.8	2.75 ± 0.7	<0.001
Lp (a) (mg/l)	131 (67, 246)	78 (37, 312)	125 (61, 202)	136 (56, 209)	NS
TG (mmol/l)	1.63 ± 0.92	1.96 ± 1.37	2.35 ± 1.45	2.01 ± 1.6	<0.001
FBG (mmol/l)	5.96 ± 1.7	6.3 ± 2.6	7 ± 2.7	6.5 ± 3.3	<0.001
WBC (×10^9)	7.5 ± 3.7	6.9 ± 2.2	8.1 ± 3.1	9.24 ± 3.2	<0.001
cTnT(ng/ml)	0.02 (0.003, 0.49)	0.07 (0.007, 2.34)	0.28 (0.01, 6.65)	1.72 (0.05, 15.1)	<0.001
hs-CRP (mg/l)	2.64 (0.58, 6.2)	2.42 (1.43, 3.83)	3.4 (1.16, 9.18)	2.43 (0.94, 11.7)	<0.001
CK-MB (U/l)	13 (8.5, 18.5)	13 (9, 26)	18 (11, 49)	31 (12, 102.8)	<0.001
eGFR (ml/min/1.73 m^2)	93.4 ± 28.9	95.3 ± 20.2	98.2 ± 19.8	96.8 ± 30.8	NS
Angiographic analysis					
Number of vessel	2.2 ± 0.6	2.13 ± 0.9	2.24 ± 0.74	1.97 ± 0.86	NS
Maximal stenosis (%)	78.3 ± 16.8	81.2 ± 20	83.3 ± 18	84.6 ± 19.1	<0.001
Gensini score	22.9 ± 18	29.9 ± 28	37.9 ± 30	43.7 ± 41	0.001
Final diagnosis					
ACS n (%)	72 (8.1)	103 (11.5)	135 (15.1)	176 (19.7)	<0.001
STEMI n(%)	11 (1.2)	31 (3.5)	60 (6.7)	92 (10.3)	<0.001
Immediate therapy					
β-Blocker n (%)	43 (19.2)	43 (19.8)	39 (17.1)	36 (16.3)	NS
Aspirin n (%)	215 (96.3)	209 (95.7)	207 (91)	211 (94.5)	NS
Stent implantation n (%)	60 (27.1)	62 (28.2)	68 (29.7)	70 (31.4)	NS

Data were expressed as the mean ± SD, median (25th-75th percentile) or %.
Q = quartile, *SBP* systolic blood pressure, *DBP* diastolic blood pressure, *HR* heart rate

higher FFAs levels remained significant between STEMI and UA + NSTEMI patients ((0.77 mmol/l (0.55, 1.1) vs. 0.58 mmol/l (0.4, 0.83), $P < 0.001$, respectively)) (Fig. 1b), which was significant after adjustment for age and gender ($P < 0.001$). Meanwhile, the FFAs levels in UA + NSTEMI patients were higher than in SCAD patients ((0.58 mmol/l (0.4, 0.83) vs. 0.44 mmol/l (0.3, 0.63), $P < 0.001$, respectively)) (Fig. 1c), and the difference still remained significant after adjustment for age and gender ($P < 0.001$), suggesting that FFAs content increased closely with the severity of coronary artery lesions in CAD.

Meanwhile, the occurrence of ACS and STEMI increased according to the FFAs quartiles (*P* value for trend = 0.003, 0.001) (Fig. 1d, e). To explore the relationship of FFAs and the prevalent ACS and STEMI, a binary logistic regression analysis was performed. After adjusted

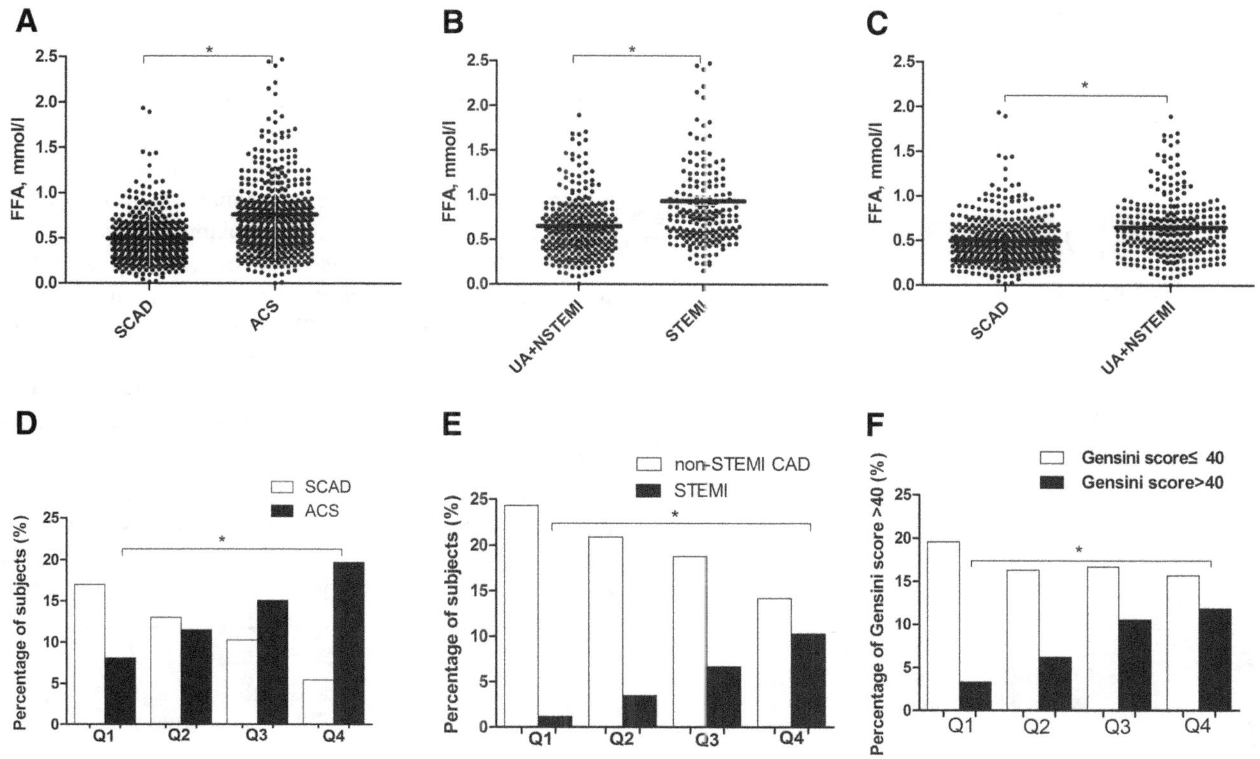

Fig. 1 Distributions of FFAs among CAD patients (**a**, **b**, **c**) and prevalence of ACS, STEMI and Gensini score more than 40 based on the FFAs quartiles (**d**, **e**, **f**). Asterisks (*) represent a *P*-value <0.05. Q = quartile.

for traditional cardiovascular risk factors including age, SBP, DBP, smoking, history of hypertension, diabetes mellitus and hyperlipidemia, the FFAs levels remained positively associated with prevalent ACS and STEMI ((for the occurrence of ACS, OR(95 % CI) = 9.956(5.21, 19.023), $P < 0.001$; for the occurrence of STEMI, OR(95 % CI) = 8.428(4.619, 15.376), $P < 0.001$)) (Tables 2 and 3).

To further explore whether the FFAs levels could reflect the severity of ischemia and necrosis focus in ACS patients, we performed Spearman's correlation analysis. It showed that FFA level was positively correlated with Gensini score and maximal stenosis (r = 0.224, $P < 0.001$ and r = 0.224, $P < 0.001$) and remained significant after adjustment for age and gender ($P = 0.001$ and $P = 0.003$). The occurrence of a higher Gensini score with more than 40 increased according to the FFAs quartiles (*P* value for trend < 0.001) (Fig. 1f), after adjusted for traditional cardiovascular risk factors including age, SBP, DBP, smoking, history of hypertension, diabetes mellitus and hyperlipidemia, the FFAs levels remained a risk factor for a higher Gensini score with more than 40 ((OR(95 % CI) = 3.741 (1.826, 7.664), $P < 0.001$)) (Table 4). Correlations of FFAs content with the infarct size in ACS patients, estimated by CK-MB and cTnT were performed, showing that FFA

Table 2 Association of FFAs levels and quartiles with prevalent ACS

	Unadjusted		Adjusted	
	OR (95 % CI)	*P*	OR (95 % CI)	*P*
FFAs	8.727 (5.331, 14.286)	<0.001	9.956 (5.21, 19.023)	<0.001
FFAs quartile				
Q1	1		1	-
Q2	1.833 (1.248, 2.693)	0.002	2.003 (1.201, 3.339)	0.008
Q3	1.811 (1.491, 2.199)	<0.001	2.081 (1.592, 2.72)	<0.001
Q4	1.988 (1.724, 2.292)	<0.001	2.189 (1.794, 2.671)	<0.001

Binary logistic regression analyses were performed. The adjusting confounders included age, gender, SBP, DBP, smoking, history of hypertension, diabetes mellitus and hyperlipidemia.
Q = quartile

Table 3 Association of FFAs levels and quartiles with prevalent STEM

	Unadjusted		Adjusted	
	OR (95 % CI)	*P*	OR (95 % CI)	*P*
FFAs	6.634 (4.269, 10.31)	<0.001	8.428 (4.619, 15.376)	<0.001
FFAs quartile				
Q1	1		1	-
Q2	3.569 (1.709, 7.453)	<0.001	5.301 (1.702, 16.509)	0.004
Q3	2.736 (1.927, 3.885)	<0.001	3.53 (2.02, 6.169)	<0.001
Q4	2.419 (1.923, 3.042)	<0.001	3.083 (2.143, 4.436)	<0.001

Binary logistic regression analyses were performed. The adjusting confounders included age, gender, SBP, DBP, smoking, history of hypertension, diabetes mellitus and hyperlipidemia.
Q = quartile

Table 4 Association of FFAs levels and quartiles with Gensini score more than 40

	Unadjusted		Adjusted	
	OR (95 % CI)	*P*	OR (95 % CI)	*P*
FFAs	2.379 (1.393, 4.062)	<0.001	3.74 (1.826, 7.664)	<0.001
FFAs quartile				
Q1	1		1	-
Q2	2.538 (1.094, 5.889)	0.03	1.934 (0.688, 5.435)	NS
Q3	2.013 (1.358, 2.984)	<0.001	1.68 (1.029, 2.743)	0.038
Q4	1.704 (1.308, 2.22)	<0.001	1.605 (1.157, 2.223)	0.005

Binary logistic regression analyses were performed. The adjusting confounders included age, gender, SBP, DBP, smoking, history of hypertension, diabetes mellitus and hyperlipidemia.
Q = quartile

levels had positively weak correlations with infarct size (r = 0.09, $P < 0.001$ and r = 0.022, $P < 0.001$).

Interaction between WBC, hs-CRP and FFAs

We constructed the multivariate linear regression analysis to elucidate the association of FFAs with inflammation parameters, after adjusting for traditional cardiovascular risk factors including age, SBP, DBP, smoking, history of hypertension, diabetes mellitus and hyperlipidemia, which showed after natural logarithm transformation that FFAs were associated with hs-CRP ($\beta = 0.003$, $p = 0.048$) and WBC ($\beta = 0.042$, $p = 0.008$), respectively.

The whole study population were divided into four groups according to the FFAs quartiles and each group was sectionalized into 2 subgroups according to their high/low levels of WBC ($\leq 10\times10^9$, $>10\times10^9$) or hs-CRP ($\leq$3.0 mg/l, >3.0 mg/l) respectively [15]. As shown in Fig. 2a, among all FFAs quartile groups, patients with hs-CRP more than 3.0 mg/l were more susceptible to

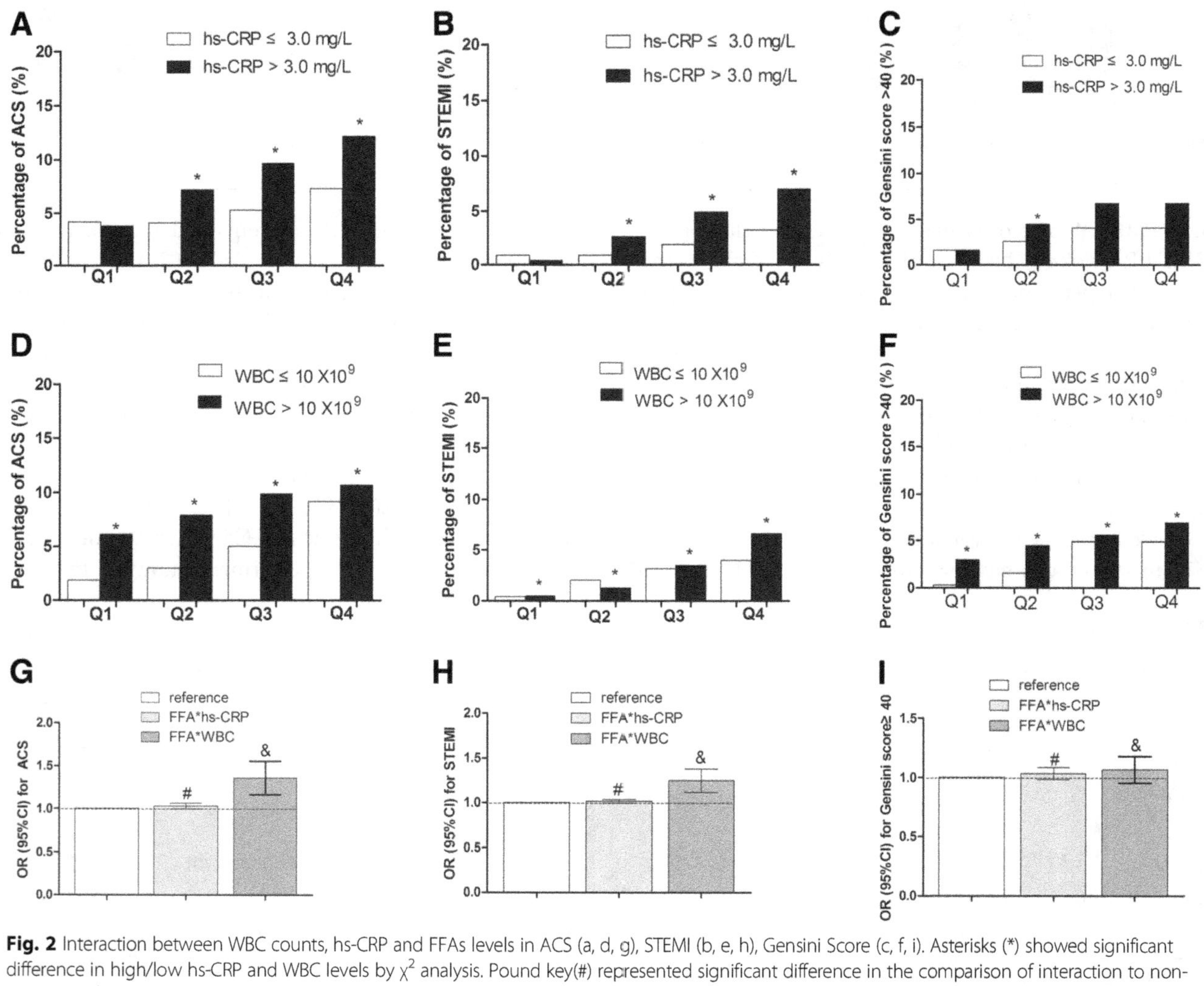

Fig. 2 Interaction between WBC counts, hs-CRP and FFAs levels in ACS (a, d, g), STEMI (b, e, h), Gensini Score (c, f, i). Asterisks (*) showed significant difference in high/low hs-CRP and WBC levels by χ^2 analysis. Pound key(#) represented significant difference in the comparison of interaction to non-interaction between FFAs and hs-CRP. Joint mark (&) showed significant difference in the comparison of interaction to non-interaction between FFAs and WBC counts. Q = quartile.

ACS, compared to patients with hs-CRP less than 3.0 mg/l (P <0.05); the trend for ACS occurrence in both high and low hs-CRP groups was significantly elevated with the distribution of higher FFA level (P value for trend < 0.05) (Additional file 1: Figure S1A). The occurrence of STEMI was elevated with higher hs-CRP, except in the lowest FFAs quartile Q1 group (P < 0.05) (Fig. 2b); a similar trend was observed in STEMI susceptibility and FFAs level in both high and low hs-CRP groups (P value for trend < 0.05) (Additional file 1: Figure S1B). Meanwhile, higher hs-CRP level was associated with a higher Gensini score in the FFAs quartile Q2 group (P < 0.05) (Fig. 2c); the percentage of Gensini score for more than 40 dramatically increased according to FFAs quartiles in both high and lowe hs-CRP groups (P value for trend <0.001) (Additional file 1: Figure S1C). The similar trendsexist in WBC counts and ACS susceptibility (Fig. 2d, Additional file 1: Figure S1D), WBC counts and STEMI susceptibility (Fig. 2e, Additional file 1: Figure S1E), WBC counts and higher Gensini score (Fig. 2f, Additional file 1: Figure S1 F), respectively.

The trend of ACS occurrence, STEMI attack and higher Gensini score with higher FFAs in high hs-CRP and WBC levels versus low hs-CRP and WBC levels were suggestive of an interaction between hs-CRP, WBC counts and FFAs in relation to the progress of myocardial ischemia. After performed by logistic regression analysis, we found a multiplicative interaction between hs-CRP, WBC and FFAs in ACS and STEMI susceptibility and a higher Gensini score ((in relation to ACS susceptibility, FFAs*hs-CRP, OR(95 % CI) = 1.029(1.016, 1.043), P < 0.001, FFAs*WBC, OR(95 % CI) = 1.357(1.281, 1.438), P < 0.001; in relation to STEMI susceptibility, FFAs*hs-CRP, OR(95 % CI) = 1.016(1.008, 1.024), FFAs*WBC, OR(95 % CI) = 1.246(1.194, 1.3), P < 0.001; in relation to a higher Gensini score, FFAs*hs-CRP, OR(95 % CI) = 1.033(1.013, 1.054), P = 0.001, FFAs*WBC, OR(95 % CI) = 1.065(1.02, 1.112), P = 0.004)) (Fig. 2g, h, i), which suggests that FFAs influence the progress of ischemia involved by inflammation processes.

Discussion

The major findings of our study confirmed that FFAs level might serve as a predictor of the severity of myocardial ischemia during the subacute onset of ACS attack. First and foremost, FFAs levels were higher in the ACS patients than the SCAD population, especially in STEMI patients. Second, the FFAs increased with the severity of necrosis and ischemia, such as cTnT and Gensini score. Moreover, we observed an association between WBC counts, hs-CRP and FFAs levels in incident ACS and higher Gensini score, which implied a possible interaction between FFAs and inflammation processes influenced the severity of ischemia.

According to the previous studies, elevated FFAs levels in AMI are associated with increased lipolytic activity, owing to an immediate increase of catecholamine with the activated sympathetic nervous system [16]. Although increasing evidence has shown that an elevation of FFAs level occurs after the onset of AMI and that higher FFAs are associated with a greater incidence of major cardiovascular events [17], no study has resolved the principal mystery whether FFAs directly trigger serious cardiovascular disease or only predict cardiometabolic dysfunction [18]. There are several mechanisms illustrating high FFAs concentration may be toxic in acute ischemic myocardium, such as mitochondrial uncoupling, activation of lipids in mitochondria, inhibition of β-oxidation, inhibition of the Na^+-K^+-ATPase pump leading to high intracellular sodium and calcium, or reduction of GLU-4 causing reduced insulin-stimulated glucose transport [19]. Therefore, it is a top priority to monitor and reduce concentrations of FFAs in the post phase of ACS [20].

Moreover, we found hs-CRP, WBC and FFAs had a multiple effect in relation to ACS susceptibility and severe myocardial ischemia (Fig. 2), which implied a possible mechanism relating FFAs together with inflammatory factors influenced the progress of ischemia. Inflammatory cytokines such as IL-6 and TNF-α were added to isolated adipocytes, resulting in increased lipolysis and FFAs levels in several in-vivo and in-vitro studies [21, 22], also, elevated circulating FFA levels led to endothelial dysfunction in-vivo via activation of PKC-mediated inflammatory pathways and excess generation of oxidants [23, 24], which would partially explain the clinically demonstrated proarrhythmogenic potential of FFAs. Further investigations in the underlying mechanisms for the joint effect of elevated FFA and inflammatory factors on myocardial ischemia are apparently warranted.

Interestingly, preexisting hypertension had been diagnosed in SCAD, ACS and STEMI patients with the prevalence of 70.5 %, 60.2 % and 48.1 %, respectively and that decreased ratio of hypertension was associated with higher occurrence of ACS and STEMI (Additional file 2). The role of hypertension history in the prevalence of ACS was difficult to explain. A large observational study showed that patients with preexisting hypertension had a more favorable in-hospital outcome [25]. Despite with a higher risk, hypertensive patients was paradoxically associated with a more favorable in-hospital diagnosis. Underlied the mystery, awareness and treatment of hypertension with potentially cardio-protective antihypertensive drugs might function as a 'protective' effect [25].

Conclusions

FFAs levels may be indicative of the severity of myocardial ischemia at subacute ACS onset and the combined

effect of FFAs and activated inflammation might play a role in myocardial ischemia of ACS.

Abbreviations

ACS: acute coronary syndrome; AMI: acute myocardial infarction; CAD: coronary artery disease; DBP: diastolic blood pressure; FBG: fasting blood glucose; FFAs: free fatty acids; FFAu: unbound FFA; HDL-C: high density lipoprotein cholesterol; HR: heart rate; hs-CRP: high-sensitivity C-reactive protein; LDL-C: low density lipoprotein cholesterol; Lp(a): lipoprotein(a); Q: quartile; SBP: systolic blood pressure; SCAD: stable coronary artery disease; STEMI: ST-segment elevation myocardial infarction; TC: total cholesterol; TG: triglyceride; UA: unstable angina; WBC: white blood cell.

Competing interests

The authors declare that they have no competing interests.

Authors' contributions

PM carried out collection of samples and data, analysis and interpretation of data, and drafting of the manuscript. LH and Z-H L participated in collection of samples and data. WC and H-HN helped in technical and material support. J-C T made critical discussion, carried out critical revision of the manuscript and obtained funding. S-M L participated in critical discussion, critical revision of the manuscript for important intellectual content. XZ: conceived of study design and participated in critical revision of the manuscript. All authors read and approved the final manuscript.

Acknowledgments

This work was supported by the National Natural Science Foundation of China (81271919, 27 81472023), the National Basic Research Program of China (973 Program) (2012CB720600, 2012CB720605) and the Special Health Standards Infrastructure Program (20120904). We thank Professor Chunhong Wang of School of Public Health, Wuhan University for assistance of statistical analysis and PhD Baozhu Wei of cardiovascular department, Zhongnan Hospital of Wuhan University for collection and interpretation of clinical data. We would like to acknowledge the reviewers for their helpful comments on this paper.

References

1. Kurien VA, Oliver MF. Serum-free-fatty-acids after acute myocardial infarction and cerebralvascular occlusion. Lancet. 1966;2:122–7.
2. Tansey MJ, Opie LH. Relation between plasma free fatty acids and arrhythmias within the first twelve hours of acute myocardial infarction. Lancet. 1983;2:419–22.
3. Oliver MF, Kurien VA, Greenwood TW. Relation between serum-free-fatty acids and arrhythmias and death after acute myocardial infarction. Lancet. 1968;1:710–4.
4. Ross R. Atherosclerosis–an inflammatory disease. N Engl J Med. 1999;340:115–26.
5. Matsuura E, Atzeni F, Sarzi-Puttini P, Turiel M, Lopez LR, Nurmohamed MT. Is atherosclerosis an autoimmune disease? BMC Med. 2014;12:47.
6. Koenig W. High-sensitivity C-reactive protein and atherosclerotic disease: from improved risk prediction to risk-guided therapy. Int J Cardiol. 2013;168:5126–34.
7. Ridker PM. Inflammation, C-reactive protein, and cardiovascular disease: moving past the marker versus mediator debate. Circ Res. 2014;114:594–5.
8. Bhardwaj A, Truong QA, Peacock WF, Yeo KT, Storrow A, Thomas S, et al. A multicenter comparison of established and emerging cardiac biomarkers for the diagnostic evaluation of chest pain in the emergency department. Am Heart J. 2011;162:276–82.
9. Li SW, Lin K, Ma P, Zhang ZL, Zhou YD, Lu SY, et al. FADS Gene Polymorphisms Confer the Risk of Coronary Artery Disease in a Chinese Han Population through the Altered Desaturase Activities: Based on High-Resolution Melting Analysis. PLoS ONE. 2013;8:e55869.
10. Shen F, Qi J, Xu F, Ning L, Pang R, Zhou X, et al. Age-related distributions of nine fasting plasma free fatty acids in a population of Chinese adults. Clin Chim Acta. 2013;415:81–7.
11. O'Gara PT, Kushner FG, Ascheim DD, Casey DJ, Chung MK, de Lemos JA, et al. 2013 ACCF/AHA guideline for the management of ST-elevation myocardial infarction: executive summary: a report of the American College of Cardiology Foundation/American Heart Association Task Force on Practice Guidelines: developed in collaboration with the American College of Emergency Physicians and Society for Cardiovascular Angiography and Interventions. 2013;82:E1-27.
12. Thygesen K, Alpert JS, Jaffe AS, Simoons ML, Chaitman BR, White HD, et al. Third universal definition of myocardial infarction. J Am Coll Cardiol. 2012;60:1581–98.
13. Braunwald E. Unstable angina and non-ST elevation myocardial infarction. Am J RespirCrit Care Med. 2012;185:924–32.
14. Gensini GG. A more meaningful scoring system for determining the severity of coronary heart disease. Am J Cardiol. 1983;51:606.
15. Ridker PM, Buring JE, Cook NR, Rifai N. C-reactive protein, the metabolic syndrome, and risk of incident cardiovascular events: an 8-year follow-up of 14719 initially healthy American women. Circulation. 2003;107:391–7.
16. Oliver MF. Sudden cardiac death: the lost fatty acid hypothesis. QJM. 2006;99:701–9.
17. Khawaja O, Bartz TM, Ix JH, Heckbert SR, Kizer JR, Zieman SJ, et al. Plasma free fatty acids and risk of atrial fibrillation (from the Cardiovascular Health Study). Am J Cardiol. 2012;110:212–6.
18. Mozaffarian D. Free fatty acids, cardiovascular mortality, and cardiometabolic stress. Eur Heart J. 2007;28:2699–700.
19. Pilz S, Marz W. Free fatty acids as a cardiovascular risk factor. ClinChem Lab Med. 2008;46:429–34.
20. Oliver MF. Control of free fatty acids during acute myocardial ischaemia. Heart. 2010;96:1883–4.
21. Mattacks CA, Pond CM. Interactions of noradrenalin and tumour necrosis factor alpha, interleukin 4 and interleukin 6 in the control of lipolysis from adipocytes around lymph nodes. Cytokine. 1999;11:334–46.
22. Van Hall G, Steensberg A, Sacchetti M, Fischer C, Keller C, Schjerling P, et al. Interleukin-6 stimulates lipolysis and fat oxidation in humans. J Clin Endocrinol Metab. 2003;88:3005–10.
23. Li H, Li H, Bao Y, Zhang X, Yu Y. Free fatty acids induce endothelial dysfunction and activate protein kinase C and nuclear factor-κB pathway in rat aorta. Int J Cardiol. 2011;152:218–24.
24. Tang Y, Li G. Chronic exposure to high fatty acids impedes receptor agonist-induced nitric oxide production and increments of cytosolic Ca2+ levels in endothelial cells. J Mol Endocrinol. 2011;47:315–26.
25. Erne P, Radovanovic D, Schoenenberger AW, Bertel O, Kaeslin T, Essig M, et al. Impact of hypertension on the outcome of patients admitted with acute coronary syndrome. J Hypertens. 2015;33:860–7.

9

The feasibility and diagnostic accuracy by multiple cardiac biomarkers in emergency chest pain patients: a clinical analysis to compare 290 suspected acute coronary syndrome cases stratified by age and gender in Taiwan

Chung-Lieh Hung[1,2], Ding-Kuo Chien[3,4,5,6], Shou-Chuan Shih[2,4,7] and Wen-Han Chang[2,3,4,5,6,8*]

Abstract

Background: Accurate diagnosis of acute coronary syndrome (ACS) in a timely fashion is challenging in the elderly population, especially elderly women, who usually exhibit atypical clinical symptoms. A multiple cardiac biomarker (MCB) based approach has been shown to improve diagnostic efficacy of ACS. However, data in various age groups and sex differences remain largely unexplored.

Methods: Point-of-care testing (POCT) was performed on 290 patients (aged ≥18 years) who were admitted to the emergency department (ED) with symptoms of acute chest pain under suspicion of acute coronary syndrome (ACS). The MCB approach in current work assessed four cardiac biomarkers: myoglobin, troponin I, creatine kinase-myocardial band isoenzyme fraction (CK-MB), and brain natriuretic peptide (BNP).

Results: Overall, the MCB approach demonstrated considerably higher sensitivity for elderly patients than for younger patients in identifying ACS (80.0 % [64.1–90.0] vs. 52.6 % [37.3–67.5] for ≥65 years and <65 years groups), with younger population showed greater specificity (44.1 % [35.3–53.4] vs. 84.9 % [76.9–90.5] for ≥65 years and <65 years groups, respectively). The highest sensitivity achieved for elderly women who reported chest pain was 87.5 % [95 % CI: 64–96.5]). In general, the sensitivity of this approach was higher for female patients than for male patients (80 % [58.4–91.9] vs. 61 % [47.8–73.0]).

Conclusions: The MCB approach can provide a quick and accurate clinical diagnosis in elderly and female patients, both of whom have traditionally proven to be challenging to diagnose from suspected acute coronary syndrome.

Keywords: Multiple cardiac biomarker, Acute coronary syndrome, Elderly

* Correspondence: branden888@gmail.com
[2]Department of Medicine, Mackay Medical College, New Taipei city, Taiwan
[3]Emergency Department, MacKay Memorial Hospital, Taipei, Taiwan
Full list of author information is available at the end of the article

Background

Acute coronary syndrome (ACS) is an extremely common condition that is one of the leading causes of death worldwide. ACS is commonly encountered in the emergency room and occurs most often in elderly patients [1, 2]; however, in recent years the average age of patients with ACS has declined due to changes in lifestyle and personal behavior.

Women who have ACS differ from their male counterparts both in terms of reported symptoms, clinical manifestations and diagnosis rates [3–5]. In terms of symptoms and clinical manifestations, female patients primarily exhibit unstable angina and non-ST-segment elevation myocardial infarction (NSTEMI), while male patients primarily exhibit STEMI [3, 5]. Regarding diagnosis, biomarker sensitivity and specificity in exercise tests have been reported to be lower in both women and men [5].

Cardiac biomarkers for acute coronary syndrome play key roles diagnosis, risk assessment, treatment, and supervision. Troponin I is a sensitive indicator of cardiomyocyte necrosis and an important biomarker for monitoring treatment. Myoglobin is the earliest biomarker of myocardial injury to appear, allowing doctors to rule out the possibility of myocardial infarction in a timely fashion. Apart from diagnostic role in heart failure, brain natriuretic peptide (BNP) is also closely related to acute coronary syndrome [6]. However, when used individually, these biomarkers are limited by several factors in clinical scenarios, especially in elderly patients [2].

Owing to differences in the diagnostic ability and performance of cardiac biomarkers across a wide range of patient population with age and gender distributions, and considering their important role in the diagnosis of acute coronary syndrome, we currently examined the accuracy of four cardiac biomarkers in the diagnosis of acute coronary syndrome in patients who experienced chest pain.

Methods

Patient enrollment

From March to November 2009, patients who visited Linkou Chang Gung Memorial Hospital, Taipei Mackey Memorial Hospital, Far Eastern Memorial Hospital, and China Medical University Hospital in Taiwan, with a primary complaint of chest pain and who were suspected of having acute coronary syndrome were recruited into this study. All enrolled patients were aged 18 years or older. Inclusion criteria includes: 1) adults ≥18 years of age and consented to participate in the study group, 2) admitted to the emergency room due to chest pains or potential acute coronary syndrome symptoms, 3) symptoms unclear or atypical but suspected to be ACS requiring further electrocardiogram analysis and blood tests. Exclusion criteria includes: 1) Pregnancy, or clinical scenarios that may cause false positive test results of elevated Troponin I or BNP, such as skeletal myopathies, or renal insufficiency [7, 8] (defined by creatinine >2.5 mg/dL), 2) Non-Taiwan residents, patients whose contact information is unavailable, patients planning to go abroad and thus would be unavailable for follow-up, and patients who had already spent more than two hours in the emergency room reception area, 3) Patients who were transferred from other hospitals, 4) Cases where written permission could not be obtained or refused to participate the study, 5) Cases in whom the symptoms were already confirmed as not the cause of acute coronary syndrome, including pneumothorax, acute pulmonary embolism, aortic dissection, acute gastroenterological diseases or chronic obstructive lung disorder, 6) Initial electrocardiogram (ECG) had shown elevated ST segment or new LBBB. Subjects with ST elevation and new left bundle branch block (LBBB) were excluded since these clearly showed the onset of AMI, and therefore did not require diagnosis by MCB test systems. Researchers then examined patients' medical records and conducted telephone interviews to identify any subsequent health issues or discomfort experienced within 45 days after diagnosis. Within 45 days of treatment, cardiologists diagnosed patients with one of the following conditions as positive for acute coronary syndrome: ST-segment elevation myocardial infarction (STEMI); non-ST segment elevation myocardial infarction (NSTEMI); sudden cardiac arrest, high-grade atrioventricular block (AVB) or ventricular arrhythmia with cardiac catheter-proven coronary occlusion by thrombus formation; emergency, urgent, or elective revascularization; and unstable angina. All study participants underwent cardiac catheter during admission to confirm the diagnosis of acute coronary syndrome by experienced interventionalists/cardiologists and patients without these conditions were not enrolled in the study.

Biochemical analysis and multi cardiac biomarker panel test

During the examination, myoglobin, creatine kinase-myocardial band isoenzyme fraction (CK-MB), troponin I, and BNP were tested using a MCB CardioProfiler Panel (Alere, San Diego, CA). Blood (3 ml) was sampled from each patient using EDTA K2 Vacuette tubes. Next, 0.25 ml of blood was siphoned from the total sample using a pipette and placed onto a test panel. The MCB test panel was then placed into a Triage MeterPro (Alere, San Diego, CA) for examination, the results of which were automatically displayed and printed after 15 min. Data were presented in quantitative form with continuous variables presented. All results were blinded to investigators. Biomarker reference values (CardioProfiler Panel) were as follows: Troponin *I* > 0.4 ng/mL, CK-MB > 4.3 ng/mL, myoglobin > 107 ng/mL, and BNP > 100 pg/mL.

Statistical analysis

Quantitative data were expressed as mean ± standard deviation. Parametric data were compared by t test, and categorical data were analyzed by the Chi-square test with Yates' correction or Fisher's exact test. Data were analyzed using SPSS® statistics software (SPSS 11.5; SPSS Inc., Chicago, IL, USA). Data were analyzed for sensitivity, specificity, positive and negative predictive values (PPV and NPV), and positive and negative likelihood ratios (LR+ and LR−). All $P < 0.05$ was considered statistically significant with two-sided analysis with $P < 0.05$ was considered statistically significant.

Results

A total of 290 patients with chest pain were enrolled in the current study with an average age of 64.5 years. Of the 290 patients, 146 were elderly (≥65 years), with an average age of 75.4 years, which represented 50.3 % of the total sample. The remaining 144 patients were <65 years of age (average age: 53.4 years) which represented 49.7 % of the total sample. Further, 109 patients were women (71 elderly and 38 young), and constituted 37.6 % of the total sample (Table 1).

A prior history of cardiovascular diseases (including prior stroke, myoacrdial infarction, history of coronary interventions or bypass graft surgery) was reported in 34.5 % of the participants (100/290). Other common comorbidities included angina (30 % [87/290]) and coronary angioplasty (22.5 % [54/290]). At baseline, elderly patients reported statistically significantly more medical conditions such as myocardial infarction, cardiovascular disease, heart failure, and stroke, compared with young patients ($p < 0.05$).

High blood pressure was found to be the most prevalent risk factor in patients with chest pain (60.7 %), followed by diabetes (30.7 %), and dyslipidemia (30.7 %). A larger proportion of elderly patients had high blood pressure and diabetes, while younger patients were more likely to have dyslipidemia, a family history of cardiovascular disease, or a history of smoking (Table 1).

A total of 73 (25.2 %) patients were diagnosed with cardiovascular disease, 35 of which were elderly (23.9 %) and 38 were young (26.4 %). Using the MCB approach in the diagnosis of acute coronary syndrome, young patients demonstrated a higher relative risk for acute coronary syndrome than elderly patients (6.25 vs. 3.16) (Table 2). In addition, 20 out of 109 (18.3 %) women were diagnosed with 53 out of 181 men (29.3 %). The MCB approach in the diagnosis of acute coronary syndrome revealed a higher relative risk in women than in men (6.17 vs. 3.36) (Table 3).

Table 1 The statistics of characters between the elderly group and younger group

Patient's group Variables	All	Patients ≥65 years	Patients <65 years	P value
Number	290	146	144	
Age (in years)	64.49 ± 13.1	75.4 ± 6.6	53.4 ± 7.6	
Female	109 (37.6 %)	71 (48.6 %)	38 (26.4 %)	
Cardiovascular Event History				
Myocardial infarction	40 (13.8 %)	21 (14.4 %)	19 (13.2 %)	0.41
Angina pectoris	87 (30 %)	44 (30.1 %)	43 (29.9 %)	0.48
Tachycardia	4 (1.4 %)	2 (1.4 %)	2 (1.4 %)	0.49
Cardiovascular diseases*	100 (34.5 %)	57 (39 %)	43 (29.8 %)	<0.05
Cardiac arrhythmia	19 (6.5 %)	12 (8.2 %)	7 (4.9 %)	0.18
Congestive heart failure*	15 (5.2 %)	13 (8.9 %)	2 (1.4 %)	<0.05
Stroke or temporal ischemia*	20 (6.9 %)	16 (10.9 %)	4 (2.8 %)	<0.05
Coronary artery bypass grafting surgery	9 (3.1 %)	6 (4.1 %)	3 (2.1 %)	0.27
Coronary angioplasty	54 (22.5 %)	30 (20.5 %)	24 (16.7 %)	0.35
Risk Factor				
High blood pressure*	176 (60.7 %)	103 (70.5 %)	73 (50.7 %)	<0.05
Diabetes*	89 (30.7 %)	53 (36.3 %)	36 (25 %)	<0.05
Lipidemia*	89 (30.7 %)	36 (24.6 %)	53 (36.8 %)	<0.05
Family history of Cardiovascular disease*	68 (23.4 %)	23 (15.7 %)	45 (31.2 %)	<0.05
Smoker*	64 (22.1 %)	7 (4.8 %)	57 (39.6 %)	<0.05

Data: mean (standard deviation), number (percentage)
*mean $P < 0.05$

Table 2 Relation between MCB tests and Cardiovascular Events by Age

Age (Patient Number)				
Acute coronary syndrome (ACS)	≧65 years (*N* = 146)		<65 years (*N* = 144)	
	Positive	Negative	Positive	Negative
MCB positive	28 (19.2 %)	62 (42.4 %)	20 (13.9 %)	16 (11.1 %)
MCB negative	7 (4.8 %)	49 (33.5 %)	18 (12.5 %)	90 62.5 %)
Odds ratio	3.161*		6.25*	

* mean $P < 0.05$

The MCB tests in the two age groups demonstrated differences in sensitivity, specificity, and PPV ($p < 0.05$). The MCB tests also demonstrated improved sensitivity (80 %) and NPV (87.5 %) for elderly patients, and higher specificity (84.9 %) and PPV (55.6 %) for younger patients. Cardiac biomarkers exhibited a higher positive likelihood ratio (LR+) in the diagnosis of acute cardiovascular syndrome in young patients (3.49 vs. 1.43) (Table 4).

Differences were also observed in the sensitivity and PPV of MCB tests across genders. The biomarkers had higher sensitivity (80 %) and NPV (93.1 %) in female patients, while the specificity (66.1 %) and PPV (43.4 %) were higher in male patients. The LR+ diagnosis of acute coronary syndrome was higher in female patients than in male patients (2.03 vs. 1.81) (Table 5).

When the efficacy of MCB tests across both age and gender groups was investigated, MCB tests showed the highest sensitivity (87.5 %) and negative likelihood ratio (LR−) in elderly female patients, and the highest specificity (91.2 %), NPV (93.9 %), and LR+ (5.67) in young female patients (Table 6).

Discussion

Acute coronary syndrome is diagnosed on the basis of typical angina, electrocardiogram (ECG) results, and cardiac enzymes analysis. Patients with positive for two out of the three clinical criteria are diagnosed with acute coronary syndrome. This study focused on patients who experienced chest pain and who were suspected of having acute coronary syndrome. If the patient demonstrated ST-segment elevation and LBBB they were diagnosed with acute coronary syndrome. In such cases, cardiac enzyme analysis was not necessary. Patients who experience chest pain without any obvious change in their electrocardiogram or patients with atypical symptoms such as chest tightness, fainting spells, sweating, and shortness of breath are confounding for clinicians. In such cases, it is necessary to examine cardiac enzymes to aid in arriving at the proper diagnosis. Thus, we investigated the diagnostic efficacy of MCB tests in patients suspected of having acute coronary syndrome.

Rapid and accurate recognition together with efficient or rapid service strategy (e.g. same-day transfer) had been shown to increase the access rate to subsequent cath-lab management and further reduced hospital stay length in ACS patients. Based on this, an efficient and cost-effective diagnostic strategy prior to optimal implementation of health care model had become a major challenge in current clinical practice. For example, Campo et al. proposed a Hub and Spoke model in intermediate-to-high risk non-ST-segment elevation ACS patients referral, while other center ever reported [9]. Previous studies have demonstrated the effects of age and gender on the diagnosis of acute coronary syndrome. The use of electrocardiograms in

Table 3 Relation between MCB tests and Cardiovascular Events By Gender

Gender (Patient Number)				
Acute coronary syndrome (ACS)	Male (*N* = 181)		Female (*N* = 109)	
	Positive	Negative	Positive	Negative
Cardiac biomarker positive	32 (17.6 %)	44 (24.3 %)	16 (14.6 %)	35 (32.1 %)
Cardiac biomarker negative	21 (11.6 %)	84 (46.4 %)	4 (3.6 %)	54 (49.5 %)
Odds ratio	3.364*		6.171*	

* mean $P < 0.05$

Table 4 Diagnostic Capabilities of MCB tests by Age

	Patient of Age		*P* value
	Patients ≥65 years	Patients <65 years	
Sensitivity	80.0 % (64.1–90.0)	52.6 % (37.3–67.5)	<0.05*
Specificity	44.1 % (35.3–53.4)	84.9 % (76.9–90.5)	<0.05*
PPV	31.1 % (22.5–41.3)	55.6 % (39.6–70.5)	<0.05*
NPV	87.5 % (76.4–93.8)	83.3 % (75.2–89.2)	0.28
LR+	1.43 (1.13–1.81)	3.49 (2.02–6.00)	
LR−	0.45 (0.22–0.91)	0.56 (0.39–0.79)	

PS: PPV, NPV, LR+ and LR− mean positive and negative predictive values, positive and negative likelihood ratios, respectively
*mean $P < 0.05$

Table 5 Diagnostic Capabilities of MCB tests by Gender

	Patient of gender		*P* value
	Men (*N* = 181)	Women (*N* = 109)	
Sensitivity	61.1 % (47.8–73.0)	80.0 % (58.4–91.9)	<0.05*
Specificity	66.1 % (57.5–73.8)	60.7 % (50.3–70.2)	0.23
PPV	43.4 % (32.9–54.6)	31.4 % (20.3–45.0)	0.07
NPV	80 % (71.4–86.5)	93.1 % (83.6–97.3)	<0.05*
LR+	1.81 (1.31–2.49)	2.03 (1.45–2.85)	
LR−	0.59 (0.41–0.84)	0.33 (0.14–0.81)	

PS: PPV, NPV, LR+ and LR− mean positive and negative predictive values, positive and negative likelihood ratios, respectively
*mean $P < 0.05$

Table 6 Diagnostic Capabilities of MCB tests by Gender and Age

	≥65 years old (*N* = 146)		<65 years old (*N* = 144)	
	Male (*N* = 75)	Female (*N* = 71)	Male (*N* = 106)	Female (*N* = 38)
Sensitivity	73.7 % (51.2–88.2)	87.5 % (64–96.5)	52.9 % (36.7–68.5)	50.0 % (15.0–85.0)
Specificity	46.4 % (34.0–59.3)	41.8 % (29.7–55.0)	81.9 % (71.5–89.1)	91.2 % (77.0–97.0)
PPV	31.8 % (20.0–46.6)	30.4 % (19.1–44.8)	58.1 % (40.8–73.6)	40.0 % (11.8–76.9)
NPV	83.9 % (71.1–89.2)	92 % (75.0–97.8)	78.7 % (68.1–86.4)	93.9 % (80.4–98.3)
LR+	1.37 (0.96–1.98)	1.50 (1.12–2.01)	2.93 (1.63–5.26)	5.67 (1.32–24.37)
LR–	0.57 (0.25–1.26)	0.29 (0.08–1.13)	0.57 (0.39–0.83)	0.55 (0.20–1.47)

PS: PPV, NPV, LR+ and LR– mean positive and negative predictive values, positive and negative likelihood ratios, respectively

elderly patients can be problematic, such as in cases when the patient has a pacemaker or relatively low ST-segment elevation [10]. Elderly patients can exhibit symptoms similar to myocardial infarction, such as with gastritis or pneumonia [11–13]. Further, only a small proportion of elderly patients with acute coronary syndrome experience typical angina symptoms [14]. Finally, patients with congestive heart failure, diabetes, or coronary artery bypass graft surgery may exhibit atypical chest pains [14]. The current study also demonstrated that elderly patients are likely to exhibit these atypical factors. In addition, patients who smoke or have dyslipidemia exhibit relatively typical chest pain symptom, leading to many cases of acute coronary syndrome in younger patients [15].

Conventionally, female patients are less likely to seek for medical help than male patients. In addition, the symptoms of myocardial ischemia with chest pain are apparent atypically and easily confused with female chest wall or breast lesions with pain [15]. A relatively low proportion of electrocardiograms in women show ST-segment elevation; thus, the use of biomarkers to analyze the probability of acute coronary syndrome in women can help overcome these difficulties in a more efficient manner. This study also demonstrated that young and female patients have a relatively higher risk of acute coronary syndrome after positive biodetection.

Troponin I is an important biomarker for diagnosing acute myocardial infarction due to its sensitivity and specificity in the detection of cardiomyocyte injury, as well as its character of remaining detectable in the blood for a continuous period of 4 days, and up to 2 weeks. However, there is also a shortcoming for clinical Troponin I use, for example, it only begins to rise 6 h after disease onset. However, patients with acute coronary syndrome will often seek for medical attention shortly after symptoms emerge, resulting in a time delay between the clinical symptoms and diagnostic results. McCord's et al. has reported that 49 % of patients with acute coronary syndrome arrive at the hospital within 4 h of disease onset, leading to a large number of patients remain undiagnosed in the emergency room for hours due to the time gap as mentioned above [16].

According to a joint European Society of Cardiology (ESC) and American College of Cardiology (ACC) committee recommendation for diagnostic indicators of myocardial infarction, the 99th percentile upper range of troponin I in normal population serves as the recommended critical value for a diagnosis of myocardial infarction and myocardial damage; however, this may cause complications for an accurate diagnosis [17]. Although troponin I demonstrates high specificity, several factors, including renal failure, sepsis, chest trauma, and anthracycline use, may generate false-positive results due to elevated troponin I levels, resulting in erroneous treatment and unnecessary hospital stays [18].

In the current study MCB tests had higher specificity in elderly women than in men (Table 6). In particular, troponin I showed high specificity in female patients, which may help to clarify the real disease in a great portion of women manifested as angina clinically. In this regard, if a patient presented with abnormal troponin *I* value, the possible misclassification as normal or false negative rate in women can be largely avoided and can be discharged from ED safely. Studies have shown that if only cardiac biomarkers are monitored within the first 6 h of onset of myocardial infarction, they are unable to provide sufficient diagnostic capability in terms of sensitivity and specificity [17]. Due to these aforementioned reasons, patients are unable to receive accurate diagnoses in a timely fashion, which not only results in overcrowded emergency rooms but also causes unnecessary hospital stays and significantly higher costs [18]. Of the 290 patients recruited in this study, 18.3 % of the women experienced cardiovascular events, which is considerably lower than the 29.3 % of men who experienced a cardiovascular event. Previous studies have demonstrated that the proportion of women with abnormal troponin I levels was relatively low because only approximately 6 % of troponin T and 3 % of troponin I exist in a free-floating state within the myocardial tissue of female gender. Since men typically have a greater number of cardiomyocytes than women, therefore the troponin I levels in men are easier to monitor or identified [19].

From the perspective of emergency room doctors, a quick and accurate diagnosis of acute coronary syndrome in elderly patients with chest pain is a major challenge. While patients' medical records and physiology can be conveniently examined, both these methods have lower sensitivity and specificity. Although electrocardiograms are continuously monitored and in general may have a diagnostic specificity of 92 %, their sensitivity is only 39 % [20]. Several studies have shown that the use of MCB tests—such as troponin I, CK-MB, and myoglobin, which are related to cardiomyocyte necrosis, or BNP, which is related to cardiomyocyte function—can effectively improve the risk classification of patients with acute coronary syndrome. Due to the traditional shortcomings of individual biomarkers, the American College of Cardiology recommends that myoglobin be included in our MCB approach to improve diagnostic capability [21]. Since myoglobin is commonly present in skeletal muscle and myocardium, its levels will elevate 1–2 h after ACS symptoms. While myoglobin has a relatively low specificity, it has a very high sensitivity. Thus, if myoglobin is added as a biomarker for the identification of acute coronary syndrome, the diagnostic workflow may be executed more quickly and accurately. Of note, the proportion of female gender varied largely in different age groups (categorized as <, or > = 65 years old) in our current work, which may potentiate the bias in the results generated.

By using a MCB approach we were able to effectively identify patients with low-risk chest pain. In particular, the MCB approach demonstrated excellent diagnostic capability in female and elderly patients, both of whom are considered to be challenging in accurate diagnosis. In our current work, both populations presented with relatively good sensitivity and NPV (> = 80 %). In particular, the sensitivity and specificity for elderly female patients were near 90 %. In light of these findings, we can not only reduce the amount of time patients spend in the emergency room but also lessen the burden on attending clinicians.

One study showed that when 1285 emergency room chest pain patients were monitored for myoglobin, CK-MB, and troponin I over 90 min, they achieved a NPV of 100 %. Of the 508 patients who were diagnosed as negative, only one returned to the emergency room with myocardial infarction 30 days after the diagnosis [22]. This demonstrates that multiple biomarker tests can effectively exclude patients with chest pains and potential acute coronary syndrome. Furthermore, non-myocardial infarction patients can be excluded when the elevation of the CK-MB level over 2 h exceeds 1.5 ng/mL or the troponin I level exceeds 0.2 ng/mL [23].

The current study demonstrates that a MCB approach is more effective in the evaluation of elderly patients than young patients. During the process of assessing and selecting potential groups and excluding potential cases, the elderly patient group showed high NPV (87.5 %) and sensitivity (80 %), both of which were statistically significant. These results showed that by using the MCB approach for elderly patients with chest pain, one can quickly and accurately exclude acute coronary syndrome and other cardiovascular diseases in 2 h. Thus, the amount of time patients spend in the emergency room is reduced and unnecessary hospital stays are avoided. A recent study showed that a MCB approach can reduce the amount of time chest pain patients spend in the emergency room from 1 to 2 days to just 3–4 h [24]. Another study shows that by expediting the diagnostic process, the MCB approach can also lessen the costs of treatment for patients with chest pain [25]. Thus, this tool may aid in reducing emergency room crowding and minimize subsequent medical expenses [25].

Moreover, by using point-of-care monitoring MCB, we can speed up report completion time and therefore improve the efficacy of clinical practice. Studies have shown that as compared with traditional testing, the reporting time in point-of-care monitoring systems can be decreased by 75–85 % [26]. Such point-of-care monitoring systems are able to aid in expediting diagnosis.

Conclusions

Our results revealed that due to the high sensitivity and NPV of MCB, the clinical implementation of such diagnostic tools can help physicians exclude acute coronary syndrome quickly and accurately in elderly patients present with atypical chest pain in the emergency department. Furthermore, we also demonstrated that MCB tests are effective in the diagnosis of acute coronary syndrome in elderly and female patients. The clinical use of MCB in high-risk, atypical chest pain or in elderly patients can therefore facilitate accurate and proper diagnosis in a more timely fashion, reduce the time spent in the emergency room, and expedite treatment delievery. Finally, MCB tests may enormously improve the clinical workflow of emergency treatment and effectively reduces the rates of diagnostic misclassification encountered in certain challenging patient populations from the emergency room.

Abbreviations

ACS: Acute coronary syndrome; BNP: Brain natriuretic peptide; CK-MB: Creatine kinase-myocardial band isoenzyme fraction; ECG: Electrocardiogram; ED: Emergency department; LBBB: Left bundle branch block; MCB: Multiple cardiac biomarker; NSTEMI: Non-ST-segment elevation myocardial infarction; POCT: Point-of-care testing; STEMI: ST-segment elevation myocardial infarction

Acknowledgement

None.

Funding

None.

Authors' contributions
WHC carried out the data collection and analysis, participated in the design alignment and drafted the manuscript. CLH carried out the edition and the draft of the manuscript. DKC participated in the manuscript drafting and the design of the study, performed the statistical analysis. SCS helped to revise the manuscript. All authors read and approved the final manuscript.

Competing interests
The authors declare that they have no competing interests.

Author details
[1]Department of Internal Medicine, Division of Cardiology, MacKay Memorial Hospital, Taipei, Taiwan. [2]Department of Medicine, Mackay Medical College, New Taipei city, Taiwan. [3]Emergency Department, MacKay Memorial Hospital, Taipei, Taiwan. [4]Department of Nursing, Mackay Junior College of Medicine, Nursing and Management, Taipei, Taiwan. [5]Graduate Institute of Injury Prevention and Control, Taipei Medical University, Taipei, Taiwan. [6]Institute of Mechatronic Engineering, National Taipei University of Technology, Taipei, Taiwan. [7]Department of Internal Medicine, Division of Gastroenterology, MacKay Memorial Hospital, Taipei, Taiwan. [8]School of Medicine, Taipei Medical University, Taipei, Taiwan.

References

1. Mehta RH, Rathore SS, Radford MJ, Wang Y, Krumholz HM. Acute myocardial infarction in the elderly: differences by age. J Am Coll Cardiol. 2001;38:736–41.
2. Wang SW, Ren GC, Shio SF, Yu SY, Zhen FY. Acute myocardial infarction in elderly Chinese. A clinical analysis of 631 cases and comparison with 389 younger cases. Jpn Heart J. 1998;29:301–7.
3. Hochman JS, Tamis JE, Thompson TD, Weaver WD, White HD, Van de Werf F, et al. Sex, clinical presentation, and outcome in patients with acute coronary syndromes. Global Use of Strategies to Open Occluded Coronary Arteries in Acute Coronary Syndromes IIb Investigators. N Engl J Med. 1999;341:226–32.
4. Hochman JS, McCabe CH, Stone PH, Becker RC, Cannon CP, DeFeo-Fraulini T, et al. Outcome and profile of women and men presenting with acute coronary syndromes: a report from TIMI IIIB. TIMI Investigators. Thrombolysis in Myocardial Infarction. J Am Coll Cardiol. 1997;30:141–8.
5. Hasdai D, Porter A, Rosengren A, Behar S, Boyko V, Battler A. Effect of gender on outcomes of acute coronary syndromes. J Am Coll Cardiol. 2003;91:1466–8.
6. Larsen AI, Dickstein K. BNP in acute coronary syndromes: the heart expresses its suffering. Eur Heart J. 2004;25:1284–6.
7. Aviles RJ, Askari AT, Lindahl B, Wallentin L, Jia G, Ohman EM, et al. Troponin T levels in patients with acute coronary syndromes, with or without renal dysfunction. N Engl J Med. 2002;346:2047–52.
8. Horwich TB, Hamilton MA, Fonarow GC. B-type natriuretic peptide levels in obese patients with advanced heart failure. J Am Coll Cardiol. 2006;47:85–90.
9. Campo G, Menozzi M, Guastaroba P, Vignali L, Belotti LM, Casella G, et al. Same-day transfer for the invasive strategy of patients with non-ST-segment elevation acute coronary syndrome admitted to spoke hospitals: Data from the Emilia-Romagna Regional Network. Eur Heart J Acute Cardiovasc Care. 2015. doi:10.1177/2048872615610867.
10. Alexander KP, Roe MT, Chen AY, Lytle BL, Pollack Jr CV, Foody JM, et al. Evolution in cardiovascular care for elderly patients with non-ST-segment elevation acute coronary syndromes: results from the CRUSADE National Quality Improvement Initiative. J Am Coll Cardiol. 2005;46:1479–87.
11. Faisal MA, Russell RM, Samloff IM, Holt PR. Helicobacter pylori infection and atrophic gastritis in the elderly. Gastroenterology. 1990;99:1543–4.
12. Walston J, McBurnie MA, Newman A, Tracy RP, Kop WJ, Hirsch CH, et al. Frailty and activation of the inflammation and coagulation systems with and without clinical comorbidities: results from the Cardiovascular Health Study. Arch Intern Med. 2002;162:2333–41.
13. Majumdar SR, Kim N, Colman I, Chahal AM, Raymond G, Jen H, et al. Incidental vertebral fractures discovered with chest radiography in the emergency department: prevalence, recognition, and osteoporosis management in a cohort of elderly patients. Arch Intern Med. 2005;165:905–9.
14. Alexander KP, Newby LK, Cannon CP, Armstrong PW, Gibler WB, Rich MW, et al. Acute coronary care in the elderly, part I: Non-ST-segment-elevation acute coronary syndromes: a scientific statement for healthcare professionals from the American Heart Association Council on Clinical Cardiology: in collaboration with the Society of Geriatric Cardiology. Circulation. 2007;115:2549–69.
15. Hung C-L, Hou CJ-Y, Yeh H-I, Chang W-H. Atypical Chest Pain in the Elderly: The Prevalence, Possible Mechanisms and Prognosis. Int J Gerontol. 2010;4:1–6.
16. McCord J, Nowak RM, McCullough PA, Foreback C, Borzak S, Tokarski G, et al. Ninety-minute exclusion of acute myocardial infarction by use of quantitative point-of-care testing of myoglobin and troponin I. Circulation. 2001;104:1483–8.
17. Thygesen K, Alpert JS, White HD, Joint ESC/ACCF/AHA/WHF Task Force for the Redefinition of Myocardial Infarction, Jaffe AS, Apple FS, et al. Universal definition of myocardial infarction. Circulation. 2007;116:2634–53.
18. Kelley WE, Januzzi JL, Christenson RH. Increases of Cardiac Troponin in Conditions other than Acute Coronary Syndrome and Heart Failure. Clin Chem. 2009;55:2098–112.
19. Elsaesser A, Hamm CE. Acute coronary syndrome: the risk of being female. Circulation. 2004;109:565–7.
20. Bhuiya FA, Pitts SR, et al. Emergency Department Visits for Chest Pain and Abdominal Pain: United States, 1999–2008. NCHS Data Brief. 2010;43:1–8.
21. Anderson JL, Adams CD, Antman EM, Bridges CR, Califf RM, Casey Jr DE. ACC/AHA 2007 guidelines for the management of patients with unstable angina/non–ST-elevation myocardial infarction: a report of the American College of Cardiology/American Heart Association Task Force on Practice Guidelines (Writing Committee to Revise the 2002 Guidelines for the Management of Patients with Unstable Angina/Non–ST-Elevation Myocardial Infarction): developed in collaboration with the American College of Emergency Physicians, American College of Physicians, Society for Academic Emergency Medicine, Society for Cardiovascular Angiography and Interventions, and Society of Thoracic Surgeons. J Am Coll Cardiol. 2007;50:e1–e157.
22. Ng SM, Krishnaswamy P, Morissey R, Clopton P, Fitzgerald R, Maisel AS. Ninety-minute accelerated critical pathway for chest pain evaluation. Am J Cardiol. 2001;88:611–7.
23. Fesmire FM. Delta CK-MB Outperforms Delta Troponin I at 2 Hours During the ED Rule Out of Acute Myocardial Infarction. Am J Emerg Med. 2000;18:1–8.
24. Than M, Cullen L, Reid CM, Lim SH, Aldous S, Ardagh MW, et al. A 2-h diagnostic protocol to assess patients with chest pain symptoms in the Asia-Pacific region (ASPECT): a prospective observational validation study. Lancet. 2011;377:1077–84.
25. Birkhahn RH, Haines E, Wen W, Reddy L, Briggs WM, Datillo PA. Estimating the clinical impact of bringing a multimarker cardiac panel to the bedside in the ED. Am J Emerg Med. 2011;29:304–8.
26. Wu AHB. Point-of-Care Testing for Conventional Cardiac markers. Point Care. 2006;5:20–4.

10

Validation study of GRACE risk scores in indigenous and non-indigenous patients hospitalized with acute coronary syndrome

Pamela J. Bradshaw[1,2*], Judith M. Katzenellenbogen[2], Frank M. Sanfilippo[1], Michael S. T. Hobbs[1], Peter L. Thompson[1,3] and Sandra C. Thompson[2]

Abstract

Background: Although cardiovascular disease is the major cause of premature death among Indigenous peoples in several advanced economies, no acute coronary syndrome (ACS) risk models have been validated in Indigenous populations. We tested the validity and calibration of three Global Registry of Acute Coronary Events (GRACE) scores among Aboriginal and non-Aboriginal Australians.

Methods: GRACE scores were calculated at admission or discharge using clinical data, with all-cause deaths obtained from data linkage. Scores for GRACE models were validated for; 1) in-hospital death, 2) death within 6 months from admission or 3) death within 6 months of discharge (this also for 1 and 5-years mortality).

Results: Aboriginal patient were younger (62 % aged <55 years versus 15 % non-Aboriginal) and their median GRACE scores lower than non-Aboriginal patients, as was crude mortality at 6 months from admission (6 % vs 10 %) and at 1 and 5 years. After age stratification, risk scores for Aboriginal patients were equivalent or higher, especially among those aged <55 years. There was a trend to more deaths after discharge among Aboriginal patients in each age group, suggesting an age-related under-estimation of risk. The c-statistics for the three GRACE models within both groups were between 0.75 and 0.79.

Conclusions: We demonstrated for the first time that while the discriminatory capacity of GRACE risk scores among Indigenous Australians is good, the models may need re-calibrating to improve risk stratification in this and other Indigenous groups, where age of onset of coronary disease is much younger than among the original reference population.

Keywords: GRACE risk score, Acute coronary syndrome, Indigenous, Mortality, Aboriginal

Background

Indigenous populations in several advanced economies experience higher rates of coronary heart disease (CHD) and mortality, starting at a younger age than the general population. The disparity, well-documented among Aboriginal and Torres Strait Islander (hereafter Aboriginal) Australians [1], has been reported among indigenous people in countries such as the United States (US), Canada and New Zealand [2–7].

Aboriginal Australians are approximately 3 % of the total population in Australia and 3.8 % of the state population of Western Australian, with around one-third living in the metropolitan area of the state capital, Perth, and 40 % living in 'remote' or 'very remote' areas during the data collection period [8]. Although this Aboriginal population is relatively young, with a median age of 21 years compared with 37 years for the non-Aboriginal population, CHD is the leading cause of death. CHD was the cause of death for 37 % of Aboriginal people aged 45 to 64 years in 2003–2007, compared with 9 % of non-Aboriginal Australians,[8] and Aboriginal people suffer coronary events at three times the age-standardised rate as other Australians, with the greatest difference among

* Correspondence: pamela.bradshaw@uwa.edu.au
[1]School of Population Health, University of Western Australia, M431, 35 Stirling Highway, Crawley, WA 6009, Australia
[2]Western Australian Centre for Rural Health, University of Western Australia, M706, 35 Stirling Highway, Crawley, WA 6009, Australia
Full list of author information is available at the end of the article

Aboriginal people aged 35–54 years [9, 10]. Aboriginal patients also suffer higher case-fatality after acute myocardial infarction than non-Aboriginals [9, 11, 12].

Among CHD risk models, only the well-validated Framingham Risk Score, used to estimate the 10-year risk for a CHD event, has been tested in indigenous groups [13, 14]. Among remote-dwelling Australian Aboriginal people, the Framingham model substantially under-estimated risk, especially for women and young adults [14].

Due to the high incidence of CHD and poorer outcomes among Aboriginal patients [9–12], accurate estimation of risk at presentation is important to ensure appropriate intervention to preserve optimal myocardial function, and to guide ongoing management. The first Global Registry of Acute Coronary Events (GRACE) score was developed to enable 'practical and accurate prediction of in-hospital mortality' for individuals presenting with symptoms of acute coronary syndrome (ACS) [15]. The data for the development of the GRACE 'in-hospital' model were gathered from hospitals in 14 countries worldwide. Two additional risk score models have been developed from the registry; to extend to the prediction of risk for death within 6 months of admission, and a score, calculated at discharge, to predict the risk for death within 6 months from discharge [16, 17]. These three models have been tested and validated in studies from several countries and retained good discriminatory capacity for predicting death, including death within one year, and out to five years [18]. A large scale review found that GRACE models performed better than similar ACS risk models. [19] The GRACE risk calculators are available online and are available for downloading to portable devices [20].

Despite the higher risk among several indigenous populations for CVD [2–7] there are no published results validating an ACS risk score in an indigenous population. As the distribution of age, sex, and risk factors contribute to the performance of risk scores among different populations, we tested three GRACE models in a cohort of Western Australian patients admitted for ACS to determine whether these prognostic models performed equally well among Aboriginal and non-Aboriginal Australians.

Methods

Study design

This retrospective cohort study used clinical data recorded in medical notes during an admission for ACS, with patients being followed up to five years to determine vital status. These clinical data were linked to public and private hospital administrative data from the Hospital Morbidity Data Collection (HMDC), one of the core administrative datasets in the Western Australian Data Linkage System in which all hospital separations in the state of Western Australia (WA) are collated for individuals under a unique identifier [21]. These linked HMDC records allow person-based analyses, where all admissions for each patient (including inter-hospital transfers) can be identified, with data from the WA Death Registry also linked to these hospital records.

Sample and case selection

The cohort of ACS patients was selected for this study from two prior studies. The first was a linked data study to validate diagnoses of acute myocardial infarction (AMI) recorded in Western Australian administrative data among patients aged 35–79 years admitted to hospitals in metropolitan Perth (the capital city) in 2003 [22]. Briefly, patients with a World Health Organisation International Classification of Disease (ICD-10 Australian Modification) code for ACS (I20.0 and I21) recorded in the principal or subsequent 'diagnosis' field, or with a positive cardiac biomarker and any other 'cardiac' or 'chest pain' diagnosis were identified (I10-I52, R07). Data were collected from patients' notes (medical records) for a sample of patients randomly selected within strata (approximately 50 % of ACS cases and 5 % of 'other' cardiac cases). The stratified sampling fractions were based on diagnosis ICD codes, admission type (emergency, booked) and cardiac biomarker status [22]. The second study extended the cohort to include all Aboriginal patients admitted to WA hospitals in 2002–2004 and a random sample of rural non-Aboriginal patients admitted in 2003 [23]. These ACS cases, including both metropolitan and rural Aboriginal and non-Aboriginal admissions over the period 2002–2004, were used in the current study. The data collection period coincides with the period of enrolment of patients to the GRACE Registry [18].

Data linkage and extraction for the studies was undertaken by the staff at the Data Linkage Unit at the Health Department of Western Australia.

To address under-identification of Aboriginal status in administrative health data, patients were classified as Aboriginal if they were flagged as Aboriginal in any hospital admission in the HMDC data [24]. The index 'episode of care' for this analysis was the first admission episode (including transfers between rural and tertiary centres, between other metropolitan hospitals and tertiary centres and between public to private hospitals) within the study period. De-identified cases were selected for the study if they met the published eligibility criteria for enrolment in the GRACE study (based on discharge diagnoses, electrocardiograph [ECG] and biomarker data), excluding those discharged from hospital within one day or who had ACS secondary to another serious condition or a procedure [16]. The selection of cases is shown in Fig. 1.

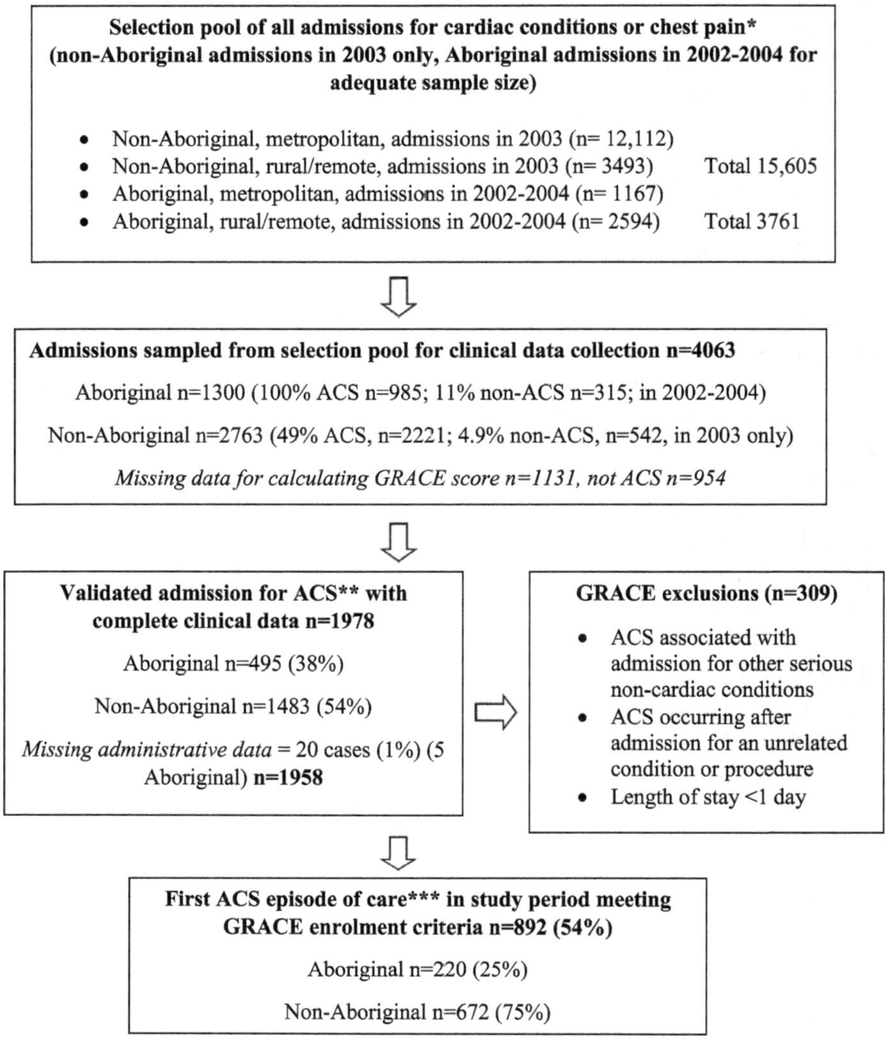

*International Classification of Diseases (ICD) 10th revision Australian Modification codes I10-I52, R07 ** Discharge diagnosis of AMI or UA (ICD-10-AM I20.0, I21) *** Includes multiple admissions associated with an episode of care e.g. transfers between rural and metropolitan, non-tertiary and tertiary, and public and private hospitals.

Fig. 1 Flow chart showing selection of 892 study cases of acute coronary syndrome admitted to hospitals in Western Australia during 2002–2004

Data collection

Clinical information was collected from patient medical records from hospitals throughout WA, including symptoms, investigations, laboratory data, medical history and procedures. The data collection has been described in detail elsewhere [22, 23]. The electrocardiogram (ECG) recordings were coded using the Minnesota system,[25] and classified according to the American Heart Association (AHA) criteria for acute coronary heart disease [26]. Cases with a principal discharge diagnosis of AMI and with AHA ECG classification of 'diagnostic, ST elevation, or evolving Q waves' were categorized as ST-elevation myocardial infarction (STEMI). Killip Class categorisation of acute heart failure (HF) (included in the two risk scores calculated on admission) was not recorded for 14 patients, but defaulted to 'class one' if they had no history of HF and no in-hospital HF on the index admission.

Risk score models

The clinical data were used to calculate the three published GRACE scores; calculated (1) on admission for risk of death in-hospital, (2) on admission for risk for death within 6 months of admission, and (3) at discharge for risk for death within 6 months of discharge [20].

All models assign a high weighting to age: for example, under the in-hospital model no points accrue for patients <40 years, but 58 points accrue to those aged

60–69 years, the same as for systolic blood pressure ≤80 mmHg, which is otherwise the highest score for any level of a factor, and greater than cardiac arrest at admission (39 points).

The risk scores from the third model (risk for death within 6-months of hospital discharge) for Aboriginal and non-Aboriginal patients were divided into tertiles for comparison with the tertiles of risk score published from the GRACE study [20]. These stratify patients into low, intermediate and high risk for death according to their diagnosis of STEMI or non-STEMI/unstable angina (UA).

The scores obtained on admission were also categorized by the probability of risk for all-cause death at 6 months estimated from the GRACE study formula,[23] for calibration against the observed proportion of deaths. We used the second model (6 months from admission model) as the number of deaths was higher.

Study endpoints

The main outcome measures were death in-hospital and 6-month mortality (from both hospital admission and discharge). One-year and five-year mortality after discharge was also measured.

Statistical analysis

Descriptive analyses were used to characterize the study cohort. Differences between groups defined by age groups (including by more or less than 55 years to account for the younger mean age of Aboriginal patients), sex and Aboriginal and non-Aboriginal status were tested using the chi-squared test for categorical data and the *t*-test for continuous variables.

As the 'c-statistic' is most frequently used to report the discriminatory capacity of prognostic GRACE risk scores, we plotted the Receiver Operating Characteristic (ROC) curve of GRACE scores against deaths at 30 days, 6 months and 1 and 5 years for the cohort overall, and for Aboriginals and non-Aboriginals separately. Calibration was tested in the 'admission to 6 months' model by comparing predicted and observed mortality at 6 months. The Hosmer-Lemeshow 'p-value' was obtained from binary logistic regression models as an indicator of the goodness of fit of the three models tested.

All analyses were carried out in IBM SPSS Statistics for Windows, Version 21.0, Armonk, NY: IBM Corp.

Ethics

The study was approved by the Human Research Ethics Committees at The University of Western Australia, the Western Australian Department of Health, the Western Australian Aboriginal Health Ethics Committee, and the Western Australian Country Health Service.

Results

Of 892 cases who would have met the GRACE study enrolment criteria, 220 (25 %) were identified as Aboriginal Australians. There was considerable disparity in age, with Aboriginal patients almost 15 years younger on average than non-Aboriginal patients, 136 (62 %) being <55 years of age compared with 99 (15 %) non-Aboriginals (Fig. 2). The demographic and clinical characteristics of the cohort are shown in Table 1.

ACS diagnoses

AMI (STEMI and non-STEMI) was the principal discharge diagnosis recorded in the HMDC for 277 (41 %) non-Aboriginal and 128 (58 %) Aboriginal patients ($p < 0.001$). Using AHA criteria, a total of 132 cases with STEMI (33 %) were identified, with a smaller proportion of Aboriginal patients meeting the criteria for STEMI (Table 1).

Coronary artery reperfusion therapy, either thrombolysis or primary percutaneous coronary intervention (PCI) was undertaken in 89 cases (Table 1), including 55 (61 %) of 90 patients with ST-segment elevation on their first ECG. The other 34 reperfusions were among 92 patients with ischaemic changes (subsequently coded as AHA 'definite' or 'probable' AMI, with evolving 'Q-waves') and 17 patients with a Minnesota suppression codes such as bundle-branch blocks (which suppress the coding of Q waves).

Reperfusion with thrombolysis was more frequent among those presenting initially to a rural hospital (58 %), with only one patient from a rural location undergoing primary PCI. AMI was also more frequently the discharge diagnosis for patients from rural locations (54 %) than from the Perth metropolitan area (40 %, $p < 0.001$).

Mortality

Total deaths in hospital, at 6 months (from admission and from discharge), and at one and five years were 39

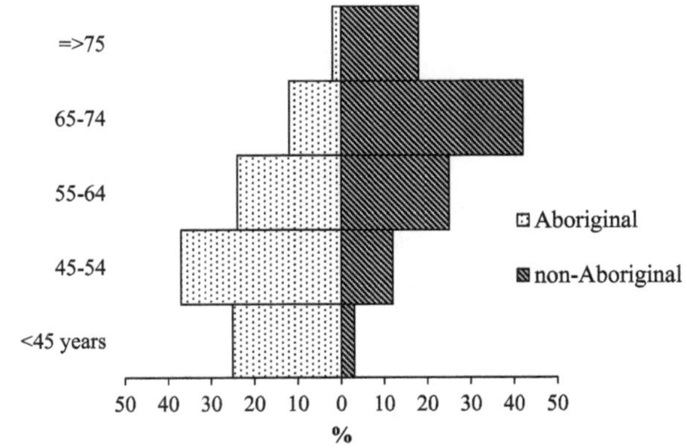

Fig. 2 Distribution by age groups among 892 Aboriginal and non-Aboriginal patients discharged with a diagnosis of ACS, Western Australia 2002–2004

Table 1 Characteristics of the cohort studied, 892 Aboriginal and non-Aboriginal patients discharged from hospital with a diagnosis of acute coronary syndrome, Western Australia 2002–2004

	Non-Aboriginal $N = 672$	Aboriginal $N = 220$	p
Males %	472 (70)	132 (60)	<0.01
Age - mean (SD)	66.4 (9.7)	52.4 (11.4)	<0.001
median (tertile cut points)	68 (63, 73)	52 (47, 57)	
Rural or remote dwelling n (%)	154 (23)	114 (52)	<0.001
On admission			
Systolic Blood Pressure – median (mmHg)	140	135	
Heart Rate - median (beats per minute)	75	86	
ST-segment deviation on ECG n (%)	199 (30)	77 (35)	0.15
Elevated initial biomarkers n (%)	241 (36)	125 (57)	<0.001
AMI	172 (64)	99 (79)	
Unstable angina	69 (17)	26 (27)	
Killip class n (%)			
1	533 (79)	185 (84)	
2	92 (14)	22 (10)	
3	44 (6)	13 (6)	
4	3 (<1)	0	
AMI (principal discharge diagnosis)	277 (41)	128 (58)	p < 0.001
STEMI AHA criteria*	102 (37)	30 (24)	
Reperfusion therapy – (N)	64	20	
Reperfusion therapy for STEMI	44 (69)	11 (55)	
Thrombolysis (% of reperfusion)	26 (59)	9 (82)	
Primary PCI (% of reperfusion)	18 (41)	2 (8)	
Reperfusion - ECG with other codes	20 (31)	9 (45)	
Thrombolysis	12 (60)	9 (100)	
Primary PCI	8 (40)	0	
History (within 5 years) n (%)			
AMI	210 (31)	65 (30)	0.86
Heart failure	69 (10)	11 (5)	<0.01
Coronary artery disease	372 (55)	108 (49)	0.15
Chronic renal failure	14 (9)	34 (16)	0.04
Diabetes	228 (34)	124 (56)	<0.001
< 55 years	22 (26)	64 (49)	0.001
≥ 55 years	206 (35)	60 (67)	<0.001
In-hospital n (%)			
Heart failure	82 (13)	11 (5)	<0.01
Arrhythmia	80 (12)	8 (4)	<0.001
PCI (excluding primary PCI)	149 (23)	36 (20)	0.22
CABG within 28 days	23 (4)	7 (3)	0.99

*Luepker R, et al. [26]

AMI acute myocardial infarction, *STEMI* ST-segment elevation myocardial infarction, *AHA* American Heart Association, *PCI* percutaneous coronary intervention, *CABG* coronary artery bypass graft surgery

(4 %), 83 (9 %), 46 (6 %), 80 (13 %) and 232 (30 %) respectively.

Total mortality at each time point favoured Aboriginal patients (Table 2). After age stratification, mortality was similar for both groups for those aged 55 years or more, but was higher among Aboriginal patients <55 years of age from 6 months after hospital discharge. However, the numbers of death were too low (except at 5 years) to show statistical difference.

GRACE scores

The mean and median scores for each of the three GRACE models (death in-hospital, from admission to 6 months, and from discharge to 6 months) were lower among Aboriginal patients (Table 2). The low scores were related to the relative youth of the Aboriginal patients, 16 % of whom did not accrue any points for age (<40 years). Additionally, only 7 %, compared with 42 % of the non-Aboriginal group, were ≥70 years, an attribute which adds 73 points to the score (in the discharge to 6 months model).

The age disparity was such that, when stratified into broad age groups (<55 and 55–79 years), GRACE scores for Aboriginal patients were equivalent or higher than those of non-Aboriginals, more noticeably in the younger group (Table 2).

Distribution of scores

Using the '6 months post-discharge' model to compare the distribution of scores with those published for the original GRACE Study cohort [20], the cut points for tertiles of risk score (0.33, 0.66) were lower for Aboriginal than non-Aboriginal patients, and lower than those

Table 2 GRACE scores from three models, and all-cause mortality, among patients discharged with a diagnosis of acute coronary syndrome for Aboriginal ($n = 220$) and non-Aboriginal ($n = 672$) patients overall and for age groups, Western Australia 2002–2004

	Non-Aboriginal	Aboriginal	Non-Aboriginal	Aboriginal	'p' (mean)
	Median (min, max)		Mean (SD)		
GRACE Score at admission for death in-hospital					
All	115 (34, 264)	100 (33, 227)	181.0 (25.8)	105.2 (38.9)	<0.001
< 55 years	75 (34, 163)	88 (33, 73)	117.3 (34.7)	90.2 (32.1)	0.03
≥ 55 years	118 (54, 212)	119 (59, 227)	122.5 (22.6)	126.8 (37.7)	0.26
Death in-hospital n (%)	*35 (5)*	*4 (2)**			
< 55 years	*2 (2)**	*1 (<1)**			
≥ 55 years	*33 (6)*	*3 (3)**			
GRACE Score at admission for 6-month mortality					
All	104 (26, 219)	83 (24, 184)	103.4 (29.5)	86.6 (33.9)	<0.001
< 55 years	63 (26, 125)	67 (24, 141)	64.9 (20.4)	70.4 (26.3)	0.11
≥ 55 years	106 (50, 176)	105 (54, 184	108.9 (26.3)	110.1 (29.6)	0.68
6-month mortality n (%)	*70 (10)*	*13 (6)*			*0.03*
< 55 years	*2 (2)**	*3 (2)**			-
≥ 55 years	*68 (12)*	*10 (11)*			*0.53*
GRACE Score at discharge for 6-month mortality					
All	109 (28,194)	89 (20,182)	108.8 (29.5)	93.0 (31.6)	<0.001
< 55 years	65 (28,103)	77 (20, 138)	68.1 (17.9)	77.0 (24.1)	0.004
≥ 55 years,	112 (54, 194)	116 (68, 182)	114.6 (26.1)	116.0 (26.5)	0.64
6-month mortality n(%)	*36 (6)*	*10 (5)*			*0.35*
< 55 years	*0 (0)**	*2 (<2)**			-
≥ 55 years	*36 (7)*	*8 (9)*			*0.32*
One-year mortality n(%)	*66 (10)*	*14 (7)*			*0.06*
< 55 years	*0 (0)**	*2 (2)**			-
≥ 55 years	*66 (12)*	*12 (14)*			*0.60*
Five-year mortality n(%)	*181 (28)*	*51 (24)*			*0.10*
< 55 years	*4 (5)*	*21 (16)*			*0.01*
≥ 55 years	*177 (32)*	*30 (34)*			*0.36*

*less than 5 cases

derived from the GRACE Study population. This was so for STEMI (0.33 corresponds to scores of 85 (Aboriginal), 95 (non-Aboriginal), 99 (GRACE), respectively, and 0.66 to score of 113, 123 and 127, respectively) and non-STEMI/UA (0.33 = 77, 96, 88 and 0.66 = 104, 121 and 118 respectively). Applying the GRACE study tertiles, >50 % of Aboriginal patients would be considered low risk for death within 6 months of discharge for both STEMI and non-STEMI/UA (Fig. 3). For non-Aboriginal patients the variations (more at low risk after STEMI, fewer after non-STEMI/UA) were less marked. The numbers of deaths in each subgroup (tertiles x Aboriginal or non-Aboriginal x AMI or non-STEMI/UA) were too few to make any comparisons of associated mortality.

Association between GRACE score and outcomes

The 'admission to 6 month' model (the highest number of end-points) was well calibrated overall, with good correlation between the predicted probability of 6-month all-cause mortality and observed deaths (Fig. 4). The fit was best for non-Aboriginals, and this resulted in good overall fit, as non-Aboriginals were 75 % of the cohort. For Aboriginal people, however, the association was less convincing, with few deaths among the 70 % in the lowest risk category (<5 % risk), and very few patients in the higher risk groups (>20 % risk). Observed deaths for the 5 Aboriginal patients estimated to be at 6-10 % risk of death to 6 months was 15 %, suggesting under-estimation of risk.

There was little difference in the discriminatory capacity of the GRACE models in both Aboriginal and non-Aboriginal groups, with the *c*-statistics ranging from 0.75 to 0.79. However, there were low numbers of deaths and broader confidence intervals throughout for the Aboriginal cohort (Table 3). Each of the three risk score models was found to demonstrate 'goodness of fit' for both groups, with Hosmer-Lemeshow 'p'-values exceeding 0.05 (Table 3).

Discussion

The GRACE risk scores for death in-hospital and to 6 months (from both admission and discharge) have proven reliable in identifying high-risk cases among patients presenting with symptoms of an ACS [18]. Testing three of the models in this population demonstrated that the models retain their prognostic capacity to discriminate between patients at different levels of risk for all-cause mortality after an admission for ACS, confirmed by *c*-statistics of 0.75 or more for both Aboriginal and non-Aboriginal patients at time points to five years.

However, in this cohort, selected 'post-hoc' to conform to the GRACE study criteria, crude mortality at each time point was lower among the Aboriginal patients, a finding at odds with the reported excess CVD mortality [1]. Such findings have been reported from studies of outcomes of AMI, where crude case-fatality after AMI for Aboriginal and non-Aboriginal patients was similar, but age-specific rate ratios for Aboriginal patients considerably

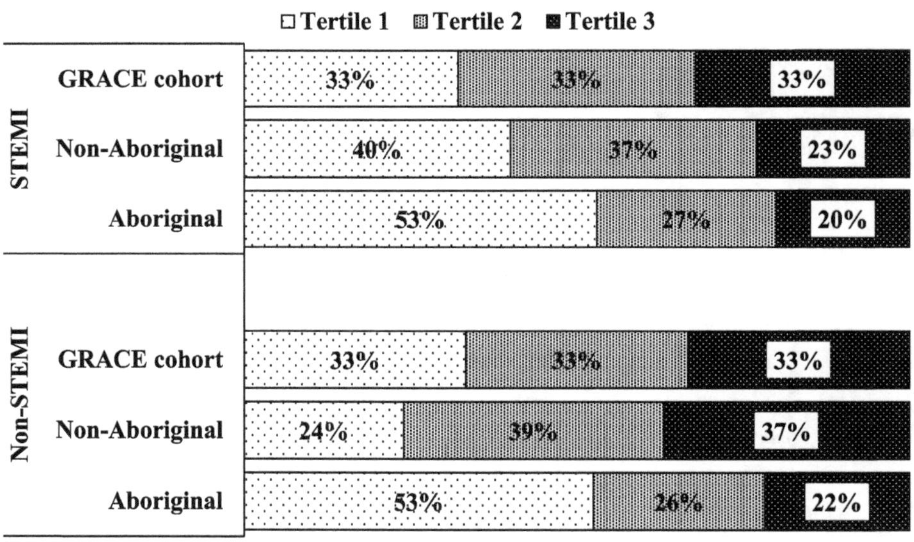

* Available at http://www.outcomes-umassmed.org/grace/
Quick Links
- GRACE Risk Score: Downloads & References
-Table showing tertiles of risk (Including absolute score and percent predicted deaths)

Fig. 3 Percentage of patients in tertiles of GRACE risk score for 'mortality to 6-month post-discharge' in the GRACE Study cohort*, and for Aboriginal and non-Aboriginal people in our study

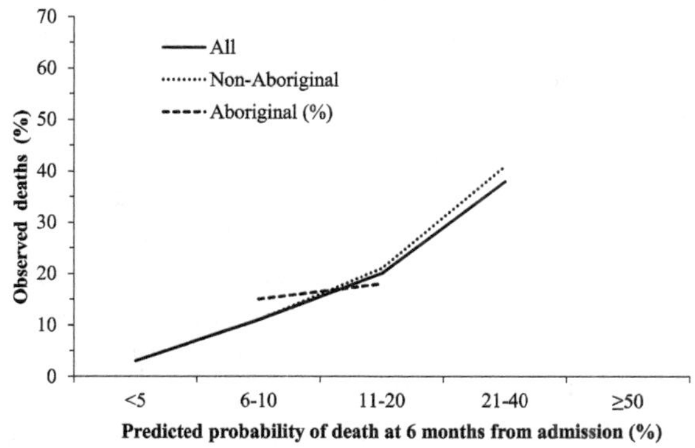

Probability of death*	<5	6-10	11-20	21-40	≥50
N (%) in risk category					
Non-Aboriginal	352 (52)	179 (27)	101 (15)	34 (5)	6 (1)
Aboriginal	157 (71)	33 (15)	22 (10)	6 (3)	2 (1)
Observed deaths n (%)					
Non-Aboriginal	12 (3)	19 (11)	21 (21)	14 (41)	4 (67)**
Aboriginal	3 (2)**	5 (15)	4 (18)**	1**	0
All	15 (30)	24 (11)	25 (20)	15 (38)	4 (50)**

*http://www.outcomes-umassmed.org/grace/
**less than 5 deaths observed in the group

Fig. 4 Observed mortality at 6 months from admission among a cohort of patients admitted with ACS including Aboriginal (n = 13 deaths) and non-Aboriginal patients (n = 70 deaths) by the probability of death indicated by the GRACE score*

higher, especially in younger age-groups [11, 12]. The Aboriginal patients in our study may have been relatively low-risk, with a smaller proportion having a diagnosis of STEMI (although more had an AMI diagnosis overall) or suffering in-hospital complications of heart failure or arrhythmia. We had too few deaths to reliably estimate any age-specific outcomes, but stratifying by age <55 years or 55 years or more, there was a trend to more deaths among young Aboriginal people after hospital discharge.

On the small numbers of deaths from admission to 6 months there was an indication of greater than predicted mortality among the 'low-risk' Aboriginal patients, and the possibility of underestimation of risk is supported by the equal or higher mean GRACE scores for both younger and older Aboriginal people after age stratification. Other than less likelihood of a history of heart failure, which contributed to lower scores for Aboriginal patients, the other elements of the GRACE scores were equivalent or attracted a higher score for Aboriginal patients. As these factors do not make as significant a contribution to the score as age, the possibility is that the dominance of age in the models contributes to an underestimation of risk, with weightings being less applicable to Aboriginal Australians.

Table 3 C-statistics* and 95 % CI for three GRACE models for prediction of death at different time points for Aboriginal and non-Aboriginal ACS patients

	c-statistic (95 % CI)			
Group(H-L p-value)*	In-hospital	6 months	One year	Five years
GRACE score on admission : death in-hospital				
Aboriginal	0.76			
(0.63)	(0.62–0.91)			
Non-Aboriginal	0.76			
(0.58)	(0.68–0.84)			
GRACE score on admission : death within 6 months of admission				
Aboriginal		0.76	0.78	0.77
(0.10)		(0.62–0.89)	(0.65–0.91)	(0.70–0.85)
Non-Aboriginal		0.79	0.76	0.75
(0.75)		(0.74–0.84)	(0.71–0.82)	(0.71–0.80)
GRACE score at discharge : death within 6 months of discharge				
Aboriginal	-	0.75	0.77	0.76
(0.30)		(0.56–0.94)	(0.63–0.92)	(0.68–0.84)
Non-Aboriginal	-	0.77	0.78	0.76
(0.87)		(0.71–0.84)	(0.72–0.83)	(0.72–0.80)

* H-L = Hosmer-Lemeshow $\chi 2$ p-value

While lacking the power to demonstrate any systematic under-estimation of risk for the GRACE models, there is some support for the caution from the GRACE investigators that the risk models may not perform as well in populations that differ substantially from the population in which the models were developed [17]. Although the GRACE risk models were developed using data from patients from over a dozen countries, minority groups may differ considerably from the study cohort. This is evident for the distribution of age in the Australian Aboriginals admitted for ACS; the mean and median ages in both the GRACE development and validation cohorts were 65 and 66 years respectively [17] ,a year or two younger than the non-Aboriginals in this study (66.4 and 68 years), but more than a decade older than Aboriginal patients at 52.4 and 52 years.

The GRACE Investigators also cautioned that socioeconomic status had not been included in the construction of the models, and may well contribute to variability in risk [17]. As Aboriginal Australians and other indigenous minorities within advanced economies are among the most socially disadvantaged [27], the potential for confounding is obvious. However, when tested among patients with AMI in a Canadian study, the GRACE score was found to be a 'robust, well-calibrated, and accurate risk-stratification tool' both within and across socioeconomic strata [28]. If the GRACE score performed well in predicting 6-month all-cause mortality among patients hospitalized with AMI, regardless of socio-economic status, the likelihood of confounding by socio-economic status is reduced. Other factors (including age) are likely to influence the capacity of the score to accurately predict the risk for death in Aboriginal patients.

The excessive reduction in Australian Aboriginal life expectancy (the mortality gap), with early CVD being the largest contributor, is a reflection of accrual of lifetime cardiovascular risk. 'Accrued risk' among Aboriginal people aged to 50 years was reported to be equivalent to that of Framingham Study participants aged to 70 years for men, and to 80 years for women [29]. Other indigenous populations in which high prevalence of CVD risk factors are reported [2, 4, 5, 7, 30, 31], and in which CVD is manifest at a younger age, include American Indians and Alaskan Natives, Canadian First Nations and Inuit peoples, and the Māori of New Zealand [2–7]. The increased rates of CVD reported for some ethnic groups, associated with changes in lifestyle with immigration, [31–34] are also likely to have distributions of risk that differ significantly from the general population. Opportunities to test the GRACE models in such populations would lead to a better understanding of risk stratification for management of ACS and, plausibly, better outcomes for minority groups.

Study limitations

Missing data for calculating the GRACE scores (e.g. initial enzyme levels and serum creatinine, ECG, medical history not recorded on data collection form) reduced the ACS cases available for both groups. Despite sampling to capture all ACS admissions among Aboriginal people in the state population across three years only 220 cases had complete data and met the criteria for this study. In addition case-fatality was low for Aboriginal patients, with only four in-hospital deaths and 10 further deaths within six months of discharge, while the rate was as predicted for the non-Aboriginal population. The resulting lack of power left us unable to undertake any analyses that might improve risk stratification among Aboriginal patients, and provide more useful estimates of low, medium and high risk in this population.

The diagnosis of AMI, ACS or unstable angina was that recorded at discharge, rather than on admission as for patients in the GRACE studies. The discharge diagnosis reflects medical decision-making using all the clinical data collected during the admission. For instance, positive biomarkers were not always associated with a discharge diagnosis of AMI, suggesting other clinical data had been taken into consideration.

Significance

This is the first study to undertake a validation of a widely-used ACS risk stratification model in an Indigenous Minority population. Australian Aboriginals are around 3 % of Australia's population while 1.7 % of the population of the United States identified as American Indian and Alaska Native, either alone or in combination with one or more other races in 2010 [35], and 4.3 % of Canadians reported an Aboriginal identity in 2011 [36]. Māori are a larger Indigenous Minority, being 15.4 % of the New Zealand population in 2012 [37]. The small size of these populations means that studies are burdened with comparatively low numbers, but the importance of the disparity in morbidity and mortality requires that attention is paid to information that may lead to improvements in disease prevention, detection, and management.

Clinical registries provide the opportunity to understand the risks for and the presentation, management and outcomes of admission of cardiovascular disease. Every effort should be made to ensure Indigenous Minorities are fully represented in such projects.

Conclusions

The GRACE risk models are useful tools for predicting the risk for in-hospital deaths and all-cause mortality at six months among patients with ACS, but may underestimate risk among Australian Aboriginals who differ significantly from the general population in the age distribution of ACS. If this is the case in other Indigenous or minority populations then re-calibration of the models is necessary to provide more accurate prognostic tools to guide intervention and ongoing management.

Abbreviations

ACS: Acute coronary syndrome; AHA: American Heart Association; CAD: Coronary heart disease; CVD: Cardiovascular disease; ECG: Electrocardiograph; GRACE: Global Registry of Acute Coronary Events; HF: Heart failure; HMDC: Hospital Morbidity Data Collection; ICD-10-AM: International Classification of Disease 10th edition Australian Modification; PCI: Percutaneous coronary intervention; ROC: Receiver Operating Characteristic; STEMI: ST-elevation myocardial infarction; UA: Unstable angina; US: United States; WA: Western Australia.

Competing interests

The authors declare that they have no competing interests

Authors' contributions

PB and JK conceptualised the study. PB undertook the analysis of the data and drafting of the manuscript. MH, ST, JK, FS, PB, and PT were investigators for the studies that contributed data to the study. Each author reviewed, edited, read and approved the manuscript.

Acknowledgements

The authors thank the staff at the Western Australian Data Linkage Branch, and the Department of Health Inpatient Data Collections for the provision of data. We also acknowledge the contribution of the data collectors, who travelled around the vast state reviewing and recording information from clinical notes.

Funding

This work was supported by the National Health and Medical Research Council of Australia Grants (Numbers 353671, 1031057). Judith Katzenellenbogen is funded by an NHMRC Early Career Fellowship (Number 037429). The Western Australian Centre for Rural Health receives funding from the Department of Health and Ageing.

Author details
[1]School of Population Health, University of Western Australia, M431, 35 Stirling Highway, Crawley, WA 6009, Australia. [2]Western Australian Centre for Rural Health, University of Western Australia, M706, 35 Stirling Highway, Crawley, WA 6009, Australia. [3]Department of Research, 2nd Floor A Block (Mailbox 26), Sir Charles Gairdner Hospital, Hospital Avenue, Nedlands 6009WA, Australia.

References

1. Mathur S, Moon L, Leigh S. Aboriginal and Torres Strait Islander people with coronary heart disease: further perspectives on health status and treatment. Canberra: Australian Institute of Health and Welfare; 2006.
2. Howard B, Lee E, Cowan L, Devereux RB, Galloway JM, Go OT, et al. Rising tide of cardiovascular disease in American Indians. The Strong Heart Study Circulation. 1999;99:2389–95.
3. Harwell TS, Oser CS, Okon NJ, Fogle CC, Helgerson SD, Gohdes D. Defining disparities in cardiovascular disease for American Indians: trends in heart disease and stroke mortality among American Indians and whites in Montana, 1991 to 2000. Circulation. 2005;112:2263–7.
4. Sewell J, Malasky B, Gedney C, Gerber T, Brody E, Pacheco E, et al. The increasing incidence of coronary artery disease and cardiovascular risk factors among a Southwest Native American Tribe. The White Mountain Apache Heart Study. Arch Intern Med. 2002;162:1368–72.
5. Heart and Stroke Heart Disease and Stroke. Position Paper July 2012. http://www.heartandstroke.com/site/apps/s/google_search.asp?q=Position+paper+aboriginal&btnG.x=19&btnG.y=11&entqr=0&sort=date%3AD%3AL%3Ad1&output=xml_no_dtd&c=iklQLcMWJtE&ie=ISO-8859-1&client=heartandstroke_frontend&b=3820995&ud=1&site=heartandstroke&oe=UTF-8&proxystylesheet=heartandstroke_frontend.
6. Wei-Randall H, Davidson M, Jin J, Mathur S, Oliver L. Acute myocardial infarction hospitalization and treatment: Areas with a high percentage of First Nations identity residents. Health Rep. 2013;24:3–10.
7. Ministry of Health. 2010. Tatau Kahukura: *Māori Health Chart Book 2010*. 2nd Edition. Wellington: Ministry of Health. http://www.health.govt.nz/publication/tatau-kahukura-maori-health-chart-book-2010-2nd-edition
8. Australian Bureau of Statistics. 4713.0 - Population Characteristics, Aboriginal and Torres Strait Islander Australians, 2006. Canberra:ABS http://www.abs.gov.au/ausstats/abs@.nsf/mf/4713.0
9. Australian Institute of Health and Welfare 2011. The health and welfare of Australia's Aboriginal and Torres Strait Islander people, an overview 2011. Cat. no. IHW 42. Canberra: AIHW; 2011.
10. Bradshaw PJ, Alfonso HS, Finn J, Owen J, Thompson PL. A comparison of coronary heart disease event rates among urban Australian Aboriginal people and a matched non-Aboriginal population. J Epidemiol Community Health. 2011;65:315–9. doi:10.1136/jech.2009.098343.
11. Katzenellenbogen J, Sanfilippo F, Hobbs M, Briffa TG, Ridout SC, Knuiman MW, et al. Incidence of and case fatality following acute myocardial infarction in Aboriginal and non-Aboriginal Western Australians (2000–2004): a linked data study. Heart Lung Circ. 2010;19:717–25. doi:10.1016/j.hlc.2010.08.009.
12. You J, Condon J, Zhao Y, Guthridge S. Incidence and survival after acute myocardial infarction in Indigenous and non-Indigenous people in the Northern Territory, 1992–2004. Med J Aust. 2009;190:298–302.
13. D'Agostino R, Grundy S, Sullivan L, Wilson P, for the CHD Risk Prediction Group. Validation of the Framingham coronary disease prediction scores. Results of a multiple ethnic groups investigation. JAMA. 2001;286:180–7.
14. Wang Z, Hoy WE. Is the Framingham coronary heart disease absolute risk function applicable to Aboriginal people? Med J Aust. 2005;182:66–9.
15. Granger C, Goldberg R, Dabbous O, Pieper KS, Eagle KA, Cannon CP, et al. Predictors of hospital mortality in the Global Registry of Acute Coronary Events. Arch Intern Med. 2003;163:2345–53.
16. Fox K, Dabbous O, Goldberg R. Prediction of risk of death and myocardial infarction in the six months after presentation with acute coronary syndrome: prospective multinational observational study (GRACE). BMJ. 2006;333:1091.
17. Eagle K, Lim M, Dabbous O, Pieper KS, Goldberg RJ, Van de Werf F, et al. A validated prediction model for all forms of acute coronary syndrome. JAMA. 2004;291:2727–33.
18. Fox K, Eagle K, Gore J, Steg P, Anderson F. The Global Registry of Acute Coronary Events, 1999 to 2009-GRACE. Heart. 2010;96:1095–15.
19. D'Ascenzo F, Biondi-Zoccai G, Moretti C, Bollati M, Omedè P, Sciuto F, et al. TIMI, GRACE and alternative risk scores in Acute Coronary Syndromes: a meta-analysis of 40 derivation studies on 216,552 patients and of 42 validation studies on 31,625 patients. Contemp Clin Trials. 2012;33:507–14.
20. Methods and formulas used to calculate the GRACE Risk Scores for patients presenting to hospital with acute coronary syndromes. Copyright 1998–2014, Center for Outcomes Research, University of Massachusetts Medical School. http://www.outcomes-umassmed.org/grace/
21. Holman CD, Bass AJ, Rouse IL, Hobbs MS. Population-based linkage of health records in Western Australia: development of a health services research linked database. Aust NZ J Public Health. 1999;23:453–9.
22. Sanfilippo FM, Hobbs MST, Knuiman MW, Ridout SC, Bradshaw PJ, Finn JC, et al. Can we monitor heart attack in the troponin era: evidence from a population-based cohort study. BMC Cardiovasc Disord. 2011;11:35. doi:10.1186/1471-2261-11-35.
23. Gausia K, Katzenellenbogen J, Sanfilippo F, Knuiman M, Thompson P, Hobbs M, et al. Evidence-based prescribing of drugs for secondary prevention of acute coronary syndrome in Aboriginal and non-Aboriginal patients admitted to Western Australian hospitals. Intern Med J. 2014;44:353–61. doi:10.1111/imj.12375.
24. Taylor L, Bentley J, Hunt J, Madden R, McKeown S, Brandt P, et al. Enhanced reporting of deaths among Aboriginal and Torres Strait Islander peoples using linked administrative health datasets. BMC Med Res Methodol. 2012; 12:91. doi:10.1186/1471-2288-12-91.
25. Prineas RJ, Crow RS, Blackburn H. The Minnesota code manual of electrocardiographic findings: standards and procedures for measurement and classification. Wright-PSG: Boston, Massachusetts; 1982.
26. Luepker R, Apple F, Christenson R, Crow RS, Fortmann SP, Goff D, et al. Case definitions for acute coronary heart disease in epidemiology and clinical research studies: a statement from the AHA Council on Epidemiology and Prevention; AHA Statistics Committee; World Heart Federation Council on Epidemiology and Prevention; the European Society of Cardiology Working Group on Epidemiology and Prevention; Centers for Disease Control and Prevention; and the National Heart, Lung, and Blood Institute. Circulation. 2003;108:2543–9.
27. Mitrou F, Cooke M, Lawrence D, Povah D, Mobilia E, Guimond E, et al. Gaps in Indigenous disadvantage not closing: a census cohort study of social determinants of health in Australia, Canada, and New Zealand from 1981–2006. BMC Public Health. 2014;14:201.
28. Alter D, Venkatesh V, Chong A, for the SESAMI Study Group. Evaluating the performance of the Global Registry of Acute Coronary Events risk-adjustment index across socioeconomic strata among patients discharged from the hospital after acute myocardial infarction. Am Heart J. 2006;1515:323–31.
29. Wang Z, Hoy W. Lifetime risk of developing coronary heart disease in Aboriginal Australians: a cohort study. BMJ Open. 2013;3, e002308. doi:10.1136/bmjopen-2012-002308.
30. Lucero A, Lambrick D, Faulkner J, Fryer S, Tarrant MA, Poudevigne M, et al. Modifiable cardiovascular disease risk factors among indigenous populations. Adv Prev Med. 2014;2014:547018. doi:10.1155/2014/547018.
31. Anand SS, Yusuf S, Vuksan V, Devanesen S, Teo KK, Montague PA, et al. Differences in risk factors, atherosclerosis, and cardiovascular disease between ethnic groups in Canada: the Study of Health Assessment and Risk in Ethnic Groups (SHARE). Lancet. 2000;356:278–84.
32. Harding S. Mortality of migrants from the Indian subcontinent to England and Wales: effect of duration of residence. Epidemiology. 2003;14:287–92.
33. Enas EA, Garg A, Davidson MA, Nair VM, Huet BA, Yusuf S. Coronary heart disease and its risk factors in first-generation immigrant Asian Indians to the United States of America. Indian Heart J. 1996;48:343–53.
34. Abdelnoor M, Eritsland J, Brunborg C, Halvorsen S. Ethnicity and acute myocardial infarction: risk profile at presentation, access to hospital management, and outcome in Norway. Vasc Health Risk Manag. 2012;8:505–15.
35. Norris T, Vines P, Hoeffel E. The American Indian and Alaska Native Population: 2010. 2010 Census Briefs, January 2012. U.S. Department of Commerce Economics and Statistics Administration U.S. Census Bureau http://www.census.gov/prod/cen2010/briefs/c2010br-10.pdf
36. Statistics Canada. Canadian Demographics at a Glance (91-003-X) http://www.statcan.gc.ca/pub/91-003-x/2014001/section03/34-eng.htm
37. Statistics New Zealand. Maori Population Estimates. June2012. http://www.stats.govt.nz/tools_and_services/media-centre/additional-releases/maori-population-estimates-15-nov-2012.aspx

11

Ethnic differences in the occurrence of acute coronary syndrome: results of the Malaysian National Cardiovascular Disease (NCVD) Database Registry (March 2006 - February 2010)

Hou Tee Lu[1,2*] and Rusli Bin Nordin[1]

Abstract

Background: The National Cardiovascular Disease (NCVD) Database Registry represents one of the first prospective, multi-center registries to treat and prevent coronary artery disease (CAD) in Malaysia. Since ethnicity is an important consideration in the occurrence of acute coronary syndrome (ACS) globally, therefore, we aimed to identify the role of ethnicity in the occurrence of ACS among high-risk groups in the Malaysian population.

Methods: The NCVD involves more than 15 Ministry of Health (MOH) hospitals nationwide, universities and the National Heart Institute and enrolls patients presenting with ACS [ST-elevation myocardial infarction (STEMI), non-ST elevation myocardial infarction (NSTEMI) and unstable angina (UA)]. We analyzed ethnic differences across socio-demographic characteristics, hospital medications and invasive therapeutic procedures, treatment of STEMI and in-hospital clinical outcomes.

Results: We enrolled 13,591 patients. The distribution of the NCVD population was as follows: 49.0% Malays, 22.5% Chinese, 23.1% Indians and 5.3% Others (representing other indigenous groups and non-Malaysian nationals). The mean age (SD) of ACS patients at presentation was 59.1 (12.0) years. More than 70% were males. A higher proportion of patients within each ethnic group had more than two coronary risk factors. Malays had higher body mass index (BMI). Chinese had highest rate of hypertension and hyperlipidemia. Indians had higher rate of diabetes mellitus (DM) and family history of premature CAD. Overall, more patients had STEMI than NSTEMI or UA among all ethnic groups. The use of aspirin was more than 94% among all ethnic groups. Utilization rates for elective and emergency percutaneous coronary intervention (PCI) and coronary artery bypass graft (CABG) were low among all ethnic groups. In STEMI, fibrinolysis (streptokinase) appeared to be the dominant treatment options (>70%) for all ethnic groups. In-hospital mortality rates for STEMI across ethnicity ranges from 8.1% to 10.1% ($p = 0.35$). Among NSTEMI/UA patients, the rate of in-hospital mortality ranges from 3.7% to 6.5% and Malays recorded the highest in-hospital mortality rate compared to other ethnic groups ($p = 0.000$). In binary multiple logistic regression analysis, differences across ethnicity in the age and sex-adjusted ORs for in-hospital mortality among STEMI patients was not significant; for NSTEMI/UA patients, Chinese [OR 0.71 (95% CI 0.55, 0.91)] and Indians [OR 0.57 (95% CI 0.43, 0.76)] showed significantly lower risk of in-hospital mortality compared to Malays (reference group).

(Continued on next page)

* Correspondence: lu.hou.tee@monash.edu

[1]Clinical School Johor Bahru, Jeffrey Cheah School of Medicine and Health Sciences, Monash University Sunway campus, 8 Jalan Masjid Abu Bakar, 80100, Johor Bahru, Johor, Malaysia

[2]Department of Cardiology, Sultanah Aminah Hospital, Jalan Abu Bakar, 80100, Johor Bahru, Johor, Malaysia

(Continued from previous page)

Conclusions: Risk factor profiles and ACS stratum were significantly different across ethnicity. Despite disparities in risk factors, clinical presentation, medical treatment and invasive management, ethnic differences in the risk of in-hospital mortality was not significant among STEMI patients. However, Chinese and Indians showed significantly lower risk of in-hospital mortality compared to Malays among NSTEMI and UA patients.

Background

Acute coronary syndrome (ACS) encompasses a spectrum of clinical entities, ranging from unstable angina (UA), non-ST-segment elevation myocardial infarction (NSTEMI) to ST-elevation myocardial infarction (STEMI) [1]. In the Western world, ACS is the most common cause of death [2]. Cardiovascular disease (CVD) mortality is on the rise in the Asia Pacific countries (including Malaysia) that were undergoing rapid urbanization, industrialization and lifestyle changes [3]. According to the Global Burden of Disease Study (GBD), ischemic heart disease (IHD) is ranked first among the leading causes of mortality for eight regions in the world [4]. The World Health Organization (WHO) estimated that CAD will be the single largest cause of disease burden in many countries world-wide by the year 2020 [5]. Similarly, in Malaysia, CVD accounted for 147,843 admissions or about 6.91% of total admissions in Ministry of Health (MOH) hospitals in year 2009 [6]. CVD accounted for approximately 24.5% of death in government hospitals in year 2010 and is the leading cause of death in Malaysia [7].

Established coronary risk factors such as cigarette smoking, diabetes mellitus (DM), hypertension, obesity, sedentary life style and dyslipidemias still play major roles in CAD [8]. While conventional cardiovascular risk factors such as smoking, blood pressure and total cholesterol predict risk within these ethnic groups, they do not fully account for the differences in risk between ethnic groups, suggesting that alternative explanations might exist [9]. Epidemiological evidence that includes cross-sectional studies, coronary angiographic studies, and registry data showed significant differences between ethnic groups who were diagnosed with ACS in terms of presentations, risk factors, coronary vessel diameters, prognoses and outcomes [10-14].

With CVD accounting for most deaths globally, eliminating ethnic disparities in cardiac care has become a new challenge in the practice of cardiology [15]. Studies have shown that CVDs present differently in between ethnic groups [16,17]. Ethnicity has been shown to be an independent predictor of adverse cardiovascular outcomes in patients with atherothrombotic disease [18] and CAD [19].

ACS registries are important tools for analyzing disease management [20,21]. Exploration of registries data may lead to changes in disease management strategies and the national health care policies [22]. The National Cardiovascular Disease (NCVD) Database Registry is one of the pioneer projects to treat and prevent CAD in Malaysia. The project is a joint effort of doctors and nurses in public, private and academic medical institutions supported by the National Heart Association, National Heart Foundation, Clinical Research Centre and the MOH, Malaysia [23].

The aim of this study is, therefore, to identify the role of ethnicity in relation to the occurrence of ACS among high-risk groups in the Malaysian population using the Malaysian NCVD.

Methods

A detailed description of NCVD has been reported elsewhere [23,24]. In brief, the NCVD for ACS is the first prospective, multi-center registry involving more than 15 MOH hospitals nationwide, universities and the National Heart Institute (IJN: *Institut Jantung Negara*). Since its establishment in 2006, all registry centers attempt to ensure the enrollment of an unbiased population. The NCVD is an observational prospective registry that collects data on 'real-life' ACS patients comprising STEMI, NSTEMI and UA according to demographic, epidemiological, management and outcome characteristics. The registry enrolls inpatients presented with ACS from January 2006 onwards and is still on-going at the time of writing.

Entry criteria of ACS include risk stratum of patients presenting with clinical features consistent with an ACS (chest pain or overwhelming shortness of breath) and defined by accompanying clinical, electrocardiographic and biochemical features. The final diagnosis of ACS was made by the attending physician using the following criteria: STEMI was diagnosed on the basis of the presence of acute chest pain with new or presumably new ST segment elevations more than 1 mm in two consecutive leads or the presence of a new left bundle branch block on the index or subsequent ECG with positive cardiac markers of necrosis [25]. NSTEMI was defined by ECG ST-segment depression or prominent T-wave inversion and/or positive biomarkers of necrosis in the absence of ST-segment elevation and in an appropriate clinical setting (chest discomfort or angina equivalent). UA was defined as angina pectoris (or equivalent type of ischemic discomfort) with any one of the three following features: a) angina occurring at rest and prolonged, usually more than 20 min; b) new-onset angina of at least Canadian Cardiovascular Society (CCS) classification III severity; c) recent acceleration of angina reflected by an increase in severity of at least one CCS class to at least CCS class III. The patient must also have normal cardiac biomarkers [26].

Demographic, significant risk factors or past medical history, anthropometric, ACS stratum, treatment, length of hospitalization, outcome (alive, dead) and complications (such as bleeding) data were obtained from the medical records and recorded on a standardized clinical research form by trained coordinators. Standardized definitions for all patient-related variables and clinical diagnoses were used [24]. Precise definition and quantification for risk factors, past medical history and ways of treatments were described in earlier publications [23,24].

Collected data were subsequently entered into a web-based centralized database with security password encryption according to individual centers. Regular data checks were performed and queries were generated for correction to ensure accuracy. Ethnicity that includes Malays, Chinese, Indians (major ethnic groups), Indigenous (Orang Asli), Kadazan, Melanau, Murut, Bajau, Bidayuh, Iban (minor ethnic groups) and other Malaysians were recorded. Ethnicity was self-reported and coded as mutually exclusive categories. We excluded 17 patients with missing ethnic information. A total of 13,591 patients were included in the analysis. The current study included ACS patients from March 2006 to February 2010 over a period of 4 years. All patients were enrolled in Malaysia at different centers as listed in Figure 1.

Statistical analysis

Data were examined for normality distribution using the stem-and-leaf plot and Kolmogorov-Smirnov test. Descriptive statistics and baseline variables were presented as numbers and percentages, means and standard deviations, or medians and interquartile ranges. A chi square test was used to assess differences between categorical variables; a one-way ANOVA with post-hoc multiple comparisons (parametric analysis) or Kruskal-Wallis test (non-parametric analysis) was used to test differences across the four ethnic groups (Malays, Chinese, Indians Others). For multivariate analysis, binary simple and multiple logistic regressions were used to model the dichotomous outcome of STEMI and NSTEMI/UA mortality among ethnic groups with adjustment for age and sex. We checked for significant interaction between age and sex and possible multicollinearity by examining the standard errors of the b coefficients. Any significant interaction should be included in the final model. Standard errors of the b coefficients that were less than 2 indicate the absence of multicollinearity. The results were reported as crude and adjusted odds ratio (OR) with 95% confidence interval for ethnicity. A p value of <0.05 was considered statistically significant. All statistical calculations were performed using the IBM SPSS Statistics 20.

Ethics approval

This NCVD study was approved by the Medical Review & Ethics Committee (MREC), MOH Malaysia in 2007 (Approval Code: NMRR-07-20-250). MREC waived informed consent for NCVD.

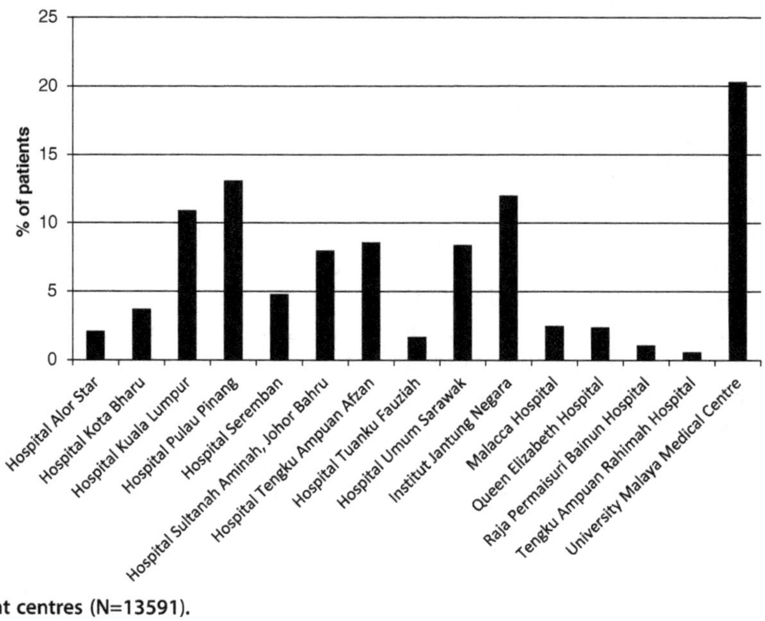

Figure 1 NCVD recruitment centres (N=13591).

Results

Socio-demographic characteristics

Socio-demographic characteristics and risk factors of the NCVD population are listed in Table 1. The distribution of the NCVD population was as follows: 49.0% Malays, 22.5% Chinese, 23.1% Indians, 5.3% Others (representing other indigenous groups and non-Malaysian nationals) and 0.1% missing data (Figure 2). The mean age of ACS patients at presentation was 59.1 (SD 12.0) years. More than 70% were males (p = 0.000). A large proportion of individuals within each ethnic group had more than two coronary risk factors including hypertension, DM and hyperlipidemia. Majority of patients were overweight [Body mass index (BMI) of more than 23 kg/m^2] in accordance with the BMI for Asian populations [27]. Malays had the highest BMI (26.0 kg/m^2) (p = 0.000). Indian had the biggest waist circumference (WC) (90.6 cm), the highest rate of DM (65.2%) and family history of premature CAD (22.2%) as compared to other ethnic groups (p = 0.000). Despite having the lowest BMI (24.8 kg/m^2), Chinese had the highest rate of hypertension (76.1%) and dyslipidemia (51.8%) (p = 0.000). Others had the highest proportion of current or former smokers (65.7%) (p = 0.000).

Table 2 shows the ethnic distribution of ACS and clearly indicated that Others (58.3%) had significantly higher STEMI (p = 0.000). Overall, more patients had STEMI than NSTEMI or UA among all the ethnic groups.

Table 3 shows that Malays had significantly higher mean total cholesterol (TC) and low density lipoprotein cholesterol (LDL) (5.5 mmol/l, 3.5 mmol/l, respectively) (p = 0.000). Indians had significantly higher mean fasting blood glucose (FBG) (8.4 mmol/l) (p = 0.000). Troponin T level was higher among Chinese (1.6 ng/ml). The level of CK is significantly higher in Others (1242 unit/l) (p = 0.000).

Hospital medications

Medication use at the time of admission is listed in Table 4. Aspirin, adenosine diphosphate antagonist, β-blockers, angiotensin-converting enzyme inhibitors, and statins were commonly prescribed to all ACS patients. The use of antiplatelet therapies, such as aspirin, was similar among all ethnic groups; more than 94% of patients in each group were taking aspirin at baseline. Malays received significantly lower proportion of low molecular weight heparin (LMWH) than other ethnic groups (p = 0.000).

Invasive therapeutic procedures

Majority of patients in the registry were recorded in centers with on-site cardiac catheterization facilities and teaching hospitals (Figure 1). For ACS patients, utilization rates for elective and emergency percutaneous coronary intervention (PCI) (13.1-16.5%) and coronary artery bypass graft (CABG) (0.7-1.8%) were generally low among all ethnic groups (Table 5). The overall rates of invasive therapeutic procedures such as PCI and CABG were slightly different across the ethnic groups. Indians and Others (16.5%, 16.5%) were likely to receive PCI than Chinese and Malays (16.0%, 13.1%) (p = 0 · 000). CABG rate was slightly higher in Others (1.8%) compared

Table 1 Socio-demographic characteristics and risk factors by ethnicity

Socio-demographic characteristics & risk factors	Ethnic group								F†	χ^{2‡}	df#	P§
	Malays		Chinese		Indians		Others*					
Age (SD) (yr)	58.3	(11.5)	62.9	(12.1)	57.7	(11.9)	56.5	(13.0)	141.2			0.000
Men (%)	5230	(78.6)	2205	(72.2)	2275	(72.0)	579	(82.0)		88.7	3	0.000
Height (SD) (cm)	161.6	(8.2)	161.7	(7.6)	162.4	(9.0)	161.3	(8.3)	3.8			0.010
Weight (SD) (kg)	68.5	(14.5)	65.3	(12.2)	68.5	(14.6)	67.2	(13.6)	24.6			0.000
WC (SD) (cm)	88.9	(15.4)	86.9	(13.2)	90.6	(15.4)	86.2	(12.7)	17.0			0.000
BMI (SD) (kg/m^2)	26.0	(4.4)	24.8	(3.7)	25.8	(4.5)	25.5	(4.1)	30.9			0.000
Smoking (%)	4141	(65.2)	1592	(55.1)	1430	(48.7)	439	(65.7)		259.0	3	0.000
Diabetes mellitus (%)	2646	(48.1)	1147	(45.0)	1780	(65.2)	200	(37.5)		315.9	3	0.000
Hypertension (%)	3859	(67.4)	2045	(76.1)	2010	(72.6)	400	(70.1)		73.9	3	0.000
Dyslipidemia (%)	2104	(48.4)	1144	(51.8)	1147	(51.2)	193	(42.6)		18.1	3	0.000
Family history of premature coronary artery disease (%)	725	(15.5)	235	(11.0)	454	(22.2)	69	(15.5)		101.1	3	0.000

*Others: Indigenous (Orang Asli), Kadazan, Melanau, Murut, Bajau, Bidayuh, Iban (minor ethnic groups) and other non-Malaysians.
†F statistics for one-way ANOVA.
‡Chi square value.
#Degree of freedom.
§P value.
WC: Waist Circumference.
BMI: Body Mass Index.
Note: We excluded 17 patients with missing ethnic information.

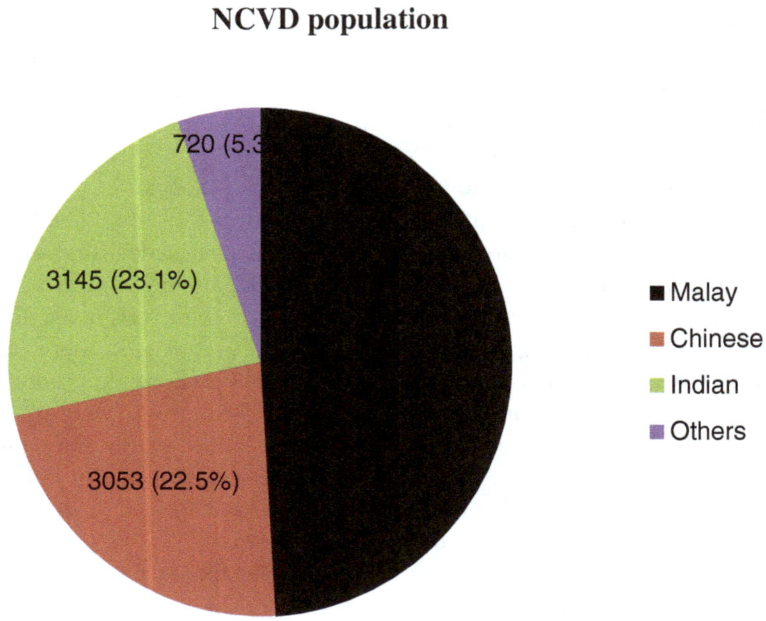

Figure 2 NVCD patients by ethnicity.

to Malays (1.4%), Chinese (1.3%) and Indians (0.7%), respectively (p = 0.006). Left anterior descending (LAD) artery was the commonest culprit artery involved in ACS among all ethnic groups followed by right coronary artery (RCA) and left circumflex (LCX) artery. However, the difference across the ethnic groups was not significant (p = 0.359).

Treatment of STEMI

Table 6 shows the reperfusion strategy for STEMI including subgroup analysis for the fibrinolytic group, door-to-needle time and door-to-balloon time. Majority of STEMI patients (≥80%) received some form of reperfusion therapy either by primary PCI or fibrinolysis. Fibrinolysis appeared to be the dominant treatment options (≥70%) for all ethnic groups. Overall, significant higher proportion of Malays (78.1%) received reperfusion therapy either by primary PCI or fibrinolysis as compared with other ethnic groups (p = 0.000). Significant higher proportion of Chinese (9.0%) received primary PCI, at the same time, no reperfusion (21.5%) was higher in Chinese than other ethnic groups (P = 0.000).

In the subset analysis for fibrinolysis, a higher proportion of Malays (8.4%) managed to achieve less than 30 minutes of door-to-needle time compared to other ethnic groups (P = 0.000) as recommended by Clinical Practice Guidelines [25,28]. Others reported higher door-to-needle time of 59 (IQR: 30–116) min compared to other ethnic groups (p = 0.013). On the other hand, in primary PCI, Others had the shortest door-to-balloon time of 81 (IQR: 48–124) min compared to other ethnic groups (p = 0.018). Overall, it is important to point out that we found a low percentage of patients achieving less than 30 minutes of door-to-needle time among all ethnic groups. Furthermore, door-to-needle and door-to-balloon time were longer than those recommended [25,28].

Table 2 Acute coronary syndrome by ethnicity

ACS stratum	Ethnic group				$\chi^{2‡}$	df[#]	P[§]
	Malays	Chinese	Indians	Others*			
STEMI**	3443(51.7)	1286(42.1)	1221(38.8)	420(58.3)	244	6	0.000
NSTEMI***	1762(26.5)	899(29.4)	972(30.9)	203(28.2)			
UA****	1451(21.8)	868(28.4)	952(30.3)	97(13.50)			

*Others: Indigenous (Orang Asli), Kadazan, Melanau, Murut, Bajau, Bidayuh, Iban (minor ethnic groups) and other non-Malaysians.
**STEMI: ST Elevation Myocardial Infarction.
***NSTEMI: Non-ST Elevation Myocardial Infarction.
****UA: Unstable Angina.
‡Chi square value.
#Degree of freedom.
§P value.

Table 3 Baseline investigation and clinical features on presentation by ethnicity

Baseline investigation & presentation	Ethnic group				F+	P#
	Malays	Chinese	Indians	Others*		
TC (mmol/l)	5.5(1.4)	5.1(1.2)	5.1(1.2)	5.3(1.3)	71.2	0.000
LDL (mmol/l)	3.5(1.3)	3.0(1.1)	3.2(1.2)	3.3(1.2)	93.7	0.000
HDL (mmol/l)	1.1(0.3)	1.2(0.4)	1.0(0.3)	1.1(0.3)	53.7	0.000
TG (mmol/l)	2.0(1.8)	2.0(1.2)	2.0(1.3)	2.0(1.1)	2.5	0.057
FBG (mmol/l)	8.0(3.7)	7.5(3.3)	8.4(3.9)	7.4(3.4)	34.7	0.000
Trop T (ng/ml)	1.5(4.6)	1.6(7.1)	1.2(3.6)	1.0(2.0)	1.2	0.300
CK (unit/l)	1075(1484)	884(1322)	789(126)	1242(1583)	36.3	0.000
Heart rate/min	83.1(21.1)	83.1(21.4)	85.9(23.1)	82.7(21.3)	14.1	0.000
SBP (mmHg)	138.9(28.9)	138.9(28.7)	140.2(27.9)	139.6(31.0)	1.8	0.153
DBP (mmHg)	80.9(16.5)	79.9(16.3)	82.2(16.0)	81.3(17.0)	9.7	0.000
Killip Class IV(%)‡	271(4.1)	100(3.3)	71(2.3)	28(3.9)	15	0.000
LVEF (%)‡	47(13)	46(13)	47(12)	47(13)	1.5	0.216

*Others: Indigenous (Orang Asli), Kadazan, Melanau, Murut, Bajau, Bidayuh, Iban (minor ethnic groups) and other Malaysians.
+Statistic for one-way ANOVA.
‡No.(%); all others: Mean (SD).
#P value.
TC: Total cholesterol.
LDL: Low density lipoprotein cholesterol.
HDL: High density lipoproteincholesterol.
TG: Triglyceride.
FBG: Fasting blood glucose.
Trop T: Troponin T.
CK: Creatinine kinase.
LVEF: Left ventricular ejection fraction.

In-hospital clinical outcomes

Indians reported significantly higher coronary care unit (CCU) days compared to Malays, Chinese and Others (3.6, 3.5, 3.2, and 2.5, respectively; p = 0.000) (Table 7). However, for total days, Malays reported significantly higher total days of admission compared to Others, Indians and Chinese (5.0, 4.9, 4.7, and 4.5, respectively; p = 0.000). Rates of major bleeding were low (≤ 0.7%) among all ethnic groups. There was no significant difference among the ethnic groups in the major or minor bleeding complication (p = 0.150) according to the Thrombolysis in Myocardial Infarction (TIMI) criteria for bleeding [29,30].

In-hospital-mortality rate for STEMI was higher than NSTEMI and UA among all ethnic groups. STEMI mortality rate ranges from 8.1 to 10.1% which was statistically insignificant (p = 0.35) across all ethnic groups. In-hospital mortality was also not significantly different across ethnic groups in a risk adjusted multivariable model that controlled for age and sex.

For NSTEMI/UA, there was statistically significant higher in-hospital-mortality (p = 0.000) among Malays (6.5%) compared to Chinese (5.6%), Others (5.4%) and Indians (3.7%). These results were persisting after age and sex adjustment. Therefore, Malays remained a positive predictor for in-hospital mortality as compared to Chinese and Indians in the NSTEMI/UA group irrespective of age and sex.

Discussion

The study has shown important ethnic differences in the demographics, comorbid coronary risk factors, clinical presentation, baseline investigations, treatments and in-hospital outcomes.

Socio-demographics and coronary risk factors

Malaysia is a multiracial South East Asian country, consisting of 28.3 million people that include 67.4% Malays, 24.6% Chinese, 7.3% Indians, and 0.7% other ethnic groups [31]. However, the percentage of Indians (majority have their origins in Southern India) captured in this registry was 23.4% which indicates an over representation of the Indian population in the NCVD.

It seems that a relatively higher proportion of Indians was being captured in the NCVD Registry. However, the causal link between ethnicity and ACS is difficult to evaluate based on cross-sectional data as the NCVD Registry consists of a well-defined population diagnosed with ACS. Therefore, based on the NCVD Registry, one cannot possibly draw any conclusion as to the higher incidence of ACS among Indians compared to other ethnic groups. The finding of over-representation of Indians in the NCVD Registry was an interesting fact that serves as a basis for a prospective cohort study to reveal the association between ethnicity and ACS. Nevertheless, people of South Asian origin such as India, Pakistan, Bangladesh, Sri

Table 4 Medication use by ethnicity

Medication use	Ethnic group				χ^{2**}	df	P#
	Malays	Chinese	Indians	Others*			
Antiplatelets							
Aspirin (%)	6092 (94.4)	2769 (94.1)	2851 (94.2)	649 (95.6)	2.6	3	0.454
Other antiplatelets (%)	4312 (68.5)	2222 (77.0)	2178 (73.0)	440 (73.0)	75.6	3	0.000
Anticoagulants							
Heparin (%)	907 (15.0)	202 (7.3)	281 (9.7)	55 (9.8)	128.9	3	0.000
LMWH (%)	3340 (54.1)	1882 (66.2)	2033 (68.6)	435 (68.5)	282.1	3	0.000
Antihypertensives							
β-blockers (%)	4238 (67.6)	2052 (71.2)	2067 (69.5)	418 (68.9)	12.3	3	0.060
ACEI (%)	3899 (62.4)	1666 (58.4)	1814 (61.1)	337 (55.9)	19.8	3	0.000
ARB (%)	468 (7.8)	242 (8.7)	304 (10.5)	59 (10.4)	20.3	3	0.000
Diuretics (%)	2016 (32.7)	798 (28.3)	888 (30.2)	196 (33.2)	19.8	3	0.000
CCB (%)	895 (14.8)	409 (14.7)	509 (17.4)	82 (14.5)	12.1	3	0.007
Anti-diabetic agents							
OHA (%)	1599 (26.1)	712 (25.4)	1157 (39.3)	112 (19.8)	217.9	3	0.000
Insulin (%)	1522 (24.7)	586 (20.8)	978 (33.1)	104 (18.2)	140.7	3	0.000
Statins							
Statins (%)	5833 (91.0)	2700 (92.1)	2737 (90.8)	646 (95.1)	16.6	3	0.001

Categorical variables are expressed as number (%).
*Others: Indigenous (Orang Asli), Kadazan, Melanau, Murut, Bajau, Bidayuh, Iban (minor ethnic groups) and other non-Malaysians.
**Pearson Chi-Square.
#P value.
LMWH: Low Molecular Weight Heparin.
ACEI: Angiotensin Converting Enzyme Inhibitors.
ARB: Angiotensin Receptor Blockers.
CCB: Calcium Channel Blockers.
OHA: Oral Hypoglycemic Agent.

Table 5 Invasive procedures and culprit arteries by ethnicity

Invasive procedures	Ethnic group				$\chi^{2‡}$	df	P#
	Malays	Chinese	Indians	Others*			
PCI (%)	874(13.1)	490(16.0)	518(16.5)	119(16.5)	27.2	3	0.000
CABG (%)	95(1.4)	41(1.3)	21(0.7)	13(1.8)	12.3	3	0.006
LMA involvement (%)	184(2.8)	82(2.7)	84(2.7)	30(4.2)	5.3	3	0.150
Culprit Artery							
LAD (%)	591(56.3)	314(56.3)	339(58.0)	81(59.6)	13.1	12	0.359
RCA (%)	318(30.3)	172(30.8)	147(25.2)	37(27.2)			
LCX (%)	103(9.8)	53(9.5)	70(12.0)	15(11.0)			
LMA (%)	18(1.7)	8(1.4)	8(1.4)	2(1.5)			
Bypass graft (%)	20(1.9)	11(2.0)	20(3.4)	1(0.7)			

Categorical variables are expressed as number (%).
*Others: Indigenous (Orang Asli), Kadazan, Melanau, Murut, Bajau, Bidayuh, Iban (minor ethnic groups) and other non-Malaysians.
‡Pearson Chi-Square.
#P value.
PCI: Percutaneous Coronary Intervention.
CABG: Coronary Artery Bypass Graft.
LMA: Left Main Artery.
LAD: Left Anterior Descending artery.
LCX: Left Circumflex artery.
RCA: Right Coronary Artery.

Table 6 Treatment of STEMI by ethnicity

Treatment of STEMI	Ethnic Group				$\chi^{2‡}$	df#	p§
	Malays	Chinese	Indians	Others*			
	No. (%)	No. (%)	No. (%)	No. (%)			
Primary PCI	188 (5.6)	111 (9.0)	93 (7.9)	30 (7.4)	40.7	6	0.000
Fibrinolysis	2607 (78.1)	858 (69.5)	878 (74.3)	307 (76.2)			
No reperfusion+	544 (16.3)	265 (21.5)	211 (17.9)	66 (16.4)			
Total	3339 (100.0)	1234 (100.0)	1182 (100.0)	403 (100.0)			
Fibrinolysis subgroup							
Type of fibrinolytic drug used							
Streptokinase	1924(97.1)	671(98.0)	661(96.2)	238(97.9)	4.3	3	0.226
Other fibrinolytic drugs	58(2.9)	14(2.0)	26(3.8)	5(2.1)			
Door-to-needle time within 30 min	559(8.4)	181(5.9)	217(6.9)	54(7.5)	20.3	3	0.000
Door-to-needle time (min)†	50(27–100)	55(30–101)	49(24–102)	59(30–116)	10.7	3	0.013¥ (0.01, 0.02)¥
Door-to-balloon time (min)†	112(78–168)	109(73–156)	96(71–165)	81(48–124)	10.4	3	0.018¥ (0.01,0.02)¥

*Others: Indigenous (Orang Asli), Kadazan, Melanau, Murut, Bajau, Bidayuh, Iban (minor ethnic groups) and other non-Malaysians.
†Median (IQR).
‡Pearson Chi-Square.
#Degree of freedom.
§P value.
+Reason for no reperfusion includes refusal, missed fibrinolysis, and contraindication.
¥Kruskal-Wallis test with Monte Carlo level of significance (99% CI).

Lanka and Nepal represents one of the largest ethnic groups in the world and also one of the regions with the highest burden of CVDs [32]. Studies on South Asian migrants in Western countries such as Canada, United Kingdom (UK) and the United States of America (USA) documented significantly higher risks of CVDs with higher morbidity and mortality than other ethnic groups [10,14,33,34]. Previous mortality statistics and cross-sectional surveys had confirmed that Indians have an increased risk of CAD compared to other ethnic groups

Table 7 In-hospital clinical outcomes by ethnicity

In-hospital clinical outcomes	Ethnic group				F†	χ^2	df	p§
	Malays	Chinese	Indians	Others*				
CCU Days‡	3.5(2.8)	3.2(2.6)	3.6(2.9)	3.2(2.5)	7.4			0.000
Total Days‡	5.0(3.7)	4.5(3.4)	4.7(3.5)	4.9(3.7)	11.3			0.000
Bleeding rate#								
Major+	44(0.7)	13(0.5)	11(0.4)	1(0.2)		13.3	9	0.150
Minor	138(2.3)	57(2.1)	43(1.6)	11(2.1)				
Minimal	6(0.1)	1(0.0)	1(0.0)	0(0.0)				
None	5777(96.8)	2617(97.4)	2683(98.0)	524(97.8)				
Mortality rate#								
STEMI	309(9.2)	125(10.1)	96(8.1)	30(8.2)		3.3	3	0.352
NSTEMI/UA	204(6.5)	97(5.6)	69(3.7)	15(5.4)		17.8	3	0.000
Adjusted OR for mortality (95% CI)¥								
STEMI	1	0.93 (0.74, 1.16)	0.93 (0.66, 1.47)	0.99 (0.66, 1.47)				
NSTEMI/UA	1	0.71 (0.55, 0.91)	0.57 (0.43, 0.76)	0.78 (0.45, 1.34)				

*Others: Indigenous (Orang Asli), Kadazan, Melanau, Murut, Bajau, Bidayuh, Iban (minor ethnic groups) and other non-Malaysians.
CCU: Coronary Care Unit.
†One-way ANOVA.
‡Mean (SD).
#Number (%).
§P value.
+TIMI (Thrombolysis In Myocardial Infarction) major bleeding involves a hemoglobin drop >5 g/dL (with or without an identified site) or intracranial hemorrhage or cardiac tamponade.
¥Binary multiple logistic regression; ORs adjusted for age and sex.

[11,35]. A cardiovascular cohort study showed that ethnicity plays a major role in CAD with Indian males found to have three times the risk of CAD as compared to Malays and Chinese in Singapore [36].

The mean age at presentation was 59.1 years among all ethnic groups. In contrast to earlier registries from developed countries, such as National Registry of Myocardial Infarction (NRMI) (mean age 68 years) [37], Global Registry of Acute Coronary Event (GRACE) registry (53% aged ≥ 65 years) [38,39] and the Euro Heart Survey I (EHS-ACS-I) (mean age 63.4 years) [40,41], our cohort was characterized by a younger age at presentation. The mean age was similar to the CREATE registry (58 years) [42] and Saudi Project for Assessment of Coronary Events (SPACE) registry (57 years) [43] that were conducted in India and Saudi Arabia, respectively. The age at presentation discrepancy observed between the European and Asian Registries should be investigated further to establish risk factors that possibly contributed toward the age difference.

Similar to ACS registries world-wide, the predominant sex was male (more than two thirds) among all ethnic groups. There were substantial differences between male and female in the presentation, diagnosis, management and outcome of CADs [44-47]. Most clinical trials have enrolled primarily men and the women have been under-represented in CAD clinical trials; further research involving larger female cohorts is required. Further, at participating centers, a lower proportion of women were found to have ischemia during the course of routine clinical care, and screening tests for ischemia were less predictive of CAD in women than those in men [48].

The patients' risk factor profiles differed significantly among the ethnic groups. For example, Malays showed significantly highest mean BMI. Chinese patients had the highest proportion of hypertension and hyperlipidemia. On the other hand, Indians had the highest mean for WC and the highest proportion for DM and family history of premature CAD. Others had significantly highest proportion of smokers. The WC recorded among all ethnic groups was generally higher than the mean WC of Malaysians [49]. The finding of high WC among Indians was similar to those previously reported in the Malaysian National Health and Morbidity Survey III [49]. The finding of high prevalence of BMI among all ethnic groups with ACS was similar to another Malaysian prevalence study on overweight and obesity among non ACS population [50]. Higher BMI among Malays with ACS was also consistent with the national study on obesity among Malaysians according to ethnicity [51]. This explains the relationship between high BMI and higher occurrence of ACS in the general population [52]. The results suggest that a higher proportion of patients with ACS also have metabolic syndrome as compared to the general population [53,54]. DM has been found to be more common in Indians. This finding was consistent with previous multi-center registries and studies in Singapore [55], Trinidad [35], Fiji [56], USA [57] and UK [33,58]. A study in Canada by the Study of Health Assessment and Risk in Ethnic Groups (SHARE) investigators also found that Indians had more plasma glucose and lipid abnormalities compared to Europeans and Chinese [16]. Indians also have higher past history of CVDs and family history of MI compared to other ethnic groups [57]. Generally, our patients had high prevalence of coronary risk factors at presentation among all ethnic groups. These findings were similar to an earlier publication using NCVD [59], Singapore population [60], Iranian population [61], Saudi Arabia population [62], and in developing countries [63].

ACS

The proportion of STEMI among all ethnic groups (38.8–58.3%) was higher compared to earlier ACS registries in developed countries: GRACE (30.0%) [38], EHS-ACS-I (42.3%) [40], NRMI (40.0%) [64], Euro Heart Survey II (EHS-ACS-II) (34.5%) [65] and Canadian Acute Coronary Syndrome Registry (27.7%) [66]. Higher proportion of STEMI compared to NSTEMI and UA in NCVD was similar to those in the CREATE registry (47.3–71.4%) [42]. In the CREATE registry, poorer socio-economic group of patients recorded a higher proportion of STEMI in India. This finding could possibly explain why Others (indigenous ethnic groups), who generally belong to the lower socioeconomic status, recorded a higher proportion of STEMI.

Lipid profile, fasting blood glucose

Our findings on serum lipid were consistent with previous studies on Indian populations living in UK and USA. Generally, Indians have lower HDL cholesterol than whites or Afro-Caribbean populations but do not have higher total or LDL cholesterol than other races [67-69].

Hospital medications

Results indicated high use of Aspirin, Beta-blockers, LMWH and Statins among all ethnic groups was in line with the Clinical Practice Guidelines [26,28,70] and comparable to those in developed countries. Religious practice could be a factor to explain the lower use of LMWH (containing porcine-related material) among Malays as the overwhelming majorities are Muslims compared to other ethnic groups.

Invasive therapeutic procedures and culprit artery

On invasive therapeutic procedures, the rate of PCI and CABG in our registry was lower than those reported in developed countries [38,40,65,66]. Our results showed disparities existed in the use of medications, PCI and CABG among ethnic groups. The finding of LAD artery as the most common culprit artery was similar to those of Yadav et al. [71] and Deshpandey and Dixit [72].

Treatment of STEMI

In STEMI, timely delivery of reperfusion therapy can reduce mortality; therefore, guidelines recommend fibrinolysis within 30 min (door-to-needle time) and primary PCI within 90 minutes (door-to-balloon-time) [25,28]. Primary PCI has been proven better than fibrinolysis in treating STEMI [73,74] and timely administration of fibrinolytic therapy significantly reduces mortality [75]. In STEMI, despite majority of patients who received reperfusion therapy, the rate of primary PCI was lower and the use of fibrinolytics was higher among all ethnic groups as compared to ACS registries in developed countries such as GRACE [38], EHS-ACS-I [40] and EHS-ACS-II [65]. In the fibrinolysis subgroup, door-to-needle time among all ethnic groups was longer than those recommended by the American and European Guidelines [25,28] and the proportion of patients achieving less than 30 minutes of door-to-needle time was low. This is one of the main concerns of our study that illustrated suboptimal care in treating STEMI. Streptokinase, the less-fibrin specific (less effective) fibrinolytic agent as compared with fibrin-selective fibrinolytic agents [76] was commonly used among all ethnic groups. Higher proportion of Chinese received less reperfusion therapy than other ethnic groups; however, the reasons for these discrepancies were unclear.

In the implementation of evidence-based reperfusion strategies, doctors have to make the best decision to allocate limited resources to patients who are at highest risk and hope to obtain the largest benefit. Many studies have found differences in the delivery of cardiac care and reperfusion procedure among different ethnic groups in ACS [77-79]. Earlier studies of ethnic variation in the treatment and outcome of ACS in USA showed that non-whites had longer door-to-needle time in the treatment of AMI [80] and were less likely to undergo invasive cardiac procedures [81,82]. However, this finding was controversial in other clinical trials [83]. Research has shown that by implementing a national quality improvement program, it is possible to reduce or eliminate the differences in care by ethnicity [84]. Considerably more effort and resources will be granted to improve the reperfusion strategies in developing countries like Malaysia for all patients regardless of their ethnic origin. Adherence to clinical practice guidelines has shown to improve quality of care and associated with significant reduction in in-hospital mortality rates [85].

In-hospital clinical outcomes

In developed countries, STEMI mortality rates were reported as 4.3–4.4% in NRMI [86], 7.0% in the GRACE Registry [38], 7.0% in the EHS-ACS-I [40] and 2.4% in the Canadian Acute Coronary Syndrome Registry [66]. In the NCVD, higher STEMI mortality rate (8.1–10.1%) in comparison with developed countries could be explained by lower use of primary PCI, higher use of less effective fibrinolytic agent (Streptokinase) and delay in door-to-needle time among all ethnic groups. In addition, LAD artery involvement as the main culprit vessel (>56%) among all ethnic groups could have contributed towards a less favorable outcome as reported earlier by Thanavaro et al. [87].

Interestingly, despite the fact that disparities exist in risk factors, clinical presentation, medical treatments and invasive management, there was no statistically significant difference in STEMI mortality among all ethnic groups. However, there are limitations in the analysis of mortality outcome comparing different ethnic groups and we advise caution in its interpretation. Firstly, it was an in-hospital mortality of STEMI and NSTEMI/UA of both genders and all age groups. As for ACS, many studies had shown higher mortality in women [88,89] and older patients [39,41,90]. Hence, the mortality outcome analyzed in this method may have over or underestimated the differences between age groups and across genders. Secondly, we used in-hospital all-cause mortality as an end point in order to minimize event misclassification. Results for cardiac-specific mortality may be different for present results. Caution should, therefore, be observed in comparing results with those from other national registries or clinical trials.

On the basis of the risk factor profiles across all ethnic groups, it would seem unreasonable for Malays to have higher NSTEMI and UA mortality. It would seem that higher mortality in Malays can be partly explained by the higher proportion of Malays receiving lower rates of PCI compared to other ethnic groups. Other possible explanations include greater cigarette consumption and higher BMI among Malays.

Earlier observational studies locally and elsewhere have shown a higher proportion of deaths in Indians with IHD compared to other ethnic groups [11,35,91]. The finding of lower in-hospital mortality in NSTEMI/UA among Indians in our study contradicted with previous studies for unexplained reasons.

There were evidences that bleeding risk in ACS differs in different type of ACS, reperfusion therapy and ethnic groups [92]. Registry data [92], prospective study [93] and randomized controlled trials (RCT) [94] of developed countries in ACS patients reported that the major bleeding risk was between 4.6–10.9%. Compared to developed countries, major bleeding in NCVD was generally low among all ethnic groups (0.2–0.7%) and this finding was similar to those in the ACS Registry in India (0.2–0.3%) (CREATE) and Middle Eastern countries

(0.83%) [95]. The finding of a lower risk of major bleeding is intriguing and possibly could be explained by the lower use of invasive cardiac procedures among all ethnic groups as compared to those in developed countries.

Strengths and limitations

The main strength of this study is the collection of data from multi centers to represent a complete and unselected group of patients in a real-world setting. Unlike restricted populations recruited in RCTs which tend to exclude high risk patients, the NCVD collects data on the full spectrum of ACS patients from a nationwide perspective. We gain insight into ACS patients that were not included in RCTs. We use a standard method across all ethnic groups in collecting data to avoid bias.

Several limitations of our study should be noted. Firstly, misclassification of ethnicity can occur as ethnicity was self-reported and mutually-exclusive. Secondly, the possibility of selection bias despite our attempt to include hospitals in different regions of the country. Many private hospitals with significant number of ACS admissions possibly with a different ethnic distribution did not participate in this registry. Ethnic minorities living in remote areas had difficulty accessing the health facilities and therefore could have been under-represented in this study. Thirdly, there may have been underreporting of risk factors such as cigarette smoking and past medical history as these measures were self-reported and this may subject to bias.

Furthermore, statistical differences are frequently observed in a large number of subjects but may not be clinically meaningful. In studies with large patient enrolment, small differences between groups will be highly significant by conventional use of the p values, and the clinical importance of these differences can only be judged with clinical insight.

Conclusions

There are two major implications of our study. First, we have shown interesting facts about the differences and similarities of demographic, risk profile, ACS stratum, treatment and outcome among different ethnic groups. Second, our study establishes a critical understanding of disease spectrum, drug usage, invasive procedures, clinical outcomes, and the overall quality of care provided to ACS patients in Malaysia. In addition, the NCVD provides insights and forms the basis for clinical investigators to design future clinical trials. The NCVD also enables clinicians and health care administrators to compare disease-specific patterns, management and outcomes which might lead to changes in national health priorities or strategies of disease management.

Abbreviations

ACS: Acute coronary syndrome; BMI: Body mass index; CABG: Coronary artery bypass graft; CCU: Coronary care unit; CREATE: Treatment and outcomes of ACS in India; CVD: Cardiovascular disease; DM: Diabetes mellitus; GRACE: Global Registry of Acute Coronary Events; IHD: Ischemic heart disease; LAD: Left anterior descending; LCX: Left circumflex; LM: Left main; LMWH: Low molecular weight heparin; LVEF: Left ventricular ejection fraction; MOH: Ministry of Health; NCVD: National Cardiovascular Disease Database Registry; NRMI: National Registry of Myocardial Infarction; NSTEMI: Non ST-segment elevation myocardial infarction; PCI: Percutaneous coronary intervention; RCA: Right coronary artery; RCT: Randomized controlled trial; SPACE: Saudi Project for Assessment of Coronary Events; STEMI: ST-elevation myocardial infarction; UA: Unstable angina; WHO: World Health Organization; TIMI: Thrombolysis in myocardial infarction; WC: Waist circumference.

Competing interests

Both authors declare that they have no competing interests.

Authors' contributions

LHT and RBN collated and analyzed the data. LHT prepared the first draft of the paper and RBN vetted the final manuscript. Both authors interpreted the results, revised the paper, and approved the final version.

Acknowledgements

The authors would like to acknowledge the Chairperson of the NCVD Governance Board for permission to use the data for this paper. We would like to thank all doctors and nurses participating in the NCVD.

References

1. Herzog E, Saint-Jacques H, Rozanki A: **The pain pathway as a tool to bridge the gap between evidence and management of acute coronary syndrome.** *Critic Path in Cardiology* 2004, **3**:20–24.
2. Rosamond W, Flegal K, Furie K, Go A, Greenlund K, Haase N, Hailpern SM, Ho M, Howard V, Kissela B, Kittner S, Donald L-J, Mary MD, James M, Claudia M, Nichol G, Donnell CO, Roger V, Sorlie P, Steinberger J, Thom T, Wilson M, Hong Y: **Heart Disease and Stroke Statistics 2008 Update. A report from the American Heart Association statistics committee and Stroke Statistics subcommittee.** *Circulation* 2008, **117**:25–146.
3. Khor GL: **Cardiovascular epidemiology in the Asia-Pacific region.** *Asia Pac J Clin Nutr* 2001, **10**(2):76–80.
4. Murray CJ, Lopez AD: **Mortality by cause for eight regions of the world: Global Burden of Disease Study.** *Lancet* 1997, **349**:1269–1276.
5. WHO: *The World Health Statistic 2012.* [http://www.who.int/gho/publications/world_health_statistics/EN_WHS2012_Full.pdf] (Accessed 15 August 2013).
6. Ministry of Health, Malaysia: *Annual Report 2009.* [http://www.moh.gov.my/images/gallery/publications/md/ar/2009-2.pdf] (Accessed 15 August 2013).
7. Health Informatics Centre, Planning and Development Division, Ministry of Health Malaysia, July 2010: *Number of discharges and deaths in government hospitals.* [http://www.moh.gov.my/images/gallery/stats/heal_fact/health_facts_2010.pdf] (Accessed 15 August 2013).
8. Kuulasmaa K, Tunstall-Pedoe H, Dobson A, *et al*: **Estimation of contribution of changes in classic risk factors to trends in coronary event rates across the WHO MONICA project populations.** *Lancet* 2000, **355**:675–687.
9. Forouhi NG, Sattar N: **CVD risk factors and ethnicity-A homogeneous relationship?** *Atherosclerosis Suppl* 2006, **S7**(1):11–19.
10. Bhopal R, Unwin N, White M, Yallop J, Walker L, Alberti KGMM, Harland J, Patel S, Ahmad N, Turner C: **Heterogeneity of coronary heart disease risk factors in Indian, Pakistani, Bangladeshi, and European origin populations: cross sectional study.** *BMJ* 1999, **319**(24):215–220.
11. Hughes K, Yeo PPB, Lun KC, Thai AC, Sothy SP, Wang KW, Cheah JS, Phoon WO, Lim P: **Cardiovascular diseases in Chinese, Malays, and Indians in Singapore. I. Differences in mortality.** *J Epid and Comm Hlth* 1990, **44**:24–28.
12. Mak KH, Chia KS, Kark JD, Chua T, Tan C, Foong BH, Lim YL, Chew SK, *et al*: **Ethnic differences in acute myocardial infarction in Singapore.** *Eur Heart J* 2003, **24**:151–160.
13. Makaryus AN, Dhama B, Raince J, Raince A, Garyali S, Labana SS, Kaplan BM, Park C, Jauhar R: **Coronary artery diameter as a risk factor for acute coronary syndromes in Asian-Indians.** *Am J Cardiol* 2005, **96**:778–780.

14. Nijjar APK, Wang H, Quan H, Khan NA: **Ethnic and sex differences in the incidence of hospitalized acute myocardial infarction: British Columbia, Canada 1995–2002.** *BMC Cardio Dis* 2010, **10**(38):1471–2261.
15. Peterson E, Yancy CW: **Eliminating racial and ethnic disparities in cardiac care.** *N Engl J Med* 2009, **360:**1172–1174.
16. Anand SS, Yusuf S, Vuksan V, Devanesen S, Teo K, Montague P, Kelemen L, Yi C, Lonn E, Gerstein H: **Differences in risk factors, atherosclerosis, and cardiovascular disease between ethnic groups in Canada: the Study of Health Assessment and Risk in Ethnic Groups (SHARE).** *Lancet* 2000, **356:**279–284.
17. Lanza GA: **Editorial. Ethnic variations in acute coronary syndromes.** *Heart* 2004, **90:**595–597.
18. Mak KH, Bhatt DL, Shao M, Hankey GJ, Easton JD, Fox KAA, Topol EJ: **Ethnic variation in adverse cardiovascular outcomes and bleeding complications in the Clopidogrel for High Atherothrombotic Risk and Ischemic Stabilization, Management, and Avoidance (CHARISMA) study.** *Am Heart J* 2009, **157**(4):658–665.
19. Shaw LJ, Shaw RS, Merz NB, Brindis RG, Klein LW, Nallamothu B, Douglas PS, Krone RJ, McKAy CR, Block PC, Hewitt K, Weintraub WS, Peterson ED on behalf of the American College of Cardiology (ACC)-National Cardiovascular Data Registry Investigators (NCDR): **Impact of ethnicity and gender differences on angiographic coronary artery disease prevalence and in-hospital mortality in the ACC-NCDR.** *Circulation* 2008, **117:**1787–1801.
20. Fox KAA: **Registries and surveys in acute coronary syndrome.** *Eur Heart J* 2006, **27:**2260–2262.
21. Alpert JS: **Editorial. Are data from clinical registries of any value?** *Eur Heart J* 2000, **21:**1399–1401.
22. Pillay MS, Noor Hisham A, Zaki M, Lim TO, Jamaiyah H, Purany SPJ: **Patient registries in Malaysia and the role of the Clinical Research Centre of the Ministry of Health.** *Med J Malaysia* 2008, **63**(Suppl C):1–4.
23. Chin SP, Jeyaindran S, Azhari R, Wan Azman WA, Omar I, Robaayah Z, Sim KH: **Acute coronary syndrome (ACS) Registry -Leading the charge for National Cardiovascular Disease (NCVD) Database.** *Med J Malaysia* 2008, **63**(Suppl C):29–36.
24. Wan Ahmad WA, Sim KH: *National Cardiovascular Disease Database (NCVD). Inaugural Report of the Acute Coronary Syndrome (ACS) Registry 2007&2008.* [http://www.acrm.org.my/ncvd/acsReport_07-08.php] (Accessed 15 August 2013).
25. Antman EM, Hand M, Armstrong PW, Bates ER, Green LA, Halasyamani LK, Hochman JS, Krumholz HM, Lamas GA, Mullany CJ, Pearle DL, Sloan MA, Smith SC: **2007 Focused Update of the ACC/AHA 2004 Guidelines for the Management of Patients With ST-Elevation Myocardial Infarction. A Report of the American College of Cardiology/American Heart Association Task Force on Practice Guidelines Developed in Collaboration With the Canadian Cardiovascular Society Endorsed by the American Academy of Family Physicians.** *J Am Coll Cardiol* 2008, **51:**200–247.
26. Jneid H, Anderson JL, Wright RS, Adams CD, Bridges CR, Casey DE Jr, Ettinger JSM, Fesmire FM, Ganiats TG, Lincoff AM, Peterson ED, Philippides GJ, Theroux P, Wenger NK, Zidar JP: **ACCF/AHA Focused Update of the Guidelines for the Management of Patients With Unstable Angina/Non–ST-Elevation Myocardial Infarction (Updating the 2007 Guidelines and Replacing the 2011 Focused Update): A Report of the American College of Cardiology Foundation/American Heart Association Task Force on Practice Guidelines.** *Circulation* 2012, **2012**(126):875–910.
27. WHO Expert Consultation: **Appropriate body-mass index for Asian populations and its implications for policy and intervention strategies.** *Lancet* 2004, **363:**157–163.
28. Steg G, James SK, Atar D, Badano LP, Blo¨mstrom-Lundqvist C, Borger MA, Mario CD, Dickstein K, Ducrocq G, Fernandez-Aviles F, Gershlick AH, Giannuzzi P, Halvorsen S, Huber K, Juni P, Kastrati A, Knuuti J, Lenzen MJ, Mahaffey KW, Valgimigli M, Hof AV, Widimsky P, Zahger D, The Task Force on the management of ST-segment elevation acute myocardial infarction of the European Society of Cardiology (ESC): **ESC Guidelines for the management of acute myocardial infarction in patients presenting with ST-segment elevation.** *Eur Heart J* 2012, **33:**2569–2619.
29. Chesebro JH, Knatterud G, Roberts R, *et al*: **Thrombolysis in Myocardial Infarction (TIMI) Trial. Phase I: a comparison between intravenous tissue plasminogen activator and intravenous streptokinase. Clinical findings through hospital discharge.** *Circulation* 1987, **76:**142–154.
30. Mehran R, Rao SV, Bhatt DL, Gibson CM, Caixeta A, Eikelboom J, Kaul S, Wiviott SD, Menon V, Nikolsky E, Serebruany V, Valgimigli M, Vranckx P, Taggart D, Sabik JF, Cutlip DE, Krucoff MW, Ohman EM, Steg PG, White H: **Standardized bleeding definitions for cardiovascular clinical trials: a consensus report from the Bleeding Academic Research Consortium.** *Circulation* 2011, **123:**2736–2747.
31. Department of Statistics, Malaysia: *Population and Demography.* 5. [http://www.statistics.gov.my/portal/index.php?option=com_content&view=article&id=1465&lang=en] (Accessed 15 August 2013).
32. Goyal A, Yusuf S: **The burden of cardiovascular disease in the Indian subcontinent.** *Indian J Med Res* 2006, **124:**235–244.
33. Cappuccio FP, Cook DG, Atkinson RW: **Prevalence, detection and management of cardiovascular risk factors in different ethnic groups in South London.** *Heart* 1997, **78:**553–563.
34. Joshi P, Islam S, Pais P, Reddy S, Dorairaj P, Kazmi K, Pandey MR, Haque S, Mendis S, Rangarajan S, Yusuf S: **Risk factors for early myocardial infarction in South Asians compared with individuals in other countries.** *JAMA* 2007, **297:**286–294.
35. Beckles GLA, Miller GJ, Kirkwood BR, Alexis SD, Carson DC, Byam NTA: **High total and cardiovascular disease mortality in adults of Indian descent in Trinidad, unexplained by major cardiovascular risk factors.** *Lancet* 1986, **327:**1298–1301.
36. Lee J, Heng D, Chia KS, Chew SK, Tan BY, Hughes K: **Risk factors and incident coronary heart disease in Chinese, Malay and Asian Indian males: the Singapore Cardiovascular Cohort Study.** *Intern J Epidem* 2001, **30:**983–988.
37. Rogers WJ, Canto JG, Lambrew CT, Tiefenbrunn AJ, Kinkaid B, Shoultz DA, Frederick PD, Every N, for the Investigators in the National Registry of Myocardial Infarction 1, 2, 3: **Temporal trend in the treatment of over 1.5 million patients with myocardial infarction in the US from 1990 through 1999.** *J Am Coll Cardiol* 2000, **36:**2056–2063.
38. Steg PG, Goldberg RJ, Gore JM, Fox KAA, Eagle KA, Sadiq I, Kasper R, Rushton-Mellor SK, Anderson FA: **Baseline characteristics, management practices, and in-hospital outcomes of patients hospitalized with acute coronary syndromes in the Global Registry of Acute Coronary Events (GRACE).** *Am J of Cardiol* 2002, **90**(4):358–363.
39. Avezum A, Makdisse M, Spencer F, Gore JM, Fox KAA, Montalescot G, Eagle KA, White K, Mehta RH, Knobel E, Collet JP: **Impact of age on management and outcome of acute coronary syndrome: observation from Global Registry of Acute Coronary Events (GRACE).** *Am Heart J* 2005, **149:**67–73.
40. Hasdai D, Behar S, Wallentin L, *et al*: **A prospective survey of the characteristics, treatments and outcomes of patients with acute coronary syndromes in Europe and the Mediterranean basin; the Euro Heart Survey of Acute Coronary Syndromes (Euro Heart Survey ACS).** *Eur Heart J* 2002, **23:**1190–1201.
41. Rosengren A, Wallentin L, Simoons M, Gitt AK, Behar S, Battler A, Hasdai D: **Age, clinical presentation, and outcome of acute coronary syndromes in the Euroheart acute coronary syndrome survey.** *Eur Heart J* 2006, **27:**789–795.
42. Xavier D, Pais P, Devereaux PJ, Xie CC, Prabhakaran D, Reddy KS, Gupta R, Joshi P, Kerkar P, Thanikachalam S, Haridas KK, Jaison TM, Naik S, Maity AK, Yusuf S, on behalf of the CREATE registry investigators: **Treatment and outcomes of acute coronary syndromes in India (CREATE): a prospective analysis of registry data.** *Lancet* 2008, **371:**1435–1442.
43. AlHabib KF, Hersi A, AlFaleh H, Kurdi M, Arafah M, Youssef M, AlNemer K, Bakheet A, AlQarni A, Soomro T, Taraben A, Malik A, Ahmed WH: **The Saudi Project for Assessment of Coronary Events (SPACE) registry: design and results of a phase I pilot study.** *Can J of Cardiol* 2009, **25**(7):255–258.
44. Leuzzi C, Modena MG: **Coronary artery disease: clinical presentation, diagnosis and prognosis in women.** *Nutr, Metab & Cardiovascular Diseases* 2010, **20:**426–435.
45. Laskey WK: **Editorial. Gender differences in the management of coronary artery disease; bias or good clinical judgment?** *Ann Intern Med* 1992, **116:**869–871.
46. Steingart RM, Packer M, Hamm P, Coglianee ME, Gersh B, Geltman E, Josephine S, *et al*: **Sex differences in the management of coronary artery disease.** *N Engl J Med* 1991, **325:**226–230.
47. Hochman JS, Tamis JE, Thompson TD, Weaver WD, White HD, Van De Werf F, Aylward P, Topol EJ, Califf RM, For the Global USe of Strategies to Open Occluded Coronary Arteries in Acute Coronary Syndrome. IIb. Investigator: **Sex, clinical presentation and outcome in patients with acute coronary syndromes.** *N Eng J Med* 1999, **341:**226–232.
48. Steingart RM, Forman S, Coglianese M, Bittner V, Mueller H, Frishman W, Handberg E, Gambino A, Knatterud G, Conti CR: **Factors Limiting the Enrollment of Women in a Randomized Coronary Artery Disease Trial.**

For the **ASYMPTOMATIC CARDIAC ISCHEMIA PILOT STUDY (ACIP) investigator.** *Clin Cardiology* 1996, **19:**614–618.

49. Kee CC, Jamaiyah H, Noor Safiza MN, Geeta A, Khor GL, Suzana S, Jamalludin AR, Rahmah R, Ahmad AZ, Ruzita AT, Wong NF, Ahmad Faudzi Y: **Abdominal obesity in Malaysian adults: National Health and Morbidity Survey III (NHMS III, 2006).** *Malaysian J Nutr* 2008, **14**(2):125–135.
50. Ismail MN, Chee SS, Nawawi H, Yusof K, Lim TO, James WPT: **Obesity in Malaysia.** *Obes Rev* 2002, **3:**203–208.
51. Rampal L, Rampal S, Geok LK, Zain AM, Ooyub S, Rahmat R, Ghani SN, Krishnan J: **A national study on the prevalence of obesity among 16,127 Malaysians.** *Asia Pacific J Clin Nutrition* 2007, **16**(3):561–566.
52. Wilson P, D'Agostino R, Sullivan L, Parise H, Kannel WB: **Overweight and obesity as determinants of cardiovscular risk. The Framingham Experience.** *Arch Intern Med* 2002, **162**(16):1867–1872.
53. Mottillo S, Filion KB, Genest J, Joseph L, Pilote L, Poirier P, Rinfret S, Schiffrin EL, Eisenberg MJ: **The metabolic syndrome and cardiovascular risk: a systematic review and meta-analysis.** *J Am Coll Cardiol* 2010, **56**(14):1113–1132.
54. Shehab A, Al-Dabbagh B, Almahmeed W, Bustani N, Nagelkerke N, Alnaeemi A, Alsheikh-Ali AA: **Prevalence, characteristics, and in-hospital outcomes of metabolic syndrome among patients with acute coronary syndrome in the United Arab Emirates.** *Open Cardiovasc Med J* 2012, **6:**81–87.
55. Hughes K, Yeo PPB, Lun KC, Thai AC, Sothy SP, Wang KW, Cheah JS, Phoon WO, Lim P: **Cardiovascular diseases in Chinese, Malays, and Indians in Singapore. II. Differences in risk factor levels.** *J Epid and Comm Health* 1990, **44:**29–35.
56. Collins VR, Dowse GK, Cabealawa S, Ram P, Zimmet PZ: **High mortality from cardiovascular disease and analysis of risk factors in Indian and Melanesian Fijians.** *Int J Epidemiol* 1996, **25**(1):59–69.
57. Meadows TA, Bhatt DL, Cannon CP, Gersh BJ, Röther J, Goto S, Liau C-S, Wilson PWF, Salette G, Smith SC, Steg G: **Ethnic differences in cardiovascular risks and mortality in atherothrombotic disease: Insights from the REduction of Atherothrombosis for Continued Health (REACH) Registry.** *Mayo Clin Proc* 2011, **86**(10):960–967.
58. Mather HM, Keen H: **The Southall Diabetes Survey: prevalence of known diabetes in Asians and Europeans.** *BMJ* 1985, **291:**1081–1084.
59. Wan Ahmad WA, Zambahari R, Ismail O, Sinnadurai J, Rosman A, Chin SP, Zainal Abidin I, Sim KH: **Malaysian National Cardiovascular Disease Database (NCVD) – Acute Coronary Syndrome (ACS) registry: How are we different?** *CVD Prevent and Control* 2011, **6**(3):81–89.
60. Tan CE, Tan BY, Emmanuel SC, Jacob E: **Prevalence of diabetes and ethnic differences in cardiovascular risk factors, The 1992 Singapore National Health Survey.** *Diabetes Care* 1999, **22:**241–247.
61. Esteghamati A, Abbasi M, Nakhjavani M, Yousefizadeh A, Basa AP, Afshar H: **Prevalence of diabetes and other cardiovascular risk factors in an Iranian population with acute coronary syndrome.** *Cardiovas Diabetol* 2006, **5:**15.
62. Al-Nuaim R: **High prevalence of metabolic risk factors for cardiovascular diseases among Saudi population, aged 30–64 years.** *Int J Cardiol* 1997, **62**(3):227–235.
63. Li N, Tuomilehto J, Dowse G, Virtala E, Zimmet P: **Prevalence of coronary heart disease indicated by electrocardiogram abnormalities and risk factors in developing countries.** *J Clin Epid* 1994, **47**(6):599–611.
64. Rogers W, Frederick PD, Stoehr E, Canto JG, Ornato JP, Gibson CM, Pollack CV, Gore JM, for the National Registry of Myocardial Infarction Investigators: **Trends in presenting characteristics and hospital mortality among patients with STEMI and NSTEMI in National Registry of Myocardial Infarction from 1990 to 2006.** *Am Heart J* 2008, **156:**1026–1034.
65. Mandelzweig L, Battler A, Boyko V, *et al*: **The second Euro Heart Survey on acute coronary syndromes: Characteristics, treatment, and outcome of patients with ACS in Europe and the Mediterranean Basin in 2004.** *Eur Heart J* 2006, **27:**2285–2293.
66. Yan AT, Tan M, Fitchett D, Chow CM, Fowlis RA, McAvinue TG, Roe MT, Peterson ED, Tu JV, Langer A, Goodman SG, Canadian Acute Coronary Syndromes Registry Investigators: **One-year outcome of patients after acute coronary syndrome (from the Canadian Acute Coronary Syndromes Registry).** *Am J Cardiol* 2004, **94**(1):25–29.
67. McKeigue PM, Adelstein AM, Shipley MJ, Riemersma RA, Marmot MG, Hunt SP, Butler SM, Turner PR, *et al*: **Diet and risk factors for CHD in Asian Indians in Northwest London.** *Lancet* 1985, **326**(8464):1086–1090.
68. Miller GJ, Kotecha S, Wilkinson WH, Wilkes H, Stirling Y, Sanders TAB, Broadhurst A, Allison J, Meade TW: **Dietary and other characteristics relevant for CHD in men of Indian, West Indian and European descent in London.** *Atherosclerosis* 1988, **70:**63–72.
69. Thomas I, Gupta S, Sempos C, Cooper R: **Serum lipids in Indian physicians living in the US compared to US born physicians.** *Atherosclerosis* 1986, **61:**99–106.
70. Hamm CW, Bassand JP, Agewall S, Bax J, Boersma E, Bueno H, Caso P, Dudek D, Gielen S, Huber K, Ohman M, Petrie MC, Sonntag F, Uva MS, Storey RF, Wijns W, Zahger D, The Task Force for the management of acute coronary syndromes (ACS) in patients presenting without persistent ST-segment elevation of the European Society of Cardiology (ESC): **ESC Guidelines for the management of acute coronary syndromes in patients presenting without persistent ST-segment elevation.** *Eur Heart J* 2011, **32:**2999–3054.
71. Yadav P, Joseph D, Joshi P, Sakhi P, Jha RK, Gupta J: **Clinical profile & risk factors in acute coronary syndrome.** *National J Comm Med* 2010, **1**(2):150–151.
72. Deshpandey JD, Dixit JV: **Hospital based study of clinical profile and risk factors for acute myocardial infarction.** *Indian Med Gazette* 2009, **Oct:**380–382.
73. Grines CL, Browne KF, Marco J, Rothbaum D, Stone GW, O'Keefe J, Everlie P, Donohue B, Chelliah N, Timmis GC: **A comparison of immediate angioplasty with thrombolytic therapy for acute myocardial infarction. The Primary Angioplasty in Myocardial Infarction Study Group.** *N Engl J Med* 1993, **328:**673–679.
74. Keeley EC, Boura JA, Grines CL: **Primary angioplasty versus intravenous thrombolytic therapy for acute myocardial infarction: a quantitative review of 23 randomized trials.** *Lancet* 2003, **361**(9351):13–20.
75. McNamara RL, Herrin J, Wang Y, Curtis JP, Bradley EH, Magid DJ, Rathore SS, Nallamothu BK, Peterson ED, Blaney ME, Frederick P, Krumholz HM: **Impact of delay in door-to-needle time on mortality in patients with ST-segment elevation myocardial infarction.** *Am J Cardiol* 2007, **100:**1227–1232.
76. The GUSTO investigator groups: **An international randomized trial comparing four thrombolytic strategies for acute myocardial infarction.** *N Engl J Med* 1993, **329:**673–682.
77. Sonel AF, Good CB, Mulgund J, Roe MT, Gibler WB, Smith SC, Cohen MG, Pollack CV, Ohman EM, Peterson ED, for the CRUSADE Investigators: **Racial variations in treatment and outcomes of Black and White patients with high-risk Non–ST-elevation acute coronary syndromes insights from CRUSADE (Can Rapid Risk Stratification of Unstable Angina Patients Suppress Adverse Outcomes With Early Implementation of the ACC/AHA Guidelines?).** *Circulation* 2005, **111:**1225–1232.
78. Feder G, Crook AM, Magee P, Banerjee S, Timmis AD, Hemingway H: **Ethnic differences in invasive management of coronary disease: prospective cohort study of patients undergoing angiography.** *BMJ* 2002, **324:**511–516.
79. Ford E, Newman J, Deosaransingh K: **Racial and ethnic differences in the use of cardiovascular procedures: findings from the California Cooperative Cardiovascular Project.** *Am J Public Health* 2000, **90**(7):1128–1134.
80. Bradley EH, Herrin J, Wang YF, McNamara RL, Webster TR, Magid DJ, Blaney M, Peterson ED, Canto JG, Pollack CV, Krumholz HM: **Racial and ethnic differences in time to acute reperfusion therapy for patients hospitalized with myocardial infarction.** *JAMA* 2004, **292**(13):1563–1572.
81. Peterson ED, Shaw LK, De Long ER, Pryor DB, Califf RM, Mark DB: **Racial variation in the use of coronary-revascularization procedures: are the differences real? Do they matter?** *N Eng J Med* 1997, **336:**480–486.
82. Chen J, Rathore SS, Radford MJ, Wang Y, Krumholz HM: **Racial differences in the use of cardiac catheterization after acute myocardial infarction.** *N Eng J Med* 2001, **344:**1443–1449.
83. Leape LL, Hilborne LH, Bell R, Kamberg C, Brook RH: **Underuse of cardiac procedures: Do women, ethnic minorities and the uninsured fail to receive needed revascularization?** *Ann Intern Med* 1999, **130:**183–192.
84. Cohen MG, Fonarow GC, Peterson ED, Moscucci M, Dai D, Hernandez AF, Bonow RO, Smith SC: **Racial and ethnic differences in the treatment of acute myocardial infarction. Findings from the Get With The Guidelines–Coronary Artery Disease Program.** *Circulation* 2010, **121:**2294–2301.
85. Peterson ED, Shah BR, Parsons L, Pollack CV, French WJ, Canto JG, Gibson CM, Rogers WJ, for the NRMI Investigators: **Trends in quality of care for patients with acute myocardial infarction in the National Registry of Myocardial Infarction from 1990 to 2006.** *Am Heart J* 2008, **156:**1045–1055.
86. Gibson CM: **NRMI and current treatment patterns for ST-elevation myocardial infarction.** *Am Heart J* 2004, **148:**29–33.
87. Thanavaro S, Kleiger RE, Province MA, Hubert JW, Miller JP, Krone RJ, Oliver GC: **Effect of infarct location on the in-hospital prognosis of patients with first transmural myocardial infarction.** *Circulation* 1982, **66**(4):742–747.
88. Weintraub WS, Vaccarino V: **Explaining racial disparities in coronary in women.** *Circulation* 2003, **108:**1041–1043.

89. Zhang Z, Fanf J, Gillespie C, Wang G, Hong Y, Yoon PW: **Age-specific gender differences in in-hospital mortality by type of AMI.** *Cardiol* 2012, **109**:1097–1103.
90. Ahmed E, El-Menyar A, Singh R, Al Binali HA, Al Suwaidi J: **Effect of age on clinical presentation and outcome of patients hospitalized with acute coronary syndrome: a 20-year registry in a middle eastern country.** *The Open Cardiovasc Med J* 2012, **6**:60–67.
91. Jeyamalar R: **Coronary artery disease in Malaysia: a perspective.** *Med J Malaysia* 1991, **46**(1):1–6.
92. Mehta R, Parson L, Rao S, Peterson ED, on behalf of National Registry of Myocardial Infarction (NRMI) Investigators: **Association of bleeding and In-hospital mortality in black and white patients with ST-segment-elevation myocardial infarction receiving reperfusion.** *Circulation* 2012, **125**:1727–1734.
93. Yan AT, Huynh RTYT, DeYoung P, Weeks A, Fitchett DH, Langer A, Goodman SG, for the INTERACT Investigators: **Bleeding and outcome in acute coronary syndrome: Insights from continuous electrocardiogram monitoring in the Integrilin and Enoxaparin Randomized Assessment of Acute Coronary Syndrome Treatment (INTERACT) trial.** *Am Heart J* 2008, **156**(4):769–775.
94. Mortensen J, Thygesen SS, Johnsen SP, Vinther PM, Kristensen SD, Refsgaard J: **Incidence of bleeding in 'real-life' acute coronary syndrome patients treated with antithrombotic therapy.** *Cardiology* 2008, **111**:41–46.
95. Shakir DK, Zubaid M, Al Mallah MH, Mahmeed WL, Alsheikhali AA, Singh R, Amin H, Rao N, Suwaidi JA: **Bleeding complications with acute coronary syndrome in six Middle Eastern countries.** *Acta Cardiol* 2011, **66**(2):203–211.

12

Pathological interactions between the endothelin-1 and the angiotensin-converting enzyme among Tunisian coronary patients

Abdelkader Chalghoum[1,2*], Yosri Noichri[1], Azza Dandana[1], Bruno Baudin[3], Abdelhédi Miled[1] and Salima Ferchichi[1]

Abstract

Background: The correct understanding of the biochemical and metabolic interactions between coronary risk factors contribute to the exploration of cardiovascular pathophysiology and improves therapeutic care.
The aim of this study was to explore the endothelin-1 (ET-1) concentration and the angiotensin converting enzyme (ACE) activity among Tunisian patients with coronary heart disease, and to investigate the metabolic relationships between these two markers,... and to assess the possible relationship between them and the different risk factors.
In this present study, ET-1 concentration was determined by an analytical method (High Performance Chromatography, coupled by Mass Spectrometry), ACE activity was measured by a kinetic method for patients and healthy controls. These subjects (157 patients and 142 controls) beneficed also by a biochemical exploration (lipid, apolipoproteins and glucose profiles) to quantify cardiovascular risk.

Results: A statistically significant increase of the ET-1 concentration was found among patients compared to healthy controls (15.2 ± 5.3 nM vs 7.1 ± 2.7 nM, p < 0,00001). For the ACE activity, in spite the treatment of the majority of patients (97%) with ACE inhibitors, this activity was statistically elevated in patients compared to healthy subjects (86.7 ± 25.4 IU/L vs 42.8 ± 12.1 IU/L, $p < 0.00001$).
Furthermore, a statistically positive correlation was identified between these two cardiac markers ($r = 0.68$ $p < 0.00001$).

Conclusion: The study of the metabolic relationship between the ET-1 and ACE among coronary patients reveals other therapeutics targets.

Keywords: Acute coronary syndrome, Endothelin-1, Angiotensin-converting enzyme, Risk factors, Metabolic interactions

Background

Acute Coronary Syndrome (ACS) is classified among the major cause of mortality and morbidity in the western countries. The diagnosis of this ischemic syndrome is essentially based on clinical examination (electrocardiogram), the biological examination (serum level of cardiac troponin) is used to identify the necrotic damage. This disease is multifactorial, complex and polygenic. The risk factors are varied and diversified, according to the Framingham reference study; these factors are classified into modifiable factors (smoking, arterial hypertension, diabetes, obesity ...) and un-modifiable factors (age, gender, heredity...). Atherosclerosis is the main etiology of this syndrome [1–4].

However, the endothelin-1 (ET-1) and the hyperactivity of the angiotensin- converting enzyme (ACE) are classified among the coronary "unconventional risk factors" [5–7].

ET-1 is an endothelium derived, potent vasoconstrictor peptide of 21 amino acids (2.5 kDa with a great structural homology with snake venom, the S6

* Correspondence: Abdelkader.chalghoum@yahoo.fr
[1]Laboratory of Biochemistry, Farhat HACHED Hospital, Street Doctor Moreau, 4000 Sousse, Tunisia
[2]Valorization and Technology Transfer Space, Center of Biotechnology of Borj Cedria, 2050 HamamLif, Tunisia
Full list of author information is available at the end of the article

sarafotoxin). It was finally isolated and sequenced from endothelial cell culture by Yanagisiwa M. in 1988. Its peptide is strongly implicated in the ACS's genesis and complications by its vasoconstrictors, pro-oxidant and thrombotic effects [7–9].

ACE (peptidyl-dipeptidase with zinc, EC, 3,4,15,1) is well known by its physiological role in the rennin angiotensin system by its role in angiotensin-I cleaving (an inactive decapeptide) to generate angiotensin II (a powerful vasoconstrictor) and its role in bradykinin hydrolysis (a potent vasodilatator). This enzyme stimulates also the release of aldosterone from the adrenal cortex, leading to sodium retention [10–12].

In this context, comes the aim of our study which is to quantify the serum concentrations of ET-1 and to measure the ECA serum activity in Tunisians coronary compared to controls subjects, investigate the impact of various risk factors on serum variation of these two parameters as well as the study of the correlation between these two vasoconstrictors.

Methods

Populations study

This is a prospective study, in which sampling was carried between January 2010 and November 2011. One hundred fifty seven Tunisian coronary patients (121 men and 36 women) middle-aged (64.8 ± 11.7 years) were recruited from the Cardiology Service of Farhat Hached, Hospital of Sousse, Tunisia. One hundred forty two healthy subjects (111 men and 31 women) middle-aged (56.8 ± 9.4 years) were considered as the control group. This age difference is unavoidable, since at a more advanced age, the risk factors accumulate, and the possibility to find healthy subjects non carriers of any risk factor becomes almost impossible (since the advanced age it is even a risk factor). So we were here between two choices: either having patients and "healthy subjects" holders of risk factors with a close age, or having a remarkable difference (not significant) of age and healthy controls without risk factors.

The patients and healthy subjects signed a free and clear consent which explains the objectives of this work with an undertaking not to publish the names of participants, their personal data including test results (following the instructions of Tunisian National Committee of Medical Ethics, consistent with the Declaration of Helsinki).

The approval of compliance with the Helsinki declaration was signed in December 2009. A datasheet had been prepared for each subject (patient or control) to identify cardiovascular risk factors and to know the susceptibility degrees to ACS. This sheet contains the anthropometric characteristics, the biological parameters, the risk factors, the treatments of patients, the exclusion factors (thyroid diseases, sarcoidosis, Gaucher disease).

Laboratory analysis

Venous blood samples were drawn after 12 h overnight fast. A collection of two tubes were made for each patient and witness: one tube without anticoagulant for determination lipid parameters, ET-1 concentration, and ACE activity and, the second one is heparinized tube for blood glucose. Serum total cholesterol (TC), triglycerides (TG), high density lipoprotein cholesterol (HDL-C) and glucose were measured with colorimetric essay using an automated system (Cx9 Pro-Beckman Coulter-Fuller-Ton CA). Low density lipoprotein cholesterol (LDL-C) was determined by Friedewald formula for TG levels below 4.5 mmol/L. Apolipoproteins (ApoA1 and Apo B) were determined by immunonephelometry (Cobas Integra 400, Roche).

After plasmatic ET-1 extraction with ethanol, the concentration was measured by High Performance Chromatography, coupled to Mass Spectrometry (3200 Q TRAP LC/MS/MS system),according the Walczak M protocol, 2010 [9],using a synthetic standard (ET-1 Sigma-Aldrich St. Louis, MO, USA) for the specific spectra identification and for the calibration curve determining. Chromatographic separation was carried out with C18 analytical column (30 mm x 2.1 mm, 3.5 µm, Waters Ireland) set at 20 °C. Two solvents mixtures were used: solvent A: Acetonitrile and solvent B: H_2O. The following gradient was used: 0–5 min 0–100% A; 5–7 min 100% A; 7–8, 100–0% A; 8–15 min, 100% B. The flow rate was set at 300 $\mu l min^{-1}$ and a sample volume of 25 µl was injected in the analytical column. The linearity zone (1.6 nM - 160 nM) is established after calibrationby a purified bovine serum (with 3 repetitions for each concentration)

ACE activity was determined by kinetic method at 340 nm, according the Chalghoum A protocol, 2012 [4], using a synthetic substrate, Furylacryloyl-phenylalanyl–glycyl-glycine (FAPGG) (Trinity Biotech,St Louis USA), with an initial measurement at $t = 0$ min and a final measurement at $t = 5$ min.

Statistical analysis

Database management and statistical analyseswere carried out using SPSS (**S**tatistical **P**ackage forthe **S**ociological **S**ciences), version 21.0 (IBM). Results are presented as means ± SD, or percentages. Means were compared using Student test. The relations between variables were assessed with Pearson's correlation analysis.

These parametric tests (means comparison, statistical correlations) were performed under of the analytical statistics conditions (Gaussian dispersion for the different parameters, $n \geq 30$ for each group and subgroup...). The significance threshold was set at 5% ($p < 0.05$).

Results

Table 1 summarizes the anthropometric and clinical data of patients and health subjects. Hypertension, diabetes, obesity, tobacco, heredity... are the majors risk factors. However our control subjects are not exposed to these factors

Biological parameters and the values of ET-1 and ACE in patients and controls subjects are shown in Table 2.

Glucose, TC, LDL-C,and apolipoprotein B(Apo B) were significantly increased in patients compared to controls. Unlike apolipoprotein A1 concentration was significantly higher among control group compared to patients. HDL-C, and TG showed no significant difference between two populations.

Figure 1 illustrates the mass spectra of the ET-1 peptide, triply ionized, 832.4 Da (M / Z).

In our study, a statistically significant elevation of the ET-1 concentration was observed among patients compared to healthy subjects. For the ACE activity, although the majority of our patients (97%) were treated with ACE inhibitors, this activity was statistically elevated in patients compared to controls subjects.

Table 1 Anthropometric characteristics and clinical data of patients and control subjects

	Patients (n = 157)	Control subjects (n = 142)
Age (x ± σ years)	64.8 ± 11.7	56.8 ± 9.4
Sex		
Men (%)	121 (77%)	111 (78.2%)
Women (%)	36 (23%)	31 (21.8%)
BMI (kg /m^2)	27.6 ± 4	23.3 ± 2.2
Hypertension (%)	88	0
Obesity (%)	52	8.5%
Diabetes (%)	64	0
Smoking (%)	62.4	7
Family cardiachistory (%)	68	6
Personnel cardiachistory (%)	66	0
Postmenopausal women (%)	100	82
Dyslipidemia (%)	40	0
Sedentary (%)	43	11
Alcohol (%)	33	14
Treatment : ACE inhibitors (%)	97	0
Statins (%)	38	0
Beta-Blockers (%)	33	
Ca-Blockers (%)	27	0
Diuretics (%)	17	0

X mean
σ standard deviation
BMI Body mass index

Table 2 The distribution of biological markers, ET-1 concentration and ACE activity in patients and control subjects

Populations Biological parameters	Patients (n = 157)	Control subjects (n = 142)	p
Glucose (x ± σmmolL/)	9.8 ± 4.2	5.40 ± 0.84	<0000.1
TC (x ± σmmol/L)	5.70 ± 3.1	4.60 ± 2.6	<0.00
HDL-C (x ± σmmol/L)	1.14 ± 0.22	1.30 ± 0.41	NS
LDL-C (x ± σmmol/L)	3.60 ± 2.16	2.80 ± 1.4	<0.001
TG (x ± σmmol/L)	1.60 ± 0.9	1.24 ± 0.3	NS
ApoA1 (x ± σ. g/L)	1.41 ± 0.62	1.80 ± 0.2	<0000.1
ApoB (x ± σ. g/L)	1.40 ± 0.81	0.70 ± 0.2	<0000.1
ET-1 (x ± σ. nM)	15.2 ± 5.3	7.1 ± 2.7	<0.00001
ACE (x ± σ. UI/L)	86.7 ± 25.4	42.8 ± 12.1	<0.00001

NS not significant ($p > 0.05$)
X mean
σ standard deviation
TC Total cholesterol
HDL-C high density lipoprotein cholesterl
LDL-C low density lipoprotein cholesterol
TG triglycerides
ApoA Apolipoprotein A
ApoB Apolipoprotein B
ET-1 Endothelin-1
ACE Angiotensin-converting enzyme

Biochemical exploration showed that these two vasoconstrictors depend on gender, arterial hypertension, tobacco, obesity and dyslipidemia, unlike diabetes, Personal cardiovascular antecedents, alcohol intake and physical inactivity (Tables 3 and 4).

Besides to that, a positive statistically correlation was founded ($r = 0.68$ $p < 0.00001$) between the ET-1 concentration and ACE activity (Fig. 2).

Discussion

Varied risk factors among patients confirm the multifactorial and polygenic origin of the ACS, well explained by the Framingham study [13, 14]. Partially balanced lipid profile in patients is caused by the diet, recommended by medical staff, by lipid-lowering therapy and in particular by the beneficial impact of the ACE inhibitors that enhance of the glucose sensitivity and the correction of lipid metabolism [14, 15].

Increased concentration of apolipoprotein B consolidates its atherogenic effects and its involvement in the genesis of ACS, although the majority of patients are under statins and anti-hypertensive medication. Unlike reversible dyslipidemia (only related to diet and lifestyle), easy to corrected by statins, mixed and genetic dyslipidemia requires a combined medication (statins + fibrates, or nicotinic acid) whereas Apo A1 (statistically higher in healthy croup) has acardio-protective effect supported by various studies. These apolipoproteins are under genetic control which showed the polygenic origin of ACS [4, 14, 16].

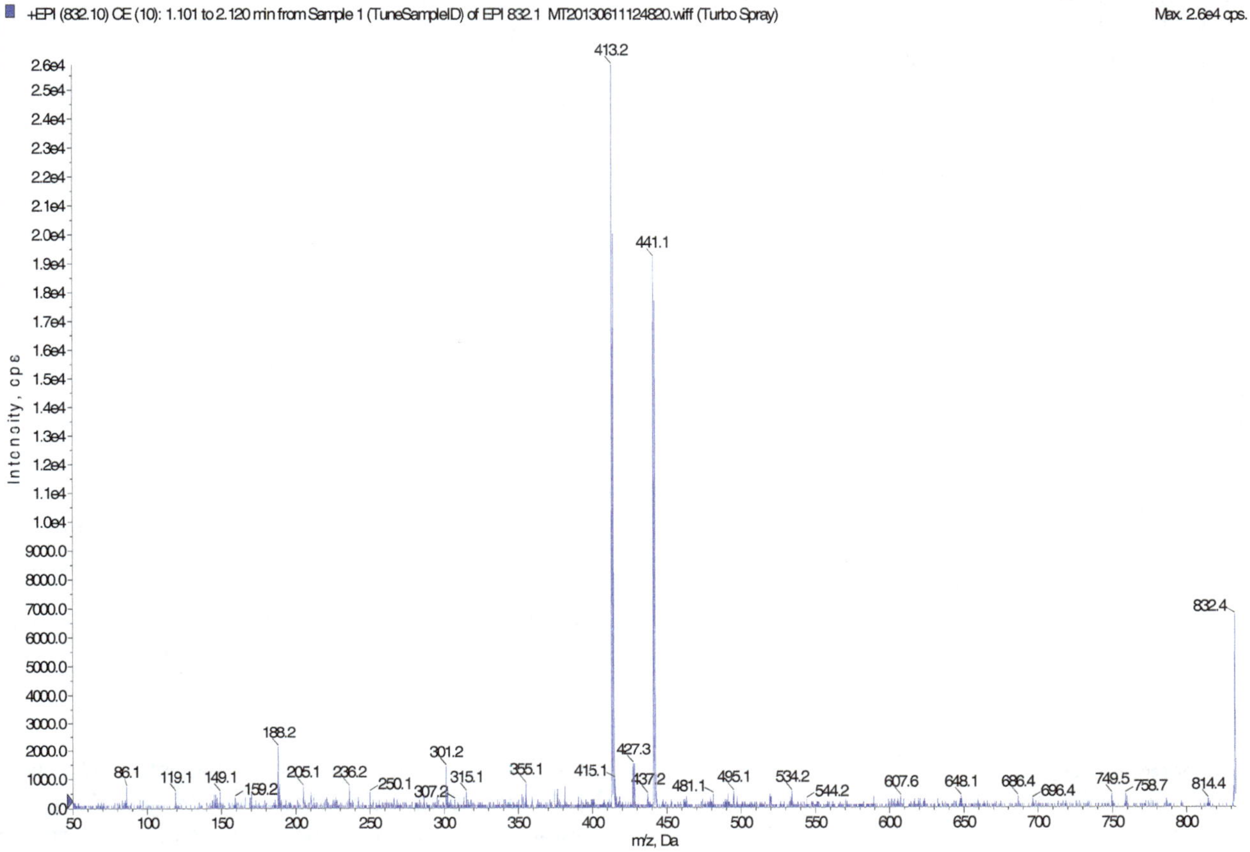

Fig. 1 The mass spectra presentation of the ET-1 peptide, triply ionized, with a peak of 832.4 Da (M / Z)

Furthermore, our study showed a statistically significant increase in the ET-1 values among patients compared to control subjects, which reflects its role not only in prolonged vasoconstriction but also in its atherogenic impact, its pro-oxidant effect (indirectly involved in the NADPH oxidase activation and radical oxygen species generation) and its pro-aggregating role (by his role in the thromboxane A2 synthesis). [8, 9, 16–18].

Although, 97% patients were under treatment with inhibitors of angiotensin-I converting enzyme, this enzyme activity was statistically higher among patients, reflecting the involvement of ACE as risk parameters for heart diseases. This role is well described in the literature and explained mainly by hypertensive and vasoconstrictor effects of this zinc-metallopeptidase. Recent studies also have been beginning the study of pro-oxidant role of this enzyme by activation of NADPH oxidase which triggers lipid peroxidation starting point for atherosclerosis. Actually vasoconstrictor and pro-oxidant effects accumulate in the pathophysiology of atherosclerosis and coronary syndromes [10, 11, 18]·

The ET-1 concentration and the ACE activity dependent, in this study on gender, hypertension, smoking,obesity and dyslipidemia, unlike diabetes, Personal cardiovascular antecedents, alcohol and physical inactivity.

The increasing concentration of ET-1 and the higher activity of the ACE in men patients is explained by hormonal and metabolic reasons (non-genetic) since they are encoded by two autosomal genes (6p24.1 for ET-1 and 17q23 for ACE), unlike the angiotensin-2 converting enzyme encoded by a gene located on the X chromosome. According to the reference Framingham study, women are protected against cardiovascular complications compared to men, this protection is manifested by blocking and inhibiting of atherogenic factors (including ET-1 and ACE) [19, 20].

The concentration and high activity in hypertensive compared with normotensive patients is explained by the vasoconstrictor effect of ET-1 and ECA and their roles in the sodium reabsorption. In hyperactivity these regulatory effects become hypertensive [9, 21, 22].

The ET-1 and the ACE inhibitions by tobacco, obesity and dyslipidemia are explained by the role of metabolic syndrome, generated by tobacco (mainly nicotine), complex lipids (among obese and dyslipidemic coronary patients). The metabolic syndrome is directly and indirectly associated with damage of the endothelial tissue, major secretory of ET-1 and ACE [23–27].

Table 3 The variation of the ET-1 concentration among patients according risk factors

Populations and risk factors	ET-1 (nM/L)		p
Gender	Men (n = 121)	17.4 ± 4.6	<0.00001
	Women (n = 36)	7.8 ± 2.3	
Hypertension	Yes (n = 138)	16.4 ± 3.3	<0.00001
	No (n = 19)	6.6 ± 1.9	
Diabetes	Yes (n = 101)	15 ± 5.1	NS
	No (n = 56)	15.6 ± 3.8	
Tobacco	Yes (n = 98)	11.6 ± 3	<0.00001
	No (n = 59)	21.2 ± 6.1	
Personal cardiovascular antecedents	Yes (n = 104)	15.3 ± 4.4	NS
	No (n = 53)	15 ± 2.8	
Obesity	Yes (n = 82)	12.2 ± 5.3	<0.001
	No (n = 75)	18.2 ± 4	
Dyslipidemia	Yes (n = 63)	11.8 ± 1.6	<0.00001
	No (n = 94)	17 .5 ± 4.6	
Alcohol	Yes (n = 52)	16 ± 4.1	NS
	No (n = 105)	14.8 ± 3.8	
Sedentarity	Yes (n = 67)	15.7 ± 3.7	NS
	No (n = 90)	14.9 ± 2.4	

NS not significant ($p > 0.05$)

Table 4 The variation of the ACE activity among patients according risk factors

Populations and risk factors	ACE (UI/L)		p
Gender	Men (n = 121)	88 ± 26.1	<0.001
	Women (n = 36)	82.4 ± 3.8	
Hypertension	Yes (n = 138)	91.8 ± 24.7	<0.00001
	No (n = 19)	49.9 ± 8.6	
Diabetes	Yes(n = 101)	86.1 ± 24.4	NS
	No (n = 56)	87.8 ± 28.2	
Tobacco	Yes(n = 98)	71.8 ± 20.1	<0.00001
	No (n = 59)	111.5 ± 27.2	
Personal cardiovascular antecedents	Yes (n = 104)	88.2 ± 26.6	NS
	No (n = 53)	83.8 ± 24.3	
Obesity	Yes(n = 82)	80.2 ± 21.4	<0.001
	No (n = 75)	93.8 ± 27.4	
Dyslipidemia	Yes(n = 63)	80.6 ± 19.7	<0.001
	No (n = 94)	90.8 ± 28.7	
Alcohol	Yes (n = 52)	85.9 ± 25.2	NS
	No (n = 105)	87.1 ± 25.9	
Sedentarity	Yes(n = 67)	87.3 ± 24.9	NS
	No (n = 90)	86.3 ± 25.6	

NS not significant ($p > 0.05$)

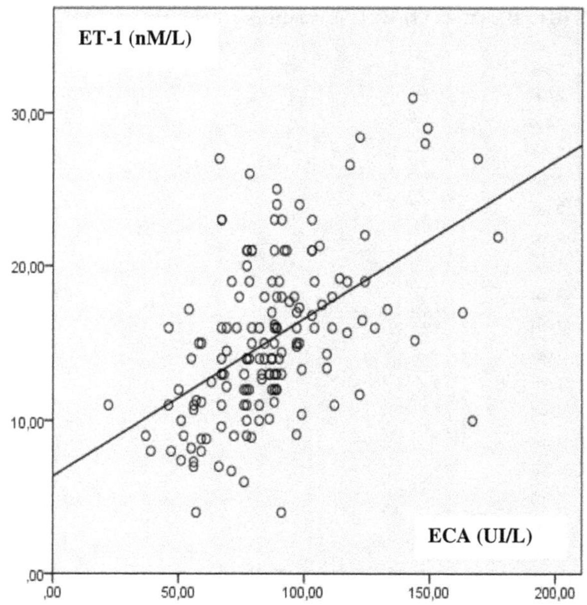

Fig. 2 The positive correlation between ET-1 concentration and ACE activity in patients population ($r = 0.68$, $p < 0.00001$)

The high percentage of diabetic patients (64%) shows the impact of this risk factor in the genesis, pathophysiology and complications of ACS, manifested at different levels (oxidative and inflammation status, metabolic and thrombotic disorders...) [24].

However, diabetes was not implicated in the change of plasmatic ET-1 and ACE activity and complications of metabolic syndrome due to the used of drug and the recommended diet [24, 25].

The difference between patients with and without cardiovascular antecedents for the two parameters is not significant given the short half time life of ET-1 and ACE, drug interactions and instant regulation of these parameters (which reaches their the highest levels during the acute phase) [7, 11, 22].

Statistically positive correlation between ET-1 concentration and ECA activity is explained by the inductive effect of the angiotensin II (generated by the ACE) in the synthesis of ET-1 and thecommon activation axis of vasoconstrictors (hypovolemia, intervention ofbaro-receptors...). This activation escapes from the regulation in these pathological situations [28–31].

A multidisciplinary study that combines the interactions between enzymes and predictive peptides according the rupture and the size of the atherosclerotic plaque (measured by appropriate technical, Optical coherence tomography) can better elucidate the complex pathophysiology of ACS and more targeted the treatment [30, 32].

Conclusion

Our study shows the impact of the ET-1 higher concentration and the ACE higher activity in the ACS predisposition and pathophysiology, seen their vasoconstrictors, pro-oxidant and pro-aggregation roles. A thorough study of each component seems important to give other therapeutic targets (ET-1 inhibitors by analogy to ACE inhibitors...). Besides to that, the study of molecular and genomics interactions between these two cardiovascular markers aim to elucidate the different metabolic cascades (activation and braking).

Abbreviations

ACE: Angiotensin-converting enzyme; ACS: Acute coronary syndrome; Apo A: Apolipoprotein A1; Apo B: Apolipoprotein B; ET-1: Endothelin-1 SPSS: Statistical package for the sociological sciences

Acknowledgments

We thank so much Mrs Ines KARKOUCH, Dr. Lamjed BOUSLAMA,and Mrs. Fatma LAZREG (English teacher), Pr. Guieder Jeridi the responsible for the ethical side of the work, the consent of patients and provided us with the clinical data and a history of each patient. We thank also the staff of the Biochemistry Laboratory and the Cardiology Department of Farhat Hached, Hospital of Sousse and the members of the platform of the Biotechnology Center of Borj Cedria,Tunisia for their valuable contribution in this work.

Funding

Our study was funded by research organizations in Tunisia (Ministry of Public Health and Ministry of Higher Education and Scientific Research) with a scientific and financial cooperation of the Laboratory of Biochemistry "A" Hospital Saint Antoine, Paris, France.

Authors' contributions

AC and YN realized of this work, patients and controls sampling, writing experimental protocols, the writing of the article and statistical analysis. BB prepared ET-1 analysis by HPLC/MS. AD and AM is responsible for apolipoproteins measurements and orientation of the results discussion. SF is the scientific director of the team that supervised and corrected the article. All authors approved the final manuscript.

Competing interests

The authors proclaim that they have no competing interests.

Author details

[1]Laboratory of Biochemistry, Farhat HACHED Hospital, Street Doctor Moreau, 4000 Sousse, Tunisia. [2]Valorization and Technology Transfer Space, Center of Biotechnology of Borj Cedria, 2050 HamamLif, Tunisia. [3]Department of Biochemistry, Saint-Antoine Hospital, 184 Street Faubourg Saint-Antoine, 75571 Paris, Cedex 12, France.

References

1. Veeranna V, Zalawadiya SK, Niraj A, Kumar A, Ference B, Afonso L. Association of level biomarkers with failure cardiovascular events is influenced by ethnicity: Result from a multi ethnic cohort. Int J Cardiol. 2013;166:487–93.
2. Reddy KS, Satija A. The Framingham heart study: Impact of the prevention and control of cardiovascular disease in India. Prog Cardiovasc Dis. 2010;53:21–7.
3. Bello N, Mosca L. Epidemiology of coronary heart disease in women. Prog Cardiovasc Dis. 2004;46:287–95.
4. Chalghoum A, Noichri Y, Chkioua L, Gammoudi I, Dandana A, Khelil S, et al. Metabolic interactions betweenthe hyperhomocysteinemia and angiotensin-1 converting enzymeactivity in Tunisian patients with coronary heart disease. Ann Biol Clin. 2012;70(5):599–604.
5. Jordan W, Reinbacher A, Cohrs S, Grunewald RW, Mayer G, Rüther E, et al. Obstructive sleep openea: Plasma endothelin-1 precursor but not endothelin-1 levels are elevated and decline with nasal continues positive airway pressure. Peptides. 2005;26:1654–60.
6. Tjam EY, Heckman GA, Smith S, Arai B, Hirdes J, Poss J, et al. Predicting heart failure mortality in frail seniors: Comparing the NYHA functional classification with the Resident Assessment Instrument (RAI) 2.0. Int J Cardiol. 2012;155:75–80.
7. Yanagisawa M, Inoue A, Ishikawa T, Kasuya Y, Kimura S, Kumagaye S, et al. Primary structure, synthesis, and biological activity of rat endothelin, an endothelium-derived vasoconstrictor peptide. Proc Natl Acad Sci. 1988;85:6964–7.
8. Yanagisawa M, Masaki T. Endothelin, a novel endothelium-derived peptide. Pharmacological activities, regulation and possible roles in cardiovascular control. Biochem Pharmacol. 1989;38(12):1877–83.
9. Walczak M, Fedorowicz A, Chłopicki S, Szymura-Oleksiak J. Determination of endothelin-1 in rats using a high-performance liquidchromatography coupled to electrospray tandem mass spectrometry. Talanta. 2010;82:710–8.
10. Akif M, Masuyer G, Schwager SL, Bhuyan BJ, Mugesh G, Isaac RE, et al. Structural characterization of angiotensin 1 converting enzyme in complex with a selenium analogue of captopril. FEBS J. 2011;278:3644–50.
11. Baudin B. New aspects on angiotensin-converting enzyme: from gene to disease. Clin Chem Lab Med. 2002;40:256–65.
12. Danilov SM, Kalinin S, Chen Z, Vinokour EI, Nesterovitch B, Schwartz E, et al. Angiotensin 1-converting enzyme Gln1069 Mutation impairs trafficking to the cell surface resulting in selective denaturation of the cell surface resulting in selective denaturation of the C Domain. PLOS One. 2010;10:10438–53.
13. Frohlich J, Sarraf AA. Cardiovascular risk and atherosclerosis prevention. Cardiovasc Path. 2013;22:16–8.
14. Hrira MY, Kerkeni M, Hamda BK, Chahed H, Ferchichi S, Addad F, et al. Apolipoprotein A-I, apolipoprotein B, high-sensitivity C-reactive protein and severity of coronary artery disease in Tunisian population. Cardiovasc Path. 2012;21:455–60.
15. Schen AJ. Renin-angiotensin system inhibition prevents type 2 diabetesmellitus. Diabetes Metab. 2004;30:498–506.
16. Demacker PN, Veerkamp MJ, Bredie SJ, Marcovina SM, de Graaf J, Stalenhoef AF. Comparison of the measurement of lipids and lipoproteins versus essay of apolipoprotein B for estimation of coronary heart disease: a study in familial combined hyperlipemia. Atherosclerosis. 2000;153:483–90.
17. Špinarová L, Špinar J, Vašků A, Goldbergová M, Ludka O, Toman J, et al. Big endothelin in chronic heart failure: marker of disease severity or genetic determination? Int J Cardiol. 2004;93:63–8.
18. Zhao W, Zhao D, Yan R, Sun Y. Cardiac oxidative stress and remodeling following infraction: role of NADPH oxidase. Cardiovasc Path. 2009;18:156–66.
19. Majed B, Tafflet M, Kee F, Haas B, Ferrieres J, Montaye M, et al. External validation of the 2008 Framingham cardiovascular risk equation for CHD and stroke events in a European population of middele-aged men. The PRIME study. Prev Med. 2013;57:49–54.
20. Russ TC, Hamer M, Stamatakis E, Starr JM, Batty GD, Kivimäki M. Does the Framingham cardiovascular disease risk score also have predictive utility for dementia death? An individual individual participant meta-analysis of 11,887 men and women. Atherosclerosis. 2013;228:256–8.
21. Gracoweski L, Stauke F, Bessard G. Endothelin-1 and cardiovascularpathology. Rev Med Interne. 1999;20:589–99.
22. Blaidi E, Ribulot DG. The endothelin system: Its involvement in the cardiovascular system. Rev Med Interne. 2010;31:792–4.
23. Matsuda M, Shimomura I. Increased oxidative stress in obesity: Implication for metabolic syndrome, diabetes, hypertension, dyslipidemia, atherosclerosis and cancer. Obes Res Clin Protect. 2013;7:330–41.
24. Kyriakides ZS, Kremastinos DT, Raptis AE, Johnston N, Raptis SA, Webb DJ, et al. Impaired effect of endothelin-1 on coronary artery stiffness in type 2

diabetes. Int J Cardiol. 2006;112:207–12.

25. Mehri S, Koubaa N, Nakbi A, Hammami S, Chaaba R, Mahjoub S, et al. Relationship between genetic polymorphism of angiotensin-converting enzyme and methylenetetrahydrofolate reductase as risk factors for type 2 diabetes in Tunisian patients. Clin Biochem. 2010;43:259–66.
26. Rashtchizadeh N, Aghaeishahsavari M, Argani H, Noroozianavval M, Veisi P, Ghorbanihaghjo A. Enalapril and lozarton effect lipids peroxidationin renal transplant recipients with renin angiotensin system polymorphism. Clin Biochem. 2007;40:194–200.
27. Kawada T, Andou T, Fukumitsu M. Metabolic syndrome showed significant relationship with carotid atherosclerosis. Heart Vessels. 2015;30:664–70.
28. Larson A, Witman MA, Guo Y, Ives S, Richardson RS, Bruno RS, et al. Acute, quercetin-induced reductions in blood pressure in hypertensive individuals are not secondary to lower plasma angiotensin-converting enzyme activity or endothelin-1: nitric oxide. Nut Res. 2012;32:557–64.
29. Chalghoum A, Noichri Y, Chkioua L, Gammoudi I, Dandana A, Chahed H, et al. Study of the intronic polymorphism of the angiotensin 1 converting enzyme among Tunisianscoronary. Ann Cardiol Angiol. 2011;60:135–40.
30. Ogoh S, Brothers RM, Barnes Q, Eubank WL, Hawkins MN, Purkayastha S, O-Yurvati A, Raven PB. Effects of changes in central blood volume on carotid-vasomotor baroreflexsensitivity at rest and during exercise. J Appl Physio. 2006;101:68–75.
31. Chalghoum A, Noichri Y, Karkouch I, Dandana A, Baudin B, Jeridi G, et al. Metabolic interactions between hyperhomocysteinemia and endothelin-1 among Tunisian patients with acute coronary diseases. Biol Res. 2015;48:32–8.
32. Iannaccone M, D'Ascenzo F, Templin C, Omedè P, Montefusco A, Guagliumi G et al. Prevalence and predictors of culprit plaque rupture at OCT in patients with coronary artery disease: a meta-analysis. Eur Heart J. 2016 doi: 10.1093/ehjci/jev283

C-Reactive protein reactions to glucose-insulin-potassium infusion and relations to infarct size in patients with acute coronary syndromes

Hadeel Alkofide[1,2], Gordon S. Huggins[3], Joni R. Beshansky[4,5], Robin Ruthazer[4,6], Inga Peter[7], Madhab Ray[1], Jayanta T. Mukherjee[1,6] and Harry P. Selker[4,6*]

Abstract

Background: Some benefits of glucose-insulin-potassium (GIK) in patients with acute coronary syndromes (ACS) may be from an anti-inflammatory effect. The primary aim of this study was to assess the impact of GIK administration early in the course of ACS on inflammatory marker C-reactive protein (CRP) levels. A secondary aim was to investigate the association between CRP and 30-day infarct size.

Methods and Results: Retrospective analysis of participants with ACS randomly assigned to GIK or placebo for at least 8 h in the IMMEDIATE Trial biological mechanism cohort ($n = 143$). High sensitivity CRP (hs-CRP) was measured at emergency department presentation, and 6 and 12 h into infusion. Logarithmically transformed hs-CRP values at 12-hours were lower with GIK vs. placebo (mean =0.65 mg/L in GIK, 0.84 mg/L in placebo), with a marginal trend toward significance ($P = 0.053$). Furthermore, using mixed models of hs-CRP, time, and study group, there was a significant increase in hs-CRP levels over time, but the rate of change did not differ between treatment arms ($P = 0.3$). Multivariable analysis showed that an elevation in hs-CRP, measured at 12 h, was an independent predictor of 30-day infarct size (β coefficient, 6.80; $P = 0.04$) using sestamibi SPECT imaging.

Conclusions: The results of this study show no significant effect of GIK on hs-CRP. In addition our results show that in patients with ACS, hs-CRP measured as early as 12 h can predict 30-day infarct size.

Keywords: Acute coronary syndromes, Glucose-insulin-potassium (GIK), Inflammation, C-reactive protein, Metabolic therapy

Backgrounds

Glucose -insulin-potassium (GIK) infusion as metabolic therapy can reduce damage to myocardial cells in the setting of ischemia or infarction [1–4]. Since its introduction in the early 1960s [5], GIK treatment has been assessed in both animal models and human studies. However, the role of GIK in patients with acute myocardial infarction (MI) remains controversial. While several clinical trials have shown no benefit of GIK treatment in patients with acute MI [6–10], other studies have reported benefit [11–15]. Most recently, the IMMEDIATE (Immediate Myocardial Metabolic Enhancement During Initial Assessment and Treatment in Emergency care) Trial failed to show significant differences in the outcome of progression to MI among patients presenting with acute coronary syndromes (ACS); but it did show that GIK was associated with lower rates of the composite outcome of cardiac arrest and/or in-hospital mortality, and with smaller infarct size [15]. The IMMEDIATE Trial is distinguished from other trials by the early administration of GIK prior to arrival at the hospital [15]. In previous studies, GIK administration was delayed until hospital admission [6–10], with a median time of

* Correspondence: hselker@tuftsmedicalcenter.org
[4]Center for Cardiovascular Health Services Research, Institute for Clinical Research and Health Policy Studies, Tufts Medical Center, Boston, MA, USA
[6]Tufts Clinical and Translational Science Institute, Tufts University, Boston, MA, USA
Full list of author information is available at the end of the article

6 h from symptom onset to GIK initiation in one study [9].

While the mechanisms underlying GIK's effects in patients with ACS are unknown, several pathways have been suggested, including a metabolic pathway by promoting of glycolysis, and reducing circulating free fatty acid (FFA) levels, and through anti-inflammatory effects [16–18]. Inflammation contributes to myocardial damage in ischemia, infarction, and reperfusion [19]. The acute phase reactant C-reactive protein (CRP) is released in response to inflammation in chronic coronary artery disease and in acute MI [19]. High CRP levels after acute MI predict infarct expansion and plaque rupture [20–22]. Whereas a reduction in the rise of CRP levels has been shown to indicate the efficacy of thrombolytic therapy and a patent infarct-related coronary artery [23, 24]. Continued elevations in CRP portend increased risk of mortality, even in the presence of currently available therapies for ACS [25].

In the setting of ACS, GIK has been demonstrated to reduce serum markers of inflammation, including CRP in one study [18] but not in others [26, 27]. Here, in the largest study to date of very early administration of GIK for ACS, the IMMEDIATE Trial, we tested the hypothesis that GIK was associated with smaller CRP elevations compared to those treated with placebo. Related to this, we further hypothesized that the changes in CRP levels following presentation with an ACS correlate with 30-day infarct size.

Methods

Study sample

This study analyzed data collected from participants enrolled in the IMMEDIATE Trial, the methodology of which has been published elsewhere [15]. In brief, it was a randomized, placebo-controlled, double-blind clinical effectiveness trial of GIK, from December 2006 through July 2011, in which paramedics, aided by electrocardiograph (ECG)-based decision support, randomized and enrolled 871 participates aged ≥30 years with high probability of ACS [15]. Participants were given either the GIK solution (30 % glucose, 50 U/L of regular insulin, and 80 mEq of KCl/L) intravenously at 1.5 mL/kg/h for 12 h, or an identical-appearing placebo as 5 % glucose solution. In the study, the median time from symptom onset to initiation of infusion was 90 min [15]. This investigation was based on the IMMEDIATE Trial biological mechanism cohort ("biocohort"), which comprised of participants who consented to participate in this biocohort, confirmed as having ACS, and treated for at least 8 h with study drug. Confirmed ACS (acute MI or angina pectoris) was determined by site investigator review and then independently adjudicated by the study clinical events committee who were blinded to study group, glucose, and potassium results. Enrolment in the biocohort began after the trial was started and only included 6 out of 13 study centers. The study protocol and analyses were approved by the Tufts Institutional Review Board (IRB) and by the IRBs responsible for each of the IMMEDIATAE Trial study sites.

Data collection

During the 12-hour infusion of study drug, glucose, insulin, FFA, and high sensitivity CRP (hs-CRP) levels were tested at three times: 1) the initial measurement, which was drawn as soon as feasible after hospital arrival; 2) 6 h after start of study drug; and 3) 12 h after start of study drug, or upon discontinuation of the infusion. Hemoglobin A1C was measured on admission and at 30 days, and infarct size was measured at 30 days by sestamibi SPECT imaging. The Trial's core laboratory interpreted the nuclear studies, and the core laboratory of Tufts Clinical and Translational Science Institute performed the hs-CRP measurements. Other covariates measured in the biocohort include demographic data, vital signs, medical history, and medications used at home, in the hospital, or upon discharge.

Data analysis

Statistical analyses were performed using R, version 2.15.2. Descriptive statistics were used to describe baseline characteristics. All tests were two-sided, using alpha <0.05 to determine statistical significance. Serum hs-CRP levels ranged widely and their distribution was highly skewed to lower levels; therefore hs-CRP concentrations were logarithmically (base 10) transformed in all further analyses. Linear regression models were used to assess the relationship between initial hs-CRP measurements and baseline characteristics; variables significantly associated with initial hs-CRP levels were adjusted-for in the analysis. The independent sample t-test was used to detect unadjusted differences in cross-sectional hs-CRP levels between GIK and placebo. In addition, using independent sample t-test, the differences between the initial and 12-hour hs-CRP measurements (delta hs-CRP) were used to assess differences by treatment arm. A mixed model was used to detect the differential effect of treatment on the rate of change in the initial, 6-, and 12-hour hs-CRP levels, adjusting for baseline and clinical characteristics associated with initial hs-CRP measurement, and accounting for repeated measures on each participant at the different time points. We also adjusted for time from symptom onset to reperfusion therapy. The linear mixed model uses a random intercept for each subject, and for within-subject correlation. The model included terms for time, from the initiation of infusion (real-time as a continuous measurement), and an interaction term between study drug and time, in order to estimate the association between treatment arms and change in the inflammatory marker over the follow-up time points. Sensitivity analysis was done by stratifying participants based on ACS diagnosis (i.e. acute MI compared to unstable angina), and by the use of statins prior to enrollment in the study.

Univariate and multivariable linear regression models were used to study the association between hs-CRP levels at the three time points (as the predictor) and infarct size (as the outcome), after adjustment for potential confounders including age, gender, and those correlated with infarct size in univariate models at a *p*-value of < 0.1. Infarct sizes ranged from 0 to 59 % of left ventricular mass, where 0 % represent those who did not develop an infarct, and 59 % was assigned to those who died ($n = 4$) before imaging, based on the fact that the largest infarct size measured in the study was 58 %. In addition, correlations between hs-CRP at the initial, 6-, and 12-hour determinations and infarct size were assessed using Spearman's rank correlation. Sensitivity analyses were performed by removing participants who had no infarct to check if the association between hs-CRP and infarct size has the same direction for those who had an infarct versus those who did not. Additional sensitivity analysis was done on participants in the placebo group only to test for the correlation between hs-CRP levels, at the three time points measured, and infarct size, without the effect of GIK. We also ran sensitivity analyses based on ACS diagnosis, and prior use of statins. Because hs-CRP baseline levels were not measured prior to study infusion initiation, but rather, after hospital arrival, the time from when the drug started and time of the first hs-CRP measurement was used as a covariate in regression models.

Results

Characteristics of study population

A total of 143 participants met the inclusion criteria for the biocohort; 68 received GIK and 75 placebo. Not all individuals had complete hs-CRP measurements; participants with at least one hs-CRP measurement available were included in the analysis ($n = 143$). Additional file 1: Figure S1 illustrates how the biocohort participants were enrolled. Their demographic and clinical characteristics by treatment arm are shown in Table 1. The average age was 64 years in both groups; 77 % of the GIK group and 70 % of the placebo group were men. Chest pain was the chief symptom of 86 % of participants, and they were randomized at a median time of 90 min after ischemic symptom onset. The median time from start of study drug to the measurement of the initial hs-CRP values was 2.5 h in the GIK group and 2.6 h in the placebo group. The entry participant characteristics were well-balanced in the GIK and placebo groups. The clinical characteristics of participants in the biocohort were similar to all IMMEDIATE Trial participants by site of enrollment. The diagnosis of ACS was more common in the biocohort, as expected because a confirmed diagnosis of ACS was a requirement for enrollment into the biocohort (Additional file 1: Table S1).

Changes in hs-CRP levels

Table 2 shows hs-CRP levels in the first 12 h of drug infusions before logarithmic transformation. Linear regression models were performed to assess the association between admission hs-CRP levels and baseline characteristics. They showed that older people, women and individuals with history of heart failure had higher hs-CRP levels upon admission (Additional file 1: Table S2). In addition the longer time from symptom onset to reperfusion therapy the higher the hs-CRP levels (Additional file 1: Table S2). These associations remained significant after adjusting for the use of study drug. No other clinical characteristics had a significant association with admission hs-CRP values.

The hs-CRP measurements increased significantly in both the control and the treatment groups by 6 and 12 h, compared with the initial measurement ($P < 0.01$ for all intragroup comparisons). Hs-CRP values were not different for those who received GIK versus placebo at the initial and 6-hour measurements; however by 12 h, the hs-CRP levels were slightly higher in placebo-treated versus GIK-treated participants ($P = 0.053$) (Fig. 1). When comparing delta hs-CRP, the differences between the initial and 12-hour hs-CRP measurements, there were no significant differences in those delta values between treatment arms (Additional file 1: Table S3). Using linear mixed model, hs-CRP levels increased significantly with time in both arms ($P < 0.01$); however, the rate of change did not differ between the GIK and placebo groups ($P = 0.30$ for time*treatment interaction). Baseline characteristics associated with initial hs-CRP were added to the model and did not change the above results. In addition, the results remained the same after adjusting for the time from symptom onset to reperfusion therapy. The results also did not change when we stratified the analysis by ACS diagnosis, and by the use of statin therapy prior to study enrollment.

Association between hs-CRP and infarct size

After adjusting for age, gender and GIK administration (variables that were associated with infarct size in univariate models), there were no significant associations between hs-CRP and infarct size at the initial and 6-hour measurements. On the other hand the 12-hour measurement and delta hs-CRP were significantly associated with infarct size (Table 3). Sensitivity analysis done by removing participants with no infarct (i.e. those with an infarct

Table 1 Baseline demographics and clinical characteristics of study participants by treatment group in the biocohort (*N* = 143)[a]

Cohort characteristics	No. (%)	
	N = 143	
	GIK (*N* = 68)	Placebo (*N* = 75)
Age, mean (SD), y	64.5 (12.9)	63.9 (12.8)
Men	52 (76.5)	52 (69.3)
Race		
White	66 (97)	71 (95)
Hispanic ethnicity	3 (4.4)	7 (9.3)
Chief complaint on presentation		
Chest pain	59 (86.8)	67 (89.3)
Shortness of breath	1 (1.5)	3 (4)
Other [b]	8 (11.7)	5 (6.7)
Medical history		
Diabetes	12 (17.6)	19 (25.3)
Heart Failure	4 (5.9)	7 (9.3)
AMI	21 (30.9)	24 (32.0)
Medication history		
Statins	30 (44.1)	29 (38.7)
Aspirin	39 (57.3)	44 (58.7)
Minutes from symptom onset to study drug, median (IQR)	86 (51.5–160.5)	81 (53–123)
Minutes from symptom onset to study drug		
0–30	1 (1.5)	0 (0)
31–60	21 (30.9)	22 (29.3)
61–90	9 (13.2)	19 (25.3)
91–180	12 (17.7)	15 (20.0)
181–360	10 (14.7)	8 (10.7)
361–24 h	6 (8.8)	5 (6.7)
Within 24 h, unspecified	3 (4.4)	4 (5.3)
>24 h	6 (8.8)	2 (2.7)
ACI-TIPI score, mean (SD), %	83 (15.7)	83.1 (12.1)
Hospital reperfusion treatment		
Thrombolytic therapy	1 (1.5)	1 (1.3)
PCI	59 (86.8)	56 (74.7)
Coronary artery bypass graft	0 (0)	2 (2.7)
Confirmed diagnosis		
Acute myocardial infarction	58 (85.3)	68 (90.7)
Any angina	10 (14.7)	7 (9.3)
Time from study drug to biomarker measurement, median (IQR), hours		
Initial	2.5 (1.3–3.3)	2.6 (1.9–3.2)
6 h	6 (6–6.3)	6 (6–6.2)
12 h	12 (12–12.2)	12.1 (12–12.3)

AMI indicates acute myocardial infarction; *ACI-TIPI* acute cardiac ischemia time-insensitive predictive instrument; *GIK* glucose-insulin-potassium; *IQR* interquartile range; *PCI* percutaneous coronary intervention; *SD* standard deviation

[a]No significant differences were noted between GIK and placebo groups

[b]Abdominal pain, back pain, dizziness, heartburn, loss of consciousness, shoulder pain and weakness

Table 2 Hs-CRP Levels in the first 12 h of emergency department admission

	GIK			Placebo		
Hs-CRP	No.	Mean (SD)	Median (IQR)	No.	Mean (SD)	Median (IQR)
Initial hs-CRP mg/L	59	8.1 (17.7)	3.1 (1.4–7.3)	61	12.3 (24.4)	3.2 (1.9–9.3)
6 h hs-CRP mg/L	58	8.6 (17.0)	3.4 (1.8–8.8)	63	15.1 (30.7)	4.2 (2.0–12.4)
12 h hs-CRP mg/L	57	9.2 (16.7)	4.5 (2.3–7.9)	64	17.6 (31.0)	5.9 (3.1–13.7)

GIK indicates glucose-insulin-potassium; *Hs-CRP* high sensitivity C-reactive protein; *IQR* interquartile range; *SD* standard deviation

size of 0, or those who died and did not have infarct size measurement available) ($n = 31$) showed the same association between hs-CRP levels and infarct size (Table 3). Also stratifying participants by ACS diagnosis and statin use prior to study enrollment did not significantly change the study results. Results from spearman's rank correlation yielded similar associations between hs-CRP and 30-day infarct size (Additional file 1: Fig. S2). When testing for the correlation between hs-CRP and infarct size in the placebo group only, we found that the 12-hour hs-CRP and the delta hs-CRP remained significantly correlated with infarct size (p-value = 0.022 and 0.049, for the 12 h and delta hs-CRP respectively).

Discussion

Our data confirm that plasma hs-CRP concentrations are increased in participants presenting to the ED with ACS, presumably reflecting a state of inflammation. However, the administration of GIK early in ACS did not have a significant impact on hs-CRP levels. Although there was a modest difference between the 12-hour hs-CRP levels with GIK, the delta hs-CRP values was not different between treatment arms. In addition, results of mixed models, adjusting for within and between subjects variability, demonstrated no effect of GIK on hs-CRP over the three time points. These results suggest that the beneficial effects of GIK in ACS observed in the main study [15], at least as reflected in the absence of an effect on hs-CRP, are less likely to be through an anti-inflammatory effect, and may be more extended through a metabolic effect.

Previous studies on the effect of GIK on CRP yielded conflicting results. In a study by Chaudhuri et al., GIK administration started in the emergency department in patients presenting with ST-segment elevation myocardial infarction (STEMI) ($n = 32$) and lasting 48 h showed significantly reduced hs-CRP values at 24 and 48 h post-infusion compared to placebo [18]. In contrast, Parikh et al., demonstrated in 25 patients with STEMI that a 24-hour infusion of GIK produced no statistically significant difference in 24 h hs-CRP levels compared with placebo [26]. Additionally a study by Hashemian et al., showed no effect of GIK on hs-CRP levels in 72 patients with STEMI treated within 12 h from symptom onset [27]. Although those studies added GIK to standard care, there are important differences in the use of GIK in the IMMEDIATE Trial. First, unlike prior clinical trials in which GIK was started typically an average of 6 h after onset of ischemic symptoms, following documentation of acute MI [6, 10, 14], in IMMEDIATE, the study drug was started prior to arrival to emergency department, upon emergency medical services (EMS) arrival in the community following a 9-1-1 call, at an average of 90 min after symptom onset [15]. Moreover, the previous studies only included participants with STEMI. In contrast, the IMMEDIATE Trial included participants with ACS, i.e., either unstable angina or acute MI (whether or not STEMI) [15].

Infarct size has shown to be a prognostic marker of adverse clinical outcomes after an acute coronary event [28]. Baseline CRP levels in healthy individuals or in patients with stable angina are independent risk factor for cardiovascular events [29]. Also the rise in CRP after acute MI or during unstable angina pectoris has been shown to be related to outcome [23, 30, 31]. In this

Table 3 Regression analysis of hs-CRP levels and 30-day infarct size[a]

	All participants			Participants with an infarct		
Regression models[b]	No.	Beta Coefficient	*P-value*	No.	Beta Coefficient	*P-value*
Initial hs-CRP mg/L[c]	83	2.3	0.46	54	3.8	0.35
6 h hs-CRP mg/L[c]	85	4.0	0.17	56	5.9	0.13
12 h hs-CRP mg/L[c]	83	6.8	0.04	56	10.6	0.02
Delta hs-CRP mg/L[d]	78	13.9	0.02	51	23.1	0.01

GIK*GIK* indicates glucose-insulin-potassium,: *Hs-CRP* high sensitivity C-reactive protein
[a]Data analyzed using logarithmically transformed hs-CRP values
[b]Adjusted for age, gender and GIK administration. In addition, the time from when the drug started to the time of the first hs-CRP measurement was used as a co-variate. The coefficient represents the fitted increase in infarct size per one unit change in logarithmically trasnformed hs-CRP.
[c]Per 1 unit increase in hs-CRP levels
[d]Difference between the initial hs-CRP and 12 h hs-CRP measurements

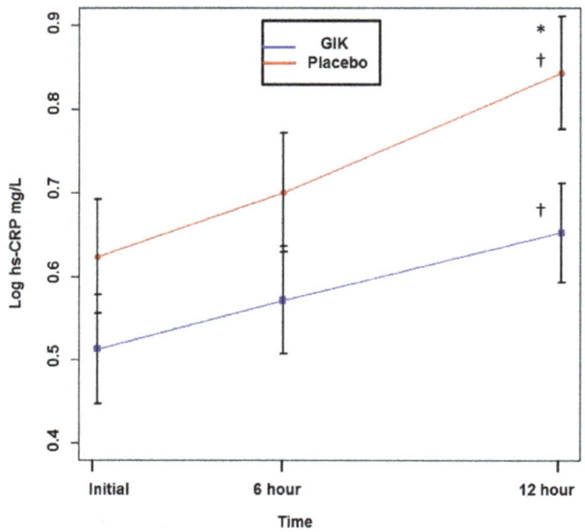

Fig. 1 hs-CRP Levels per Treatment Arm. Time course of mean ± SEM hs-CRP at initial, 6 h and 12 h per treatment arm. *GIK* indicates glucose-insulin-potassium; *Hs-CRP* high sensitivity C-reactive protein. *$P = 0.053$ between groups at 12 h (independent sample t-test). † P˂0.01 within group differences between initial and 6 h, 6 h and 12 h, and initial and 12 h (paired sample t-test). Initial time represents the first hs-CRP measurement (median = 2.5 h)

study on participants presenting to EMS with ACS, we document a relationship between hs-CRP level measured at 12 h and 30-day infarct size. In addition, the magnitude of change in hs-CRP levels, between the initial and 12-hour values, was related to infarct size. Limiting the analysis to those participants with a documented infarct size measurement, and also to those in the placebo group only, showed similar results. Previous studies have shown no clear relationship between CRP levels on hospital admission and infarct size in patients with acute coronary events [32]; but nevertheless, cumulative or peak CRP levels have been correlated with infarct size [33]. Peak CRP levels are reached by no earlier than 24 h after infarction [34]. Adding to that picture, our hs-CRP measurements reflect that an early rise, within 12 h of ACS symptom onset, correlates with 30-day infarct size. Imaging studies in IMMEDIATE Trial biocohort participants at 30 days showed an 80 % reduction infarct size associated with GIK, both for the entire ACS cohort ($n = 110$) and in those presenting with STEMI ($n = 75$) [15]. Therefore the modest reduction seen in hs-CRP levels at 12 h between the two groups may be indirectly related to infarct size.

This study has several limitations. First, although our sample is larger than previous studies on the effect of GIK on hs-CRP levels [18, 26, 27]. the size of the IMMEDIATE Trial biocohort may have limited our power to detect treatment interactions. Second, CRP levels prior to the onset of GIK infusion and after the 12 h infusion were not available. Finally, although CRP is commonly used as an inflammatory biomarker, it is somewhat non-specific and other biomarkers have been considered as an alternative to CRP. For instance, serum amyloid A, interleukin-6, and adhesion molecules such as soluble intercellular adhesion molecule type 1, similar to CRP, are markers of inflammation that are produced by the liver [35]. Therefore, if GIK exerts an anti-inflammatory effect it may be reflected through biomarkers other than CRP. Nevertheless this study has several strengths including serial hs-CRP levels measurements within 12 h after GIK initiation, compared to other studies, in which the effect of GIK on CRP was assessed at 24–48 h following treatment. Moreover, our data were collected in a randomized placebo-controlled trial, with both GIK and placebo participants having balanced characteristics.

Conclusions

In patients with an ACS, early administration of GIK appears to have no significant effect on hs-CRP levels measured in the first 12 h of treatment infusion. This is consistent with a model that the primary immediate benefits of GIK are more likely metabolic rather than anti-inflammatory. Nevertheless, in order to more fully understand the mechanisms by which GIK exert its potential benefits in patients with an ACS, future research should consider markers of endothelial dysfunction, microvascular dysfunction, and coagulation. Our findings of a possible association between the early rise in hs-CRP levels and infarct size, are consistent with the role of inflammation in extent of infarction, an effect that deserves further investigation as a marker of acute myocardial damage and inflammation.

Abbreviations

ACS: Acute coronary syndromes; CRP: C-reactive protein; EMS: Emergency medical services; FFA: Free fatty acid; GIK: Glucose-insulin-potassium; hs-CRP: High sensitivity C-reactive protein; IMMEDIATE: Immediate Myocardial Metabolic Enhancement During Initial Assessment and Treatment in Emergency care; MI: Myocardial infarction; STEMI: ST-segment elevation myocardial infarction.

Competing interests

The authors declare that they have no competing interest.

Authors' contribution

All authors contributed extensively to the work presented in this paper. Dr. Harry Selker and Joni Beshansky ran the IMMEDIATE Trial and the biomarker analysis for this project, as well as guided in the interpretation of data analysis, and writing of the manuscript. Dr. Gordon Huggins supervised the project and provided guidance on the interpretation of data analysis and writing of the manuscript. Robin Ruthazer contributed extensively to the analysis of the data, interpretation of results and writing of the manuscript. Dr. Inga Peter, Dr. Madhab Ray, and Dr. Jayanta T Mukherjee helped in interpretation of results and manuscript writing. Hadeel Alkofide ran the analysis and wrote the manuscript. All authors read and approved the final manuscript.

Acknowledgements

The MMEDIATE Trial was funded by the National Institutes of Health cooperative agreement from National Heart, Lung and Blood Institute (U01HL077821, U01HL077826, U01HL077823). The IMMEDIATE Trial is registered at www.ClinicalTrials.gov (NCT00091507). The project described was supported by the National Center for Advancing Translational Sciences, National Institutes of Health (Grant Numbers UL1 TR000073 and UL1 TR001064). The content is solely the responsibility of the authors and does not necessarily represent the official views of the NIH. Hadeel Alkofide is supported by a scholarship from King Saud University, Riyadh, Saudi Arabia.

Author details

[1]Clinical and Translational Science Graduate Program, Sackler School of Biomedical Sciences, Tufts Clinical and Translational Science Institute, Tufts University, Boston, MA, USA. [2]Department of Clinical Pharmacy, College of Pharmacy, King Saud University, Riyadh, Saudi Arabia. [3]MCRI Center for Translational Genomics, Molecular Cardiology Research Institute, Tufts Medical Center, Boston, MA, USA. [4]Center for Cardiovascular Health Services Research, Institute for Clinical Research and Health Policy Studies, Tufts Medical Center, Boston, MA, USA. [5]Regulatory and Clinical Research Management, Department of Health Sciences, Regis College, Weston, MA, USA. [6]Tufts Clinical and Translational Science Institute, Tufts University, Boston, MA, USA. [7]Department of Genetics and Genomic Sciences, Icahn School of Medicine at Mount Sinai, New York, NY, USA.

References

1. Lee L, Horowitz J, Frenneaux M. Metabolic manipulation in ischaemic heart disease, a novel approach to treatment. Eur Heart J. 2004;25(8):634–41. doi:10.1016/j.ehj.2004.02.018.
2. Hadj A, Pepe S, Marasco S, Rosenfeldt F. The principles of metabolic therapy for heart disease. Heart Lung Circ. 2003;12 Suppl 2:S55–62.
3. Schofield RS, Hill JA. Role of metabolically active drugs in the management of ischemic heart disease. Am J Cardiovasc Drugs. 2001;1(1):23–35.
4. Hadj A, Pepe S, Rosenfeldt F. The clinical application of metabolic therapy for cardiovascular disease. Heart Lung Circ. 2007;16 Suppl 3:S56–64. doi:10.1016/j.hlc.2007.04.001.
5. Sodi-Pallares D, Testelli MR, Fishleder BL, Bisteni A, Medrano GA, Friedland C, et al. Effects of an intravenous infusion of a potassium-glucose-insulin solution on the electrocardiographic signs of myocardial infarction. A preliminary clinical report. Am J Cardiol. 1962;9:166–81.
6. Apstein CS, Opie LH. Glucose-insulin-potassium (GIK) for acute myocardial infarction: a negative study with a positive value. Cardiovasc Drugs Ther. 1999;13(3):185–9.
7. Opie LH, Bruyneel K, Owen P. Effects of glucose, insulin and potassium infusion on tissue metabolic changes within first hour of myocardial infarction in the baboon. Circulation. 1975;52(1):49–57.
8. Malmberg K, Ryden L, Efendic S, Herlitz J, Nicol P, Waldenstrom A, et al. Randomized trial of insulin-glucose infusion followed by subcutaneous insulin treatment in diabetic patients with acute myocardial infarction (DIGAMI study): effects on mortality at 1 year. J Am Coll Cardiol. 1995;26(1):57–65.
9. Mehta SR, Yusuf S, Diaz R, Zhu J, Pais P, Xavier D, et al. Effect of glucose-insulin-potassium infusion on mortality in patients with acute ST-segment elevation myocardial infarction: the CREATE-ECLA randomized controlled trial. JAMA. 2005;293(4):437–46. doi:10.1001/jama.293.4.437.
10. Timmer JR, Svilaas T, Ottervanger JP, Henriques JP, Dambrink JH, van den Broek SA, et al. Glucose-insulin-potassium infusion in patients with acute myocardial infarction without signs of heart failure: the Glucose-Insulin-Potassium Study (GIPS)-II. J Am Coll Cardiol. 2006;47(8):1730–1. doi:10.1016/j.jacc.2006.01.040.
11. Oliver MF, Opie LH. Effects of glucose and fatty acids on myocardial ischaemia and arrhythmias. Lancet. 1994;343(8890):155–8.
12. Malmberg K. Prospective randomised study of intensive insulin treatment on long term survival after acute myocardial infarction in patients with diabetes mellitus. DIGAMI (Diabetes Mellitus, Insulin Glucose Infusion in Acute Myocardial Infarction) Study Group. BMJ. 1997;314(7093):1512–5.
13. Apstein CS. Glucose-insulin-potassium for acute myocardial infarction: remarkable results from a new prospective, randomized trial. Circulation. 1998;98(21):2223–6.
14. van der Horst IC, Zijlstra F. van 't Hof AW, Doggen CJ, de Boer MJ, Suryapranata H et al. Glucose-insulin-potassium infusion inpatients treated with primary angioplasty for acute myocardial infarction: the glucose-insulin-potassium study: a randomized trial. J Am Coll Cardiol. 2003;42(5):784–91.
15. Selker HP, Beshansky JR, Sheehan PR, Massaro JM, Griffith JL, D'Agostino RB, et al. Out-of-hospital administration of intravenous glucose-insulin-potassium in patients with suspected acute coronary syndromes: the IMMEDIATE randomized controlled trial. JAMA. 2012;307(18):1925–33. doi:10.1001/jama.2012.426.
16. Grossman AN, Opie LH, Beshansky JR, Ingwall JS, Rackley CE, Selker HP. Glucose-insulin-potassium revived: current status in acute coronary syndromes and the energy-depleted heart. Circulation. 2013;127(9):1040–8. doi:10.1161/CIRCULATIONAHA.112.130625.
17. Addo TA, Keeley EC, Cigarroa JE, Lange RA, de Lemos JA, Dobbins RL, et al. Effect of glucose-insulin-potassium infusion on plasma free fatty acid concentrations in patients undergoing primary percutaneous coronary intervention for ST-elevation myocardial infarction. Am J Cardiol. 2004; 94(10):1288–9. doi:10.1016/j.amjcard.2004.07.115.
18. Chaudhuri A, Janicke D, Wilson MF, Tripathy D, Garg R, Bandyopadhyay A, et al. Anti-inflammatory and profibrinolytic effect of insulin in acute ST-segment-elevation myocardial infarction. Circulation. 2004;109(7):849–54. doi:10.1161/01.CIR.0000116762.77804.FC.
19. Spagnoli LG, Bonanno E, Sangiorgi G, Mauriello A. Role of inflammation in atherosclerosis. J Nucl Med. 2007;48(11):1800–15. doi:10.2967/jnumed.107.038661.
20. Sano T, Tanaka A, Namba M, Nishibori Y, Nishida Y, Kawarabayashi T, et al. C-reactive protein and lesion morphology in patients with acute myocardial infarction. Circulation. 2003;108(3):282–5. doi:10.1161/01.CIR.0000079173.84669.4F.
21. Pietila K, Harmoinen A, Hermens W, Simoons ML, Van de Werf F, Verstraete M. Serum C-reactive protein and infarct size in myocardial infarct patients with a closed versus an open infarct-related coronary artery after thrombolytic therapy. Eur Heart J. 1993;14(7):915–9.
22. Anzai T, Yoshikawa T, Shiraki H, Asakura Y, Akaishi M, Mitamura H, et al. C-reactive protein as a predictor of infarct expansion and cardiac rupture after a first Q-wave acute myocardial infarction. Circulation. 1997;96(3):778–84.
23. Pietila KO, Harmoinen AP, Jokiniitty J, Pasternack AI. Serum C-reactive protein concentration in acute myocardial infarction and its relationship to mortality during 24 months of follow-up in patients under thrombolytic treatment. Eur Heart J. 1996;17(9):1345–9.
24. Andreotti F, Hackett DR, Haider AW, Roncaglioni MC, Davies GJ, Beacham JL, et al. Von Willebrand factor, plasminogen activator inhibitor-1 and C-reactive protein are markers of thrombolytic efficacy in acute myocardial infarction. Thromb Haemost. 1992;68(6):678–82.
25. Armstrong EJ, Morrow DA, Sabatine MS. Inflammatory biomarkers in acute coronary syndromes: part II: acute-phase reactants and biomarkers of endothelial cell activation. Circulation. 2006;113(7):e152–5. doi:10.1161/CIRCULATIONAHA.105.595538.
26. Parikh SV, Abdullah SM, Keeley EC, Cigarroa JE, Addo TA, Warner JJ, et al. Effect of glucose-insulin-potassium (GIK) infusion on biomarkers of cardiovascular risk in ST elevation myocardial infarction (STEMI): insight into the failure of GIK. Diab Vasc Dis Res. 2007;4(3):222–5. doi:10.3132/dvdr.2007.043.
27. Hashemian MVA, Akaberi A. Effect of glucose–insulin–potassium on Plasma concentrations of C-reactive protein in acute ST- Elevation Myocardial Infarction; A Randomized Clinical Trial. Pak J Med Sci. 2011;27(3):4.
28. Hombach V, Grebe O, Merkle N, Waldenmaier S, Hoher M, Kochs M, et al. Sequelae of acute myocardial infarction regarding cardiac structure and function and their prognostic significance as assessed by magnetic resonance imaging. Eur Heart J. 2005;26(6):549–57. doi:10.1093/eurheartj/ehi147.
29. Lagrand WK, Visser CA, Hermens WT, Niessen HW, Verheugt FW, Wolbink GJ, et al. C-reactive protein as a cardiovascular risk factor: more than an epiphenomenon? Circulation. 1999;100(1):96–102.
30. Suleiman M, Khatib R, Agmon Y, Mahamid R, Boulos M, Kapeliovich M, et al. Early inflammation and risk of long-term development of heart failure and mortality in survivors of acute myocardial infarction

predictive role of C-reactive protein. J Am Coll Cardiol. 2006;47(5):962–8. doi:10.1016/j.jacc.2005.10.055.
31. Ohlmann P, Jaquemin L, Morel O, El Behlgiti R, Faure A, Michotey MO, et al. Prognostic value of C-reactive protein and cardiac troponin I in primary percutaneous interventions for ST-elevation myocardial infarction. Am Heart J. 2006;152(6):1161–7. doi:10.1016/j.ahj.2006.07.016.
32. Haase J, Bayar R, Hackenbroch M, Storger H, Hofmann M, Schwarz CE, et al. Relationship between size of myocardial infarctions assessed by delayed contrast-enhanced MRI after primary PCI, biochemical markers, and time to intervention. J Interv Cardiol. 2004;17(6):367–73. doi:10.1111/j.1540-8183.2004.04078.x.
33. Orn S, Manhenke C, Ueland T, Damas JK, Mollnes TE, Edvardsen T, et al. C-reactive protein, infarct size, microvascular obstruction, and left-ventricular remodelling following acute myocardial infarction. Eur Heart J. 2009;30(10):1180–6. doi:10.1093/eurheartj/ehp070.
34. Gruzdeva O, Uchasova E, Dyleva Y, Belik E, Shurygina E, Barbarash O. Insulin resistance and inflammation markers in myocardial infarction. J Inflamm Res. 2013;6:83–90. doi:10.2147/JIR.S43081.
35. Ridker PM, Rifai N, Stampfer MJ, Hennekens CH. Plasma concentration of interleukin-6 and the risk of future myocardial infarction among apparently healthy men. Circulation. 2000;101(15):1767–72.

14

Glucose–insulin–potassium therapy in patients with acute coronary syndrome

Pei-Yin Jin[1*], Hai-San Zhang[2], Xiao-Yan Guo[1], Wei-Fang Liang[1] and Qin-Fu Han[1]

Abstract

Background: Glucose-insulin-potassium (GIK) has been advocated in the setting of acute coronary syndrome (ACS) to reduce ischemia-related arrhythmias and myocardial injury. We conducted a meta-analysis of randomized controlled trials (RCTs) to assess whether the use of GIK infusions >3 or <3 hours after the onset of symptoms reduce mortality or cardiac arrest.

Methods: Electronic databases (Medline, EMBASE, and Cochrane Central Register of Controlled Trials) and references of retrieved articles were searched for RCTs evaluating the effect of GIK infusions, <3 hours or >3 hours after the onset of symptoms, on mortality and/or cardiac arrest. Pooled odds ratios (ORs) with 95% confidence intervals (CIs) were calculated for each outcome.

Results: Nine trials were identified and eligible for review. The summary OR for in-hospital mortality was 1.01 (95% CI 0.94 to 1.09), based on 2,542 deaths among 27,294 patients. The subgroup analysis according to the study enrollment time (within 3 hours [OR, 0.77, 95% CI 0.50-1.16], vs. >3 hours [OR, 0.90; 95% CI, 0.67-1.21]) did not reveal any difference in mortality.

Conclusions: Administration of GIK in ACS patients does not significantly reduce mortality whether or not GIK administration >3 or <3 hours after the onset of symptoms.

Keywords: Glucose–insulin–potassium, Acute coronary syndrome, Meta-analysis

Background

Glucose–insulin–potassium (GIK) has long been advocated as an adjunctive treatment for patients with cardiac dysfunction during episodes of ischemia and reperfusion. Experimental and clinical studies have demonstrated that GIK could improve the efficiency of energy use, reduce circulating free fatty acids, and be anti-apoptotic [1,2]. GIK has now been commonly applied in patients with acute coronary syndrome (ACS) as a metabolic support to ischemic myocardium.

Since the first application of GIK in the setting of cardiac ischemic disease in the 1962 [3], GIK therapy has gone through alternating periods of varying attention. Early trials in the setting of acute myocardial infarction (AMI) suggested a benefit from GIK therapy (6). However, a recent large, randomized, placebo-controlled trial [4] has failed to show any survival benefit, even revealed increased morbidity. A 2010 meta-analysis of eight randomized trials that involved >22,000 patients did not reveal any mortality benefit with GIK therapy in ST-segment–elevation AMI. However, all the studies examined AMI patients ≥3 hours after the onset of symptoms except for Glucose-Insulin-Potassium Study-1 (GIPS-1), which accounted for only 3% of the total population in the meta-analysis [4]. The most recent completed IMMEDIATE trial [5]. Their hypothesis was that the timing of GIK-infusion was responsible for the inconsistent results of prior GIK-trials. Therefore, 871 patients with a suspected acute coronary syndrome (ACS) were randomized to GIK infusion or placebo in the ambulance, thereby significantly shortening system delay. So there is still uncertainty regarding GIK clinical effectiveness according to the study enrollment time

*Correspondence: 13323729039@189.cn
[1]Department of Cardiovascular Medicine, The People's Hospital of Anyang, Anyang, Henan, China
Full list of author information is available at the end of the article

(within 3 hours vs. >3 hours). The objective of this analysis was to systematically review randomized trials to assess the effectiveness of GIK in ACS patients.

Methods

We followed the preferred reporting items for systematic reviews and meta-analyses guidelines (PRISMA) to report our study findings [6].

Eligibility criteria

The study's eligibility criteria were as follows: (1) RCT, (2) comparison of GIK as adjunctive therapy, (3) report of a risk estimate (relative risk, odds ratio, or data from which it could be calculated), and (4) report of all-cause mortality.

Data sources and search strategies

The PubMed (1966 to May 2014), EMBASE (1966 to May 2014) and the Cochrane Central Register of Controlled Trials (CENTRAL, 1996 to May 2014) were searched for randomized, placebo controlled trials that examined the adjunctive use of GIK in the setting of ACS using the Cochrane randomized controlled trial filter and the following MeSH headings/text words: coronary artery disease, acute coronary syndrome, myocardial infarction, AMI, ACS, glucose-insulin-potassium and GIK Electronic searches were supplemented with a review of the reference lists of retrieved articles and by contacting experts in the field. The electronic search was up to date as of May 2014 and no language restrictions were applied.

Data extraction

Two individuals (Wei-Fang Liang and Qin-Fu Han) independently extracted data from eligible articles. Data extracted included GIK protocol (dose and infusion method), demographic data, trial characteristics, outcome data (all-cause mortality).

Quality assessment

We evaluated the quality of the evidence by using the GRADE (Grades of Recommendation, Assessment, Development and Evaluation) approach [7,8]. In addition, the GRADE profiler 3.6 software was used to create the evidence profile. GRADE Working Group grades of evidence were as follows: High quality: Further research is very unlikely to change our confidence in the estimate of effect. Moderate quality: Further research is likely to have an important impact on our confidence in the estimate of effect and may change the estimate. Low quality: Further research is very likely to have an important impact on our confidence in the estimate of effect and is likely to change the estimate. Very low quality: We are very uncertain about the estimate.

Subgroup analysis

Subgroup analyses of the time of GIK administration (before or after reperfusion) were performed because Dr. Opie suggests that GIK infusion in A MI is more likely to be beneficial when given before reperfusion therapy [9]. Further subgroup analyses of studies comparing GIK with standard therapy were performed according to duration of therapy from AMI onset (<3 hours and >3 hours) [2].

Statistical analyses

Categorical variables were reported as frequency and proportions. Relative estimate was presented by using odd ratios (ORs) with 95% CI, calculated by using the fixed effects model. The heterogeneity among the studies was assessed by using the I^2 statistic and the Cochran Q statistic for each outcome [10]. A P value of less than 0.10 of the Cochran Q test suggests that the heterogeneity is beyond random error or chance [10]. Meta-regression was performed to assess the influence of duration of therapy from AMI onset on the pooled estimate of effect. P values were considered significant for $P < 0.05$. Statistical analyses were performed using Review Manager (RevMan) Version 5.1 and STATA (StataCorp LP, USA) version 11.0.

Ethics

This meta analysis didn't require ethical approval.

Results

Identification of eligible studies

A total of 567 unique records were identified through comprehensive database search, and 1 additional article was identified from other sources. Of these citations, nine trials [4,5,11-17] met the inclusion criteria in our meta-analysis (see Figure 1 for the preferred reporting items for systematic reviews and meta-analyses guidelines (PRISMA) flow diagram).

Characteristics of eligible studies

The studies used different perioperative GIK protocols. Study protocols and participant characteristics are presented in Table 1. Three trials did not report time from onset of symptom to treatment [14,16,17]. Two trials reported time from onset of symptom to treatment within 3 hours [5,13], while four trials reported time from onset of symptom to treatment >3 hours [4,11,12,15]. No included trials were at low quality, and the GRADE assessment of strength of evidence varied from moderate to high quality (Additional file 1) because of unclear reporting of allocation concealment and blinding in many studies.

Mortality and subgroup analysis

In nine RCTs studying GIK in patients with AMI or ACS, meta analysis did not demonstrate a significant reduction in mortality (OR 1.04, 95% CI 0.85 to 1.27, p = 0.70,

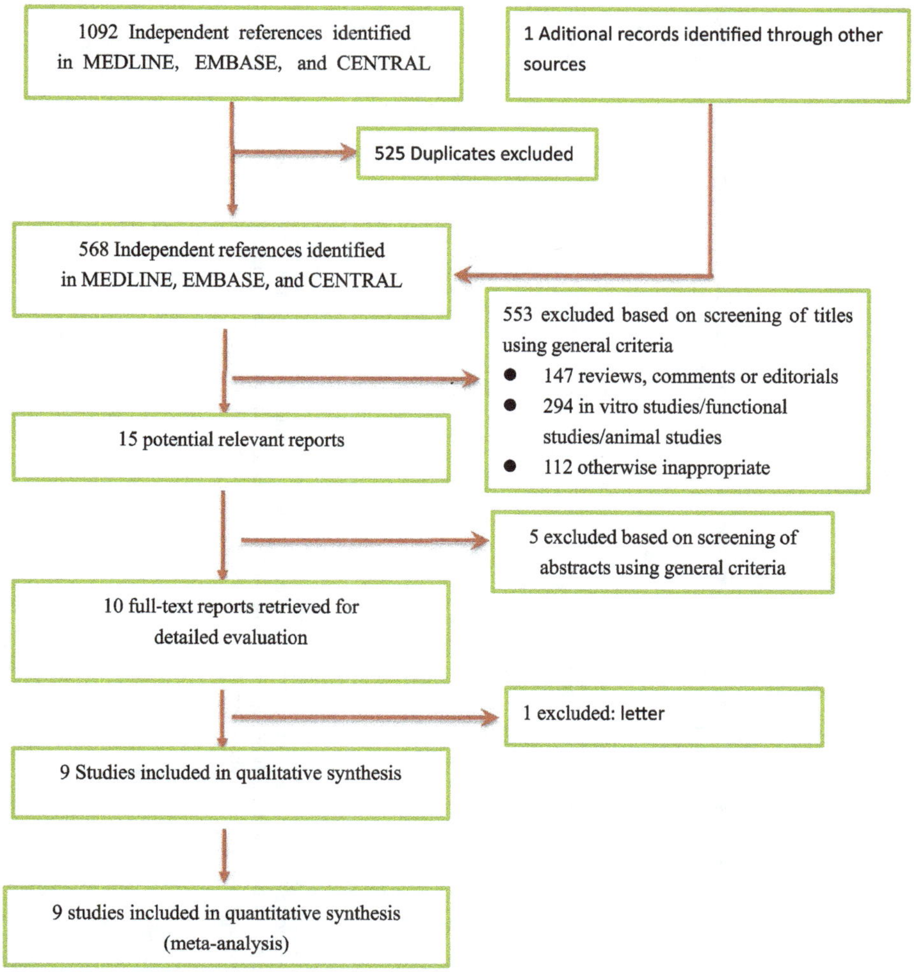

Figure 1 Identification of eligible studies.

although there was still considerable heterogeneity between trials ($I^2 = 47.0\%$, $p = 0.06$, Figure 2).

Because the effect of GIK on AMI might vary depending upon the time of GIK treatment (before and after reperfusion), [9] we performed a subgroup analysis to examine the heterogeneity of the results. Five Trial [5,11,13,15,16] and combined CREATE-ECLA and OASIS-6 subgroup analysis [9] evaluated the effect of receiving GIK before reperfusion and found no significant reduction in mortality (OR 0.89, 95% CI 0.70 to 1.13, $p = 0.35$). The trial by Krljanac et al. [15] showed the largest effect of treatment but it was also the smallest trial. Exclusion of this trial removed the statistical heterogeneity ($I^2 = 0\%$, p = 0.43) and did not affect the lack of effect on mortality (OR 0.95; 95% CI 0.84 to 1.03, $p = 0.447$). Two trials [12,14] and combined CREATE-ECLA and OASIS-6 subgroup analysis [9] studied the effect of GIK after reperfusion. Overall, there was no significant reduction in mortality (OR 1.36, 95% CI 0.92 to 2.02, $p = 0.12$).

The potential benefit of GIK is thought to be related to timeliness of administration after onset of cardiac ischemia, so we did subgroup analysis according to time from onset of symptom to treatment (with 3 hours *vs.* >3 hours). Two RCTs [5,13] evaluated the effect of receiving GIK within 3 hours from onset of symptom to treatment and found no significant reduction in mortality (OR 0.77, 95% CI 0.50 to 1.16, $p = 0.21$). Four trials [4,11,12,15] studied the effect of GIK >3 hours from onset of symptom to treatment. Overall, there was no significant reduction in mortality (OR 0.90; 95% CI, 0.67-1.21, $p = 0.48$) (Figure 3).

Meta-regression and sensitivity analyses

Only six [4,5,11-13,15] of the eligible nine studies reported data on time from onset of symptom to treatment. Meta-regression was used to assess the possible influence of time from onset of symptom to treatment of the six studies [4,5,11-13,15] on the mortality outcome (Figure 4). This analysis showed that heterogeneity could not be

Table 1 Characteristics of included studies

Study	No. of patients	Age*	Male(%)*	Killip I (%)*	Diabetes (%)*	Glucose (%)	Insulin (U/500 ml)	Potassium (%)	Infusion rate (ml/kg/h)	Time from onset of symptom to treatment (h)*	24-h glucose (mmol/L)*
ECLA (1998))	470	58.2/60.5	77/68.3	84.4/86.3	18.5/18	25	50	0.3	1.5	11.4/10.6	4.25/4.04
POL-GIK (1999)	954	62/60	70/67.2	94.1/97	6.5/6.1	10	32	0.3	42 ml/h	5	5.9/6.2
GIPS-I (2003)	940	59.9/60.8	73.7/79.3	89.5/92.7	10.5/10.6	20	7-11	0.3	3	2.75-2.78/ 2.75-2.82	7.7/8.1*
REVIAL (2004)	312	60.8/64.1	71.6/72.6	67.7/69.4	22.6/23.6	20	40	0.25	1.8	-	-
CREATE-ECLA (2005)	20201	58.6/58.6	77.6/77.6	84.2/85.1	17.6/17.8	25	50	0.3	1.5	4.7/4.7¶	8.6/7.5
Krljanac G (2005)	118	56.6/56.7	66.7/72.5	-	17/17	25	50	0.3	1	3.1/3.2	-
GIPS-II (2006)	889	61.8/61.2	73/74	100/100	9/10	20		0.3	2	-	-
OASIS-6 (2007)	2748	61.5/62.1	73.1/71.7	-	14.9/14.0	25	50	0.3	1.5	-	8.5/7.5
IMMEDIATE (2012)	871	63.9/63.3	72.5/69.6	-	29.4/26.3	30	25	0.6	1.5	1.5/1.5	-

ECLA = Estudios Cardiologicos Latinoamerica; *POL-GIK* = Polish-Glucose-Insulin-Potassium; *GIPS-I* = Glucose–insulin–potassium study-I; *GIPS-II* = Glucose–insulin–potassium study-II; *REVIVAL* = The Reevaluation of Intensified Venous Metabolic Support for Acute Infarct Size Limitation; *OASIS-6* = Organization to Assess Strategies for Ischemic Syndromes; DIGAMI = the Diabetes and Insulin-Glucose Infusion in Acute Myocardial Infarction; HI-5 = The hyperglycemia: intensive insulin infusion in infarction; IMMEDIATE = the Immediate Myocardial Metabolic Enhancement During Initial Assessment and Treatment in Emergency care Trial.
*numerator/denominator indicates treatment group/control group.
¶median, Glucose (%) and potassium (%) mass concentration.

Study or Subgroup	GIK Events	GIK Total	Control Events	Control Total	Weight	Odds Ratio M-H, Random, 95% CI	Year
1.1.1 GIK before reperfusion							
ECLA 1998	10	135	16	139	4.9%	0.61 [0.27, 1.41]	1998
GIPS-I 2003	23	476	27	464	8.9%	0.82 [0.46, 1.46]	2003
Krljanac G 2005	2	78	4	40	1.2%	0.24 [0.04, 1.35]	2005
GIPS-II 2006	13	444	8	445	4.3%	1.65 [0.68, 4.02]	2007
CREATE-ECLA And OASIS-6	438	4990	453	5051	30.4%	0.98 [0.85, 1.12]	2007
IMMEDIATE 2012	18	411	28	460	8.1%	0.71 [0.38, 1.30]	2012
Subtotal (95% CI)		6534		6599	58.0%	**0.89 [0.70, 1.13]**	
Total events	504		536				
Heterogeneity: Tau² = 0.02; Chi² = 6.28, df = 5 (P = 0.28); I² = 20%							
Test for overall effect: Z = 0.94 (P = 0.35)							
1.1.2 GIK after reperfusion							
POL-GIK 1999	44	494	22	460	10.0%	1.95 [1.15, 3.30]	1999
REVIVAL 2004	7	155	5	157	2.6%	1.44 [0.45, 4.63]	2004
CREATE-ECLA and OASIS-6	380	4373	335	4314	29.4%	1.13 [0.97, 1.32]	2005
Subtotal (95% CI)		5022		4931	42.0%	**1.36 [0.92, 2.02]**	
Total events	431		362				
Heterogeneity: Tau² = 0.06; Chi² = 3.86, df = 2 (P = 0.15); I² = 48%							
Test for overall effect: Z = 1.54 (P = 0.12)							
Total (95% CI)		11556		11530	100.0%	**1.04 [0.85, 1.27]**	
Total events	935		898				
Heterogeneity: Tau² = 0.03; Chi² = 15.18, df = 8 (P = 0.06); I² = 47%							
Test for overall effect: Z = 0.39 (P = 0.70)							
Test for subgroup differences: Chi² = 3.27, df = 1 (P = 0.07), I² = 69.4%							

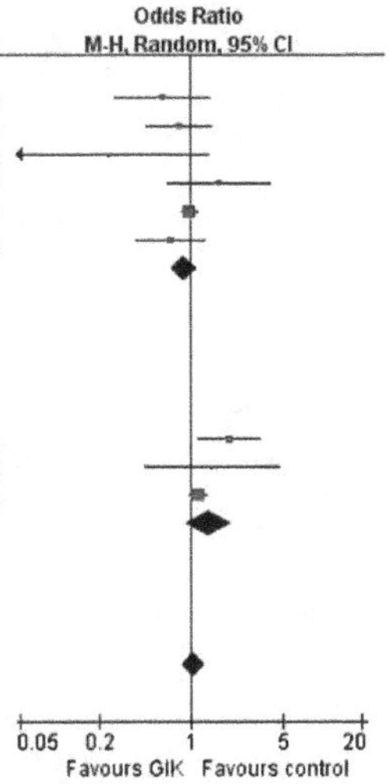

Figure 2 Forest plot for in-hospital mortality according to before or after reperfusion.

explained by time from onset of symptom to treatment (coefficient =0.032, $p = 0.639$).

The two trials showing the largest effect of treatment [11,15] were also the two smallest, and together accounted for 2% of patients in this analysis. This systematic review did not find any corresponding small negative trials, and thus there is suggestion of publication bias. Although publication bias could result in an overestimation of treatment effect, this would not likely produce a qualitative change in the results of this analysis, given the relatively large number of patients in this analysis. Indeed, a sensitivity analysis, which excluded all reports of <500 patients, still found a significant reduction in mortality, but the apparent treatment effect was considerably smaller (OR: 0.96; 95% CI 0.85 to 1.10, $p = 0.58$).

Discussion

Our meta-analysis of 9 trials assessing the use of GIK infusions in AMI patients reveals no benefit with these therapies in mortality. Furthermore, subgroup analysis indicates that the GIK is not effective in reducing the mortality of AMI whether reperfusion strategy (before or after reperfusion) or timeliness of symptom to treatment (within 3 hours or >3 hours).

A 2010 meta-analysis by Zhao et al. confirmed that GIK, aiming at the administration of large doses of glucose and insulin without paying attention to an increase in plasma glucose does not improve mortality [18]. The untoward effects of secondary hyperglycemia have been given a plausible explanation. These assumptions were, however, questioned by Selker et al. [9] and Grossman [2] referring to experimental evidence that insulin reduces reperfusion-induced myocar injury. Grossman advocated that to be effective GIK has to be instituted very early after the onset of symptoms indicating myocardial ischemia, which would be the true test of the GIK hypothesis. However, all the studies examined AMI patients ≥3 hours after the onset of symptoms except for Glucose –Insulin - Potassium Study - 1 (GIPS-1) and IMMEDIATE trial.

Further subgroup analysis and meta regression of trials refuted the possibility that GIK would benefit patients when initiated from symptom to treatment within 3 hours, [2] although preclinical studies suggested that GIK could suppress ischemia reperfusion injury [19-21]. There are several possible explanations for the discordance between the positive findings in preclinical studies and the predominantly negative RCTs.

As one interprets the findings of our systematic review, a distinction should be made between the use of GIK and tight glycemic control. The studies reviewed in the present meta-analysis examined the benefit of GIK when administered as metabolic support. That is, these solutions were administered at a set concentration and rate to enhance glucose uptake and utilization within ischemic myocardium. It has been postulated that studies that use GIK as a metabolic 'cocktail' were negative because of this lack of attention to glycemic control. It has been established that hyperglycemia at the time of myocardial ischemia is associated with increased mortality in both diabetic and nondiabetic individuals [22]. There is also evidence that acute hyperglycemia is associated with increased platelet and leukocyte activation [23,24]. It has been speculated that in the CREATE trial, the potential benefits.

Study or Subgroup	GIK Events	GIK Total	Control Events	Control Total	Weight	Odds Ratio M-H, Random, 95% CI	Year
1.6.1 Time from symptom onset to GIK <3 hour							
GIPS-I 2003	23	476	27	464	6.5%	0.82 [0.46, 1.46]	2003
IMMEDIATE 2012	18	411	28	460	5.8%	0.71 [0.38, 1.30]	2012
Subtotal (95% CI)		**887**		**924**	**12.3%**	**0.77 [0.50, 1.16]**	
Total events	41		55				
Heterogeneity: Tau² = 0.00; Chi² = 0.13, df = 1 (P = 0.72); I² = 0%							
Test for overall effect: Z = 1.26 (P = 0.21)							
1.6.2 Time from symptom onset to GIK > 3 hour							
ECLA 1998	13	135	15	139	3.6%	0.88 [0.40, 1.93]	1998
POL-GIK 1999	98	494	103	460	16.8%	0.86 [0.63, 1.17]	1999
CREATE-ECLA 2005	1004	10088	976	10107	43.5%	1.03 [0.94, 1.13]	2005
Krljanac G 2005	2	78	6	40	0.9%	0.15 [0.03, 0.78]	2005
Subtotal (95% CI)		**10795**		**10746**	**64.8%**	**0.90 [0.67, 1.21]**	
Total events	1117		1100				
Heterogeneity: Tau² = 0.04; Chi² = 6.58, df = 3 (P = 0.09); I² = 54%							
Test for overall effect: Z = 0.71 (P = 0.48)							
1.6.3 Did not report time							
REVIVAL 2004	7	155	5	157	1.7%	1.44 [0.45, 4.63]	2004
GIPS-II 2006	13	444	8	445	2.9%	1.65 [0.68, 4.02]	2007
OASIS-6 2007	104	1374	92	1374	18.3%	1.14 [0.85, 1.53]	2007
Subtotal (95% CI)		**1973**		**1976**	**22.9%**	**1.19 [0.91, 1.56]**	
Total events	124		105				
Heterogeneity: Tau² = 0.00; Chi² = 0.69, df = 2 (P = 0.71); I² = 0%							
Test for overall effect: Z = 1.29 (P = 0.20)							
Total (95% CI)		**13655**		**13646**	**100.0%**	**0.98 [0.84, 1.14]**	
Total events	1282		1260				
Heterogeneity: Tau² = 0.01; Chi² = 10.58, df = 8 (P = 0.23); I² = 24%							
Test for overall effect: Z = 0.26 (P = 0.80)							
Test for subgroup differences: Chi² = 3.74, df = 2 (P = 0.15), I² = 46.6%							

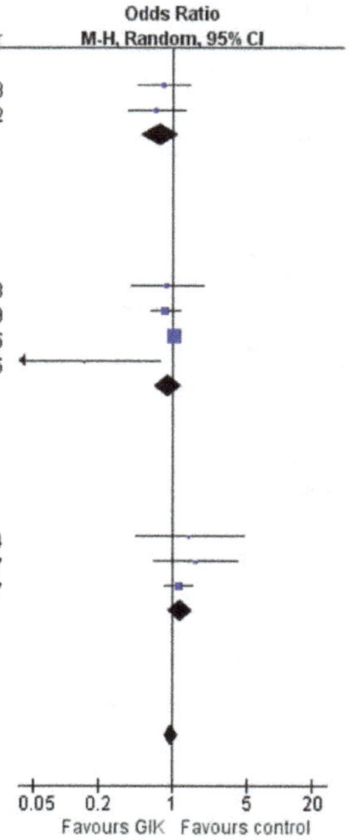

Figure 3 Forest plot for in-hospital mortality according to timeliness from symptom to treatment (<3 hour or >3 hour).

In addition, the concomitant medications used during current clinical practice, which are typically absent in experimental studies, may influence the effectiveness of agents directed against reperfusion injury.

Limitations

The present meta-analysis highlights several shortcomings in the perioperative GIK literature. Many trials examining the use of GIK infusions in AMI are not adequately powered to examine mortality end point. Indeed, mortality was not the primary outcomes in many of the studies analyzed in the present review. In addition, a potential limitation of our meta-analysis is that it was based on trial-specific rather than patient-specific data. Its most important limitation, many trials didn't report the timeliness from symptom to treatment.

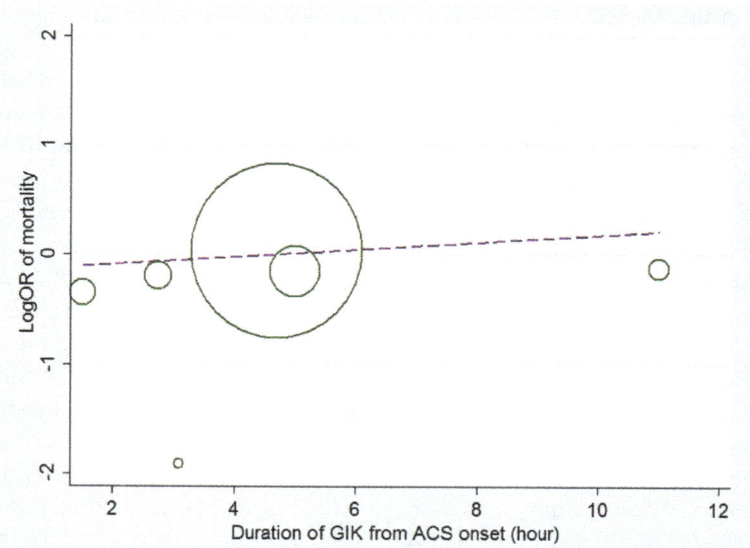

Figure 4 Meta regression for mortality according to timeliness from symptom to treatment (hours).

Conclusions

In summary, this systematic review and meta-analysis showed that administration of GIK in ACS patients does not significantly reduce mortality whether or not GIK administration >3 or <3 hours after the onset of symptoms.

Abbreviations

GIK: Glucose-insulin-potassium; ACS: Acute coronary syndrome; OR: Odd ration; CI: Confidence interval; ECLA: Estudios Cardiologicos Latinoamerica; POL-GIK: Polish-Glucose-Insulin-Potassium; GIPS-I: Glucose–insulin–potassium study-I; GIPS-II: Glucose–insulin–potassium study-II; REVIVAL: The Reevaluation of Intensified Venous Metabolic Support for Acute Infarct Size Limitation; OASIS-6: Organization to Assess Strategies for Ischemic Syndromes; DIGAMI: The Diabetes and Insulin-Glucose Infusion in Acute Myocardial Infarction; HI-5: The hyperglycemia: intensive insulin infusion in infarction; IMMEDIATE: The Immediate Myocardial Metabolic Enhancement During Initial Assessment and Treatment in Emergency care Trial; PRISMA: Preferred reporting items for systematic reviews and meta-analyses guidelines; RCT: Randomized controlled trial.

Competing interests

The authors declare that they have no competing interests.

Authors' contributions

PYJ conceived the study, participated in the design, collected the data, performed statistical analyses, and drafted the manuscript. HSZ and XYG collected the data, performed statistical analyses, and helped to draft the manuscript. WFL and QFH collected the data, performed statistical analyses, helped to revise the manuscript critically for important intellectual content. All authors read and approved the final manuscript.

Acknowledgements

This research received no specific grant from any funding agency in the public, commercial or not-for-profit sectors.

Author details

[1]Department of Cardiovascular Medicine, The People's Hospital of Anyang, Anyang, Henan, China. [2]The Second Affiliated Hospital of Xinxiang Medical University, Xinxiang 453002, Henan, China.

References

1. Goodwin GW, Ahmad F, Doenst T, Taegtmeyer H: **Energy provision from glycogen, glucose, and fatty acids on adrenergic stimulation of isolated working rat hearts.** *Am J Physiol* 1998, **274**(4 Pt 2):H1239–H1247.
2. Grossman AN, Opie LH, Beshansky JR, Ingwall JS, Rackley CE, Selker HP: **Glucose-insulin-potassium revived: current status in acute coronary syndromes and the energy-depleted heart.** *Circulation* 2013, **127**(9):1040–1048.
3. Sodi-Pallares D, Testelli MR, Fishleder BL, Bisteni A, Medrano GA, Friedland C, De Micheli A: **Effects of an intravenous infusion of a potassium-glucose-insulin solution on the electrocardiographic signs of myocardial infarction. A preliminary clinical report.** *Am J Cardiol* 1962, **9**:166–181.
4. Mehta SR, Yusuf S, Diaz R, Zhu J, Pais P, Xavier D, Paolasso E, Ahmed R, Xie C, Kazmi K, Tai J, Orlandini A, Pogue J, Liu L: **Effect of glucose-insulin-potassium infusion on mortality in patients with acute ST-segment elevation myocardial infarction: the CREATE-ECLA randomized controlled trial.** *JAMA* 2005, **293**(4):437–446.
5. Selker HP, Beshansky JR, Sheehan PR, Massaro JM, Griffith JL, D'Agostino RB, Ruthazer R, Atkins JM, Sayah AJ, Levy MK, Richards ME, Aufderheide TP, Braude DA, Pirrallo RG, Doyle DD, Frascone RJ, Kosiak DJ, Leaming JM, Van Gelder CM, Walter GP, Wayne MA, Woolard RH, Opie LH, Rackley CE, Apstein CS, Udelson JE: **Out-of-hospital administration of intravenous glucose-insulin-potassium in patients with suspected acute coronary syndromes: the IMMEDIATE randomized controlled trial.** *JAMA* 2012, **307**(18):1925–1933.
6. Liberati A, Altman DG, Tetzlaff J, Mulrow C, Gotzsche PC, Ioannidis JP, Clarke M, Devereaux PJ, Kleijnen J, Moher D: **The PRISMA statement for reporting systematic reviews and meta-analyses of studies that evaluate healthcare interventions: explanation and elaboration.** *BMJ* 2009, **339**:b2700.
7. Higgins JP, Altman DG, Gotzsche PC, Juni P, Moher D, Oxman AD, Savovic J, Schulz KF, Weeks L, Sterne JA: **The Cochrane Collaboration's tool for assessing risk of bias in randomised trials.** *BMJ* 2011, **343**:d5928.
8. Guyatt GH, Oxman AD, Vist GE, Kunz R, Falck-Ytter Y, Alonso-Coello P, Schunemann HJ, Group GW: **GRADE: an emerging consensus on rating quality of evidence and strength of recommendations.** *BMJ* 2008, **336**(7650):924–926.
9. Opie LH: **Glucose-insulin-potassium therapy in patients with STEMI.** *JAMA* 2008, **299**(20):2385–2386. author reply 2387-2388.
10. Higgins JP, Thompson SG, Deeks JJ, Altman DG: **Measuring inconsistency in meta-analyses.** *BMJ* 2003, **327**(7414):557–560.
11. Diaz R, Paolasso EA, Piegas LS, Tajer CD, Moreno MG, Corvalan R, Isea JE, Romero G: **Metabolic modulation of acute myocardial infarction. The ECLA (Estudios Cardiologicos Latinoamerica) collaborative group.** *Circulation* 1998, **98**(21):2227–2234.
12. Ceremuzynski L, Budaj A, Czepiel A, Burzykowski T, Achremczyk P, Smielak-Korombel W, Maciejewicz J, Dziubinska J, Nartowicz E, Kawka-Urbanek T, Piotrowski W, Hanzlik J, Cieslinski A, Kawecka-Jaszcz K, Gessek J, Wrabec K: **Low-dose glucose-insulin-potassium is ineffective in acute myocardial infarction: results of a randomized multicenter Pol-GIK trial.** *Cardiovasc Drugs Ther* 1999, **13**(3):191–200.
13. van der Horst IC, Zijlstra F, Hof AW V 'T, Doggen CJ, De Boer MJ, Suryapranata H, Hoorntje JC, Dambrink JH, Gans RO, Bilo HJ: **Glucose-insulin-potassium infusion inpatients treated with primary angioplasty for acute myocardial infarction: the glucose-insulin-potassium study: a randomized trial.** *J Am Coll Cardiol* 2003, **42**(5):784–791.
14. Pache J, Kastrati A, Mehilli J, Bollwein H, Ndrepepa G, Schuhlen H, Martinoff S, Seyfarth M, Nekolla S, Dirschinger J, Schwaiger M, Schomig A: **A randomized evaluation of the effects of glucose-insulin-potassium infusion on myocardial salvage in patients with acute myocardial infarction treated with reperfusion therapy.** *Am Heart J* 2004, **148**(1):e3.
15. Krljanac G, Vasiljevic Z, Radovanovic M, Stankovic G, Milic N, Stefanovic B, Kostic J, Mitrovic P, Radovanovic N, Dragovic M, Marinkovic J, Karadzic A: **Effects of glucose-insulin-potassium infusion on ST-elevation myocardial infarction in patients treated with thrombolytic therapy.** *Am J Cardiol* 2005, **96**(8):1053–1058.
16. Timmer JR, Svilaas T, Ottervanger JP, Henriques JP, Dambrink JH, van den Broek SA, van der Horst IC, Zijlstra F: **Glucose-insulin-potassium infusion in patients with acute myocardial infarction without signs of heart failure: the Glucose-Insulin-Potassium Study (GIPS)-II.** *J Am Coll Cardiol* 2006, **47**(8):1730–1731.
17. Diaz R, Goyal A, Mehta SR, Afzal R, Xavier D, Pais P, Chrolavicius S, Zhu J, Kazmi K, Liu L, Budaj A, Zubaid M, Avezum A, Ruda M, Yusuf S: **Glucose-insulin-potassium therapy in patients with ST-segment elevation myocardial infarction.** *JAMA* 2007, **298**(20):2399–2405.
18. Zhao YT, Weng CL, Chen ML, Li KB, Ge YG, Lin XM, Zhao WS, Chen J, Zhang L, Yin JX, Yang XC: **Comparison of glucose-insulin-potassium and insulin-glucose as adjunctive therapy in acute myocardial infarction: a contemporary meta-analysis of randomised controlled trials.** *Heart* 2010, **96**(20):1622–1626.
19. De Leiris J, Opie LH, Lubbe WF: **Effects of free fatty acid and enzyme release in experimental glucose on myocardial infarction.** *Nature* 1975, **253**(5494):746–747.
20. Oates A, Nubani R, Smiley J, Kistler L, Hughey S, Theiss P, Perez-Tamayo RA, Eiferman D, Lonchyna V, Higgins RS: **Myocardial protection of insulin and potassium in a porcine ischemia-reperfusion model.** *Surgery* 2009, **146**(1):23–30.
21. Suranadi IW, Demaison L, Chate V, Peltier S, Richardson M, Leverve X: **An increase in the redox state during reperfusion contributes to the cardioprotective effect of GIK solution.** *Br J Haematol (1985)* 2012, **113**(5):775–784.

22. Capes SE, Hunt D, Malmberg K, Gerstein HC: **Stress hyperglycaemia and increased risk of death after myocardial infarction in patients with and without diabetes: a systematic overview.** *Lancet* 2000, **355**(9206):773–778.
23. Desai MY, Dalal D, Santos RD, Carvalho JA, Nasir K, Blumenthal RS: **Association of body mass index, metabolic syndrome, and leukocyte count.** *Am J Cardiol* 2006, **97**(6):835–838.
24. Sudic D, Razmara M, Forslund M, Ji Q, Hjemdahl P, Li N: **High glucose levels enhance platelet activation: involvement of multiple mechanisms.** *Br J Haematol* 2006, **133**(3):315–322.

15

Two parameters reflect lipid-driven inflammatory state in acute coronary syndrome: atherogenic index of plasma, neutrophil–lymphocyte ratio

Youqin Zhan, Tan Xu and Xuerui Tan*

Abstract

Background: Atherosclerosis is a systemic, lipid-driven immune-inflammatory disease.

Methods: We retrospectively reviewed institutional electronic medical records to seek chest pain patients who were suspicious of acute coronary syndrome (ACS) between January 2011 and December 2013. All the patients were identified by undergoing coronary angiography. On admission white blood cell and its subtypes were measured as part of the automated complete blood count and fasting venous blood samples were obtained and analyzed for lipids profiles used automated analysis.

Results: A total of 376 consecutive patients with ACS were investigated. In the same period, 378 patients admitted with chest pain suspicious of ACS were also included in this study for control. Blood glucose, serum creatinine, white blood cell, neutrophil and monocyte were insignificantly higher in the ACS group. ACS group had higher total cholesterol and lower high density lipid-cholesterol. However, triglyceride and low density lipid-cholesterol were similar between ACS and control groups. Atherogenic index of plasma (AIP) was significantly higher in ACS group compared to control group ($p = 0.029$). Similarly, ACS group had higher neutrophil–lymphocyte ratio (NLR) than those in control group. In the subgroups, the NLR were significantly higher in the STEMI group ($p < 0.001$). However, AIP were similar between the three subgroups ($p = 0.748$).

Conclusions: Our data firstly investigated the lipid-driven inflammatory state in acute coronary syndrome through two easily feasible parameters. There suggest that there are higher AIP and NLR in the ACS patients. Moreover, ACS subgroups are all lipid-driven states, but inflammation levels are different in the entity ACS subgroups.

Keywords: Acute coronary syndrome, Inflammation, Lipid profile, Atherogenic index of plasma, Neutrophil–lymphocyte ratio

Background

Coronary heart disease (CHD) is leading cause of morbidity and mortality worldwide [1]. CHD is mainly caused by coronary atherosclerosis with or without luminal thrombosis and vasospasm [2]. Atherosclerosis is a systemic, lipid-driven immune-inflammatory disease [3]. The function of inflammation in the development and progression of atherosclerosis has been clarified [4]. The presence of inflammation at the site of the atherosclerotic lesion has a critical pathophysiological role in acute rupture [5].

In recent years, several studies have been demonstrated that White blood cell (WBC) count and its subtypes are also known as classic markers of inflammation in cardiovascular diseases [6–9]. Palmerini T showed that a high neutrophil–lymphocyte ratio (NLR) is a strong and independent predictor of in-hospital cardiovascular mortality due to ST-segment elevation myocardial infarction (STEMI) [6].

Dyslipidemia is a well-established risk factor for the development of atherosclerosis which is lipid-driven

* Correspondence: tanxuerui@vip.sina.com
Department of Cardiology, First Affiliated Hospital of Shantou University Medical College, Shantou, Guangdong 515041, China

disease [10, 11]. The common combined occurrence of high fasting blood concentrations of triglycerides (TG) and low levels of high density lipoprotein cholesterol (HDL-c) has been referred to as atherogenic dyslipidemia [12]. Dobiasova and Frohlich have referred to this $\log_{10}$ [TG/HDL-c] as the atherogenic index of plasma (AIP) that allows the demonstration of a correlation with smaller low-density lipoprotein- cholesterol (LDL-c) particles and increased fractional esterification rate for cholesterol in plasma [13, 14]. Interestingly, AIP is associated more strongly with elevated C-reactive protein levels [12]. However, fewer studies evaluate AIP and classic markers of inflammation together. There may be links between NLR and AIP in patients with acute coronary syndrome (ACS) according to the pathophysiologic of atherosclerosis, lipid-driven immune-inflammatory disease [3].

We, therefore, aimed to determine the relationships between classic markers of inflammation (white blood cell and its subtypes) and AIP in acute coronary syndrome, also to evaluate the value the aforementioned parameters in the differential diagnoses of chest pain patients.

Methods

Study design and definition

We retrospectively reviewed institutional electronic medical records to seek chest pain patients who were suspicious of acute coronary syndrome between January 2011 and December 2013. All the patients were identified by undergoing coronary angiography. ACS group included STEMI, non-ST elevated myocardial infarction (NSTEMI) and unstable angina (UA) that were defined based on the criteria formulated by updated guidelines [15, 16]. Patients in the control group were certified the coronary artery normal by angiography. The chief complaint of all the included patients was chest pain. All the patients' medical records were reviewed to extract the demographic and clinical data by two physicians (Youqin Zhan and Tan Xu).

Hypertension was determined if the systolic BP (SBP) was ≥140 mm Hg and/or the diastolic BP (DBP) was over 90 mm Hg and/or use of antihypertensive medication [17]. Individuals with type 2 diabetes were diagnosed according to the criteria of the American Diabetes Association, [18] namely when plasma fasting glucose was more than 7.0 mmol/L (or 2-h postprandial glucose ≥11.1 mmol/L) and/or if there was current use of diabetes medication.

Patients with clinical evidence of active infection, cancer, hematological disease, systemic inflammatory conditions, autoimmune disease, liver disease, and renal failure were excluded from the study. As well as, patients with a history of prior myocardial infarction (MI), cerebrovascular event, peripheral arterial disease, percutaneous coronary intervention, coronary bypass surgery, and treatment with anti-platelet or statins were also excluded.

Laboratory analysis

On admission WBC and its subtypes were measured as part of the automated complete blood count (Beckman counter LH780, USA). Fasting venous blood samples were obtained and analyzed for lipids, liver and kidney function used automated analysis (Beckman counter AU5800, USA). The NLR and AIP was calculated by EXCEL (Microsoft Excel). The NLR was calculated as the ratio of the neutrophils and lymphocytes, both obtained from the same automated blood sample at admission. AIP was defined as logarithm of this ratio (TG/HDL-C]) on the base of 10, which corrects for the lack of normative distribution of the ratio [14].

Statistical analysis

The data were stored using the MS Excel program. The statistical analysis was carried out using SPSS for Windows release 13.0. Continuous variables are expressed as means and SD, as counts and percentages for Categorical variables. The conformity of all parameters to a normal distribution was tested using the Kolmogorov-Smirnov test. The independent t test and oneway ANOVA test were used for continuous variables. The x^2 test was performed for the comparison of categorical variables. A value of $p < .05$ on the two-sided test was considered statistically significant.

This study was submitted to and approved by the Research and Ethics Committee of First Affiliated Hospital of Shantou University Medical College.

Results

Baseline characteristics

In this case-control retrospective study, a total of 376 consecutive patients with ACS were investigated. In the same period, 378 patients admitted with chest pain suspicious of ACS were also included in this study for control. Comparison of clinical and biochemical variables in the ACS and control groups are shown in Table 1. All the Subjects hadn't the history of previous use of statin. The patients in the ACS group were older than those in the control group. Body mass index, rate of smoking, history of hypertension were not different between the ACS and control groups. Blood glucose, serum creatinine, white blood cell, neutrophil and monocyte were insignificantly higher in the ACS group. On lipid profiles, ACS group had higher total cholesterol and lower HDL-c. However, TG and LDL-c were similar between ACS and control groups.

Lipid-driven inflammatory state-AIP and NLR

All the included patients were suspicious of acute coronary syndrome: lipid-driven inflammatory state. Two

Table 1 Comparison of clinical and biochemical variables in the ACS and control groups

	ACS group ($n = 376$)	Control group ($n = 378$)	p value
Age (years)	63.60 ± 11.74	59.81 ± 9.47	<0.001[b]
Male gender (%)	206 (54.79)	199 (52.65)	0.560[a]
BMI (kg/m^2)	23.51 ± 2.08	22.76 ± 1.18	0.510[b]
Smoker (%)	250 (66.49)	174 (46.03)	0.070[a]
History of hypertension (%)	168 (44.68)	184 (48.68)	0.275[a]
History of diabetes mellitus (%)	84 (22.34)	46 (12.17)	<0.001[a]
SBP (mmHg)	130.99 ± 24.26	136.54 ± 20.48	0.001[b]
DBP (mmHg)	80.60 ± 14.50	82.54 ± 12.66	0.050[b]
Blood glucose (mmol/L)	9.23 ± 11.03	5.96 ± 1.84	<0.001[b]
Serum creatinine (ummol/L)	101.84 ± 38.57	88.17 ± 29.99	<0.001[b]
WBC (*10^9/L)	10.83 ± 3.65	7.60 ± 2.49	<0.001[b]
Neutrophil (*10^9/L)	7.98 ± 3.44	5.33 ± 10.25	<0.001[b]
Lymphocyte (*10^9/L)	1.93 ± 0.92	2.08 ± 0.74	0.016[b]
Monocyte (*10^9/L)	0.68 ± 0.33	0.513 ± 0.213	<0.001[b]
Hemoglobin (g/L)	138.62 ± 66.94	134.27 ± 14.21	0.217[b]
TC (mmol/L)	5.09 ± 1.30	4.86 ± 1.20	0.015[b]
TG (mmol/L)	1.62 ± 1.15	1.83 ± 5.13	0.402[b]
HDL-c (mmol/L)	1.11 ± 0.34	1.24 ± 0.62	<0.001[b]
LDL-c (mmol/L)	3.31 ± 1.09	3.67 ± 7.37	0.367[b]

BMI body mass index, *SBP* systolic blood pressure, *DBP* diastolic blood pressure, *WBC* white blood cell, *TC* total cholesterol, *TG* triglyceride, *HDL-c* high density lipid-cholesterol, *LDL-c* low density lipid-cholesterol. [a]Chi-square test. [b]Independent *t* test

parameters, AIP and NLR, maybe reflect the state. As was to be expected, AIP was significantly higher in ACS group compared to control group ($p = 0.029$, shown in Fig. 1a). Similarly, ACS group had higher NLR than those in control group ($p < 0.001$, shown in Fig. 1b).

In order to further analyze the lipid-driven inflammatory state in ACS, the ACS groups were divided into three subgroups, namely, STEMI, NSTEMI and UA groups. Of the 376 ACS patients included, 237 (63.03 %) had STEMI, 74 (19.68 %) had NSTEMI and 65 (17.29 %) had UA. Table 2 shows the baseline characteristic of the aforementioned three groups. Mean ages, male genders and body mass index were similar in the three groups ($p = 0.234$, $p = 0.078$ and $p = 0.172$, respectively). Smoking was more frequently in the STEMI group ($p = 0.033$). Rate of hypertension was higher in the UA groups ($p = 0.002$). However, the frequencies of diabetes mellitus were similar between the three groups ($p = 0.194$). On the inflammation profiles, white blood cell, neutrophil and monocyte were lower in the UA groups than the other two groups ($p < 0.001$, $p < 0.001$ and $p = 0.004$, respectively). On the lipid profiles, there were no differences in total cholesterol, triglyceride, high density lipid-cholesterol and low density lipid-cholesterol between the three subgroups ($p = 0.189$, $p = 0.578$, $p = 0.702$, and $p = 0.574$, respectively). In the subgroups, the NLR were significantly higher in the

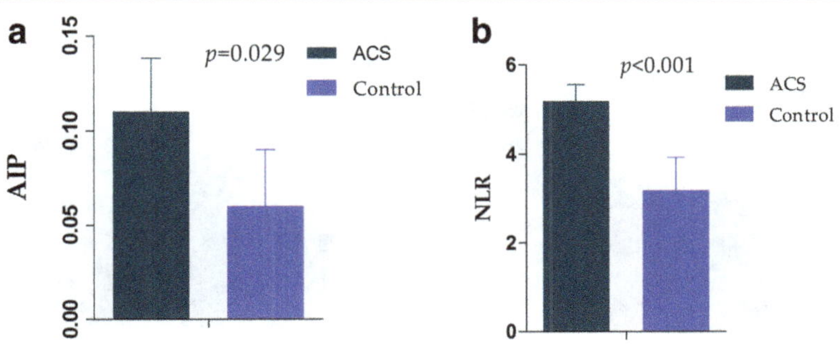

Fig. 1 Comparison AIP (1**a**), NLR (1**b**) between the ACS and control groups

Table 2 The baseline characteristic of STEMI, NSTEM and UA groups

	STEMI group $n = 237$	NSTEMI group $n = 74$	UA group $n = 65$	p value
Age (years)	62.81 ± 11.45	64.91 ± 13.05	64.98 ± 11.11	0.234[b]
Male gender (%)	129 (54.43)	39 (52.70)	38 (58.46)	0.078[a]
BMI (kg/m^2)	23.66 ± 1.99	23.16 ± 2.28	23.38 ± 2.22	0.172[b]
Smoker (%)	169 (71.31)	42 (56.76)	39 (60.00)	0.033[a]
History of hypertension (%)	90 (37.97)	39 (52.70)	39 (60.00)	0.002[a]
History of diabetes mellitus (%)	48 (20.25)	16 (21.62)	20 (30.77)	0.194[a]
SBP (mmHg)	127.07 ± 21.54	134.45 ± 30.66	141.34 ± 22.07	<0.00 [b]
DBP (mmHg)	79.00 ± 13.49	82.42 ± 17.48	84.37 ± 13.53	0.014[b]
Blood glucose (mmol/L)	9.94 ± 13.60	8.55 ± 3.33	7.40 ± 3.57	0.218[b]
Serum creatinine (ummol/L)	101.50 ± 37.56	104.78 ± 43.93	99.75 ± 36.06	0.727[b]
WBC (*10^9/L)	11.45 ± 3.56	11.14 ± 3.82	8.16 ± 2.43	<0.00 [b]
Neutrophil (*10^9/L)	8.63 ± 3.35	8.18 ± 3.60	5.32 ± 2.15	<0.00 [b]
Lymphocyte (*10^9/L)	1.88 ± 0.94	1.98 ± 0.94	2.07 ± 0.81	0.302[b]
Monocyte (*10^9/L)	0.70 ± 0.34	0.74 ± 0.38	0.56 ± 0.24	0.004[b]
Hemoglobin (g/L)	136.67 ± 16.70	150.49 ± 147.18	132.13 ± 15.24	0.210[b]
TC (mmol/L)	5.14 ± 1.29	5.08 ± 1.27	4.92 ± 1.35	0.189[b]
TG (mmol/L)	1.59 ± 1.12	1.75 ± 1.39	1.59 ± 0.94	0.578[b]
HDL-c (mmol/L)	1.11 ± 0.31	1.14 ± 0.47	1.10 ± 0.27	0.702[b]
LDL-c (mmol/L)	3.36 ± 1.07	3.24 ± 1.14	3.23 ± 1.08	0.574[b]

BMI body mass index, *SBP* systolic blood pressure, *DBP* diastolic blood pressure, *WBC* white blood cell, *TC* total cholesterol, *TG* triglyceride, *HDL-c* high density lipid-cholesterol, *LDL-c* low density lipid-cholesterol. [a]Chi-square test. [b]oneway ANOVA test

STEMI group ($p < 0.001$, shown in Fig. 2a). However, AIP were similar between the three subgroups ($p = 0.748$, shown in Fig. 2b).

Discussion

Our data firstly investigated the lipid-driven inflammatory state in acute coronary syndrome through two easily feasible parameters. Retrospective evaluation of the AIP and NLR as a lipid and inflammation profiles in ACS patients yielded the following salient information. The main conclusions were that: (i) there were higher AIP and NLR in the ACS patients compared with other chest pain patients suspicious of ACS; and (ii) In the ACS subgroups, the NLR were significantly higher in the STEMI group, however, AIP were similar.

Regarding lipids profiles in ACS patients, there has been accumulated several clinical trials to demonstrate the potential role of lipid in the development of ACS. A statistically significant association between thrombosis caused by plaque rupture and high TC, low high-density lipoprotein cholesterol, and high TC/HDL-C ratio in men has been evaluated by Burke et al. [19]. In this study, there found that significantly higher TC and lower HDL-c in ACS group.

Recently, more studies have been focused on the parameter-AIP, which is a surrogate of small LDL particle size. Altan O. et al found that high AIP is a strong risk factor for CAD in both Turkish men and women [12]. Similarly, in the present study, AIP also was also higher in the ACS groups compared with control groups.

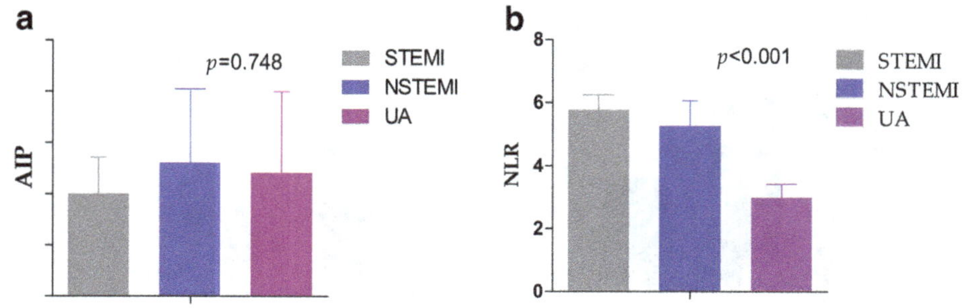

Fig. 2 Comparison AIP (2**a**), NLR (2**b**) between the ACS subgroups

However, between the subgroups of ACS, there were no difference in TC, HDL-c and AIP, which may reflects the coherence of ACS subgroups. Otherwise, a recent study [20] showed that the TC/HDL ratio was a marker of severity of CAD in relation to the number of vessels affected in patients with ACS without ST-segment elevation.

On the inflammation of ACS, it has been shown to play a role in the pathogenesis of coronary atherosclerosis [21]. In recent years, higher white blood cell [22] (WBC), and neutrophil [23, 24], have been evaluated to be associated with ACS. It has been shown that elevated baseline WBC count was associated with higher short-term mortality in UA and NSTEMI [25]. A recent study [22] presented that WBC was strongly associated with CHD. In terms of neutrophil, more studies described that elevated neutrophil may predict worse outcomes, such as chronic heart failure, [24] cardiogenic death [23]. Our study shows that a significantly higher WBC and neutrophil in the ACS group, and there also exists significantly differences in WBC and neutrophil between the ACS subgroups.

Moreover, NLR was introduced as a potential marker to determine inflammation in cardiac disorder and shown as a predictor of long-term mortality in ACS patients [26, 27]. Ramazan C. O. et al reported that NLR was significantly associated with adverse in-hospital outcomes, independent of GRACE risk score in STEMI patients. In the present study, ACS patients also had higher NLR compared to angiographic normal patients. Moreover, the NLR had significant differences in the ACS subgroups, highest in the STEMI subgroup.

The most challenging finding of the present study was to demonstrate the lipid-driven inflammation state in ACS patients used two combination parameters- AIP and NLR. To the best of our knowledge, no studies have assessed the potential role of AIP and NLR together in ACS patients to evaluate the lipid-driven inflammation state. Unlikely many other marker and bioassays, AIP and NLR are inexpensive and readily available markers that provides an additional level of risk scores in predicting short and long term outcomes in ACS patients. In this study, there are differences of AIP and NLR between ACS and control groups. However, in the ACS subgroups, although no difference found in AIP, yet there were differences in NLR. In the view of above differences, there may interpret as the following in leading pathological terms. Firstly, ACS is a systemic, lipid-driven inflammatory disease. Therefore, compared to angiographic normal patients, ACS groups had higher AIP and NLR, which reflect the lipid and inflammation status. Secondly, in the ACS groups, there are all lipid-driven states, so there is no difference in AIP. However, there may be different inflammation levels in the ACS groups. Lastly, coincidence may exist in the differences.

Study limitations

The present study must be interpreted within the context of its potential limitations. First, this was a retrospective and single-center pilot study. Further prospective multicenter studies with a larger sample size may be needed. Second, the patients in NSTEMI and UA subgroups were smaller compared with the STEMI subgroups which may disturb the results. Third, we could not compare AIP and NLR with other lipid and inflammatory markers, because they were not routinely assessed in our study population.

Conclusion

Our data suggest that there are higher AIP and NLR in the ACS patients, which evaluate the lipid-driven inflammation state, used two inexpensive parameters. Moreover, ACS subgroups are all lipid-driven states, but inflammation levels are different in the entity ACS subgroups. One challenge of the study is that we firstly evaluate the lipid-driven inflammation state of ACS used two ratio parameters together, AIP and NLR. Further studies are required to confirm the clinical relevance of these findings by comparing the association of AIP and NLR together with clinical outcomes.

Abbreviations

CHD: coronary heart disease; ACS: acute coronary syndrome; STEMI: ST-segment elevation myocardial infarction; NSTEMI: non-ST elevated myocardial infarction; UA: unstable angina; MI: myocardial infarction; WBC: white blood cell; NLR: neutrophil–lymphocyte ratio; TG: triglycerides; HDL-c: high density lipoprotein cholesterol; AIP: atherogenic index of plasma; LDL-c: low-density lipoprotein- cholesterol.

Competing interests

The authors declare that they have no competing interests.

Authors' contributions

YZ and TX performed the survey and wrote the draft of manuscript. XT designed the study, helped interpret the analysis results, and assisted in modifying the manuscript. All authors read and approved the final manuscript.

Acknowledgements

None.

Funding

The study was partially supported by the National Natural Science Foundation of China; (NO.81473063).

References

1. Kaya MG, Uyarel H, Akpek M, Kalay N, Ergelen M, Ayhan E, et al. Prognostic value of uric acid in patients with ST-elevated myocardial infarction undergoing primary coronary intervention. Am J Cardiol. 2012;109(4):486–91.
2. Libby P, Theroux P. Pathophysiology of coronary artery disease. Circulation. 2005;111(25):3481–8.
3. Falk E, Nakano M, Bentzon JF, Finn AV, Virmani R. Update on acute coronary syndromes: the pathologists' view. Eur Heart J. 2013;34(10):719–28.

4. Libby P. Inflammation in atherosclerosis. Nature. 2002;420(6917):868–74.
5. Fiechter M, Ghadri JR, Jaguszewski M, Siddique A, Vogt S, Haller RB, et al. Impact of inflammation on adverse cardiovascular events in patients with acute coronary syndromes. J Cardiovasc Med (Hagerstown). 2013;14(11):807–14.
6. Palmerini T, Brener SJ, Mehran R, Dangas G, Genereux P, Riva DD, et al. Leukocyte count is a modulating factor for the mortality benefit of bivalirudin in ST-segment-elevation acute myocardial infarction: the HORIZONS-AMI trial. Circ Cardiovasc Interv. 2013;6(5):518–26.
7. Yilmaz M, Tenekecioglu E, Arslan B, Bekler A, Ozluk OA, Karaagac K, Agca FV, Peker T, Akgumus A. White Blood Cell Subtypes and Neutrophil-Lymphocyte Ratio in Prediction of Coronary Thrombus Formation in Non-ST-Segment Elevated Acute Coronary Syndrome. Clin Appl Thromb Hemost. 2015;21(5):446–452.
8. Horne BD, Anderson JL, John JM, Weaver A, Bair TL, Jensen KR, et al. Which white blood cell subtypes predict increased cardiovascular risk? J Am Coll Cardiol. 2005;45(10):1638–43.
9. Kounis NG, Soufras GD, Tsigkas G, Hahalis G. White blood cell counts, leukocyte ratios, and eosinophils as inflammatory markers in patients with coronary artery disease. Clin Appl Thromb Hemost. 2015;21(2):139–143.
10. Smith Jr SC, Jackson R, Pearson TA, Fuster V, Yusuf S, Faergeman O, et al. Principles for national and regional guidelines on cardiovascular disease prevention: a scientific statement from the World Heart and Stroke Forum. Circulation. 2004;109(25):3112–21.
11. LaRosa JC. Prevention and treatment of coronary heart disease: who benefits? Circulation. 2001;104(14):1688–92.
12. Onat A, Can G, Kaya H, Hergenc G. "Atherogenic index of plasma" (log10 triglyceride/high-density lipoprotein-cholesterol) predicts high blood pressure, diabetes, and vascular events. J Clin Lipidol. 2010;4(2):89–98.
13. Frohlich J, Dobiasova M. Fractional esterification rate of cholesterol and ratio of triglycerides to HDL-cholesterol are powerful predictors of positive findings on coronary angiography. Clin Chem. 2003;49(11):1873–80.
14. Dobiasova M, Frohlich J. The plasma parameter log (TG/HDL-C) as an atherogenic index: correlation with lipoprotein particle size and esterification rate in apoB-lipoprotein-depleted plasma (FER(HDL)). Clin Biochem. 2001;34(7):583–8.
15. O'Gara PT, Kushner FG, Ascheim DD, Casey Jr DE, Chung MK, de Lemos JA, et al. 2013 ACCF/AHA guideline for the management of ST-elevation myocardial infarction: a report of the American College of Cardiology Foundation/American Heart Association Task Force on Practice Guidelines. Circulation. 2013;127(4):e362–425.
16. Hamm CW, Bassand JP, Agewall S, Bax J, Boersma E, Bueno H, et al. ESC Guidelines for the management of acute coronary syndromes in patients presenting without persistent ST-segment elevation: The Task Force for the management of acute coronary syndromes (ACS) in patients presenting without persistent ST-segment elevation of the European Society of Cardiology (ESC). Eur Heart J. 2011;32(23):2999–3054.
17. Chobanian AV, Bakris GL, Black HR, Cushman WC, Green LA, Izzo Jr JL, et al. The Seventh Report of the Joint National Committee on Prevention, Detection, Evaluation, and Treatment of High Blood Pressure: the JNC 7 report. JAMA. 2003;289(19):2560–72.
18. Kerner W, Bruckel J. Definition, classification and diagnosis of diabetes mellitus. Exp Clin Endocrinol Diabetes. 2014;122(7):384–386.
19. Burke AP, Farb A, Malcom GT, Liang YH, Smialek J, Virmani R. Coronary risk factors and plaque morphology in men with coronary disease who died suddenly. N Engl J Med. 1997;336(18):1276–82.
20. Penalva RA, Huoya Mde O, Correia LC, Feitosa GS, Ladeia AM. Lipid profile and intensity of atherosclerosis disease in acute coronary syndrome. Arq Bras Cardiol. 2008;90(1):24–30.
21. Libby P, Ridker PM, Maseri A. Inflammation and atherosclerosis. Circulation. 2002;105(9):1135–43.
22. Cavusoglu E, Chopra V, Gupta A, Ruwende C, Yanamadala S, Eng C, et al. Usefulness of the white blood cell count as a predictor of angiographic findings in an unselected population referred for coronary angiography. Am J Cardiol. 2006;98(9):1189–93.
23. Huang G, Zhong XN, Zhong B, Chen YQ, Liu ZZ, Su L, et al. Significance of white blood cell count and its subtypes in patients with acute coronary syndrome. Eur J Clin Invest. 2009;39(5):348–58.
24. Kyne L, Hausdorff JM, Knight E, Dukas L, Azhar G, Wei JY. Neutrophilia and congestive heart failure after acute myocardial infarction. Am Heart J. 2000;139(1 Pt 1):94–100.
25. Sabatine MS, Morrow DA, Cannon CP, Murphy SA, Demopoulos LA, DiBattiste PM, et al. Relationship between baseline white blood cell count and degree of coronary artery disease and mortality in patients with acute coronary syndromes: a TACTICS-TIMI 18 (Treat Angina with Aggrastat and determine Cost of Therapy with an Invasive or Conservative Strategy-Thrombolysis in Myocardial Infarction 18 trial)substudy. J Am Coll Cardiol. 2002;40(10):1761–8.
26. Tamhane UU, Aneja S, Montgomery D, Rogers EK, Eagle KA, Gurm HS. Association between admission neutrophil to lymphocyte ratio and outcomes in patients with acute coronary syndrome. Am J Cardiol. 2008;102(6):653–7.
27. Duffy BK, Gurm HS, Rajagopal V, Gupta R, Ellis SG, Bhatt DL. Usefulness of an elevated neutrophil to lymphocyte ratio in predicting long-term mortality after percutaneous coronary intervention. Am J Cardiol. 2006;97(7):993–6.

16

Chest pain in the emergency department: risk stratification with Manchester triage system and HEART score

Luís Leite[1*], Rui Baptista[1], Jorge Leitão[2], Joana Cochicho[2], Filipe Breda[2], Luís Elvas[1], Isabel Fonseca[3], Armando Carvalho[2] and José Nascimento Costa[2]

Abstract

Background: Fast and accurate chest pain risk stratification in the emergency department (ED) is critical. The HEART score predicts the short-term incidence of major adverse cardiac events (MACE) in this population, dividing it in three risk categories. We aimed to describe the population with chest pain, to characterize the subgroup of patients with acute coronary syndrome (ACS) and to assess the prognostic value of Manchester triage system and of HEART score.

Methods: Retrospective observational study including patients admitted to the ED of a tertiary hospital with chest pain as the presenting symptom. The primary outcome was a composite of all-cause mortality, myocardial infarction or unscheduled revascularization at 6 weeks.

Results: We enrolled 233 patients (age 58 ± 19; 55.4 % males). The most common final diagnosis was non-specific chest pain ($n = 86$, 36.9 %), followed by ACS ($n = 22$, 9.4 %). Male gender, smoking and chronic kidney disease were associated with higher risk of ACS. According to Manchester triage system, chest pain patients stratified with red or orange priority had a higher incidence of ACS (16.5 % vs. 3.8 %, $p = 0.006$). The application of HEART score showed that most patients were in low risk category (56.3 %). The six-week incidence of MACE in each category was 2 %, 15.6 % and 76.9 % ($p < 0.001$). HEART score accurately predicted the short-term incidence of MACE in chest pain patients (c-statistic 0.880; 95 % CI, 0.807–0.950, $p < 0.001$).

Conclusions: Chest pain patients have very different levels of severity and the discriminatory power of Manchester triage system should be used in the assessment of this population. The HEART score seems to be an effective tool for risk stratification in the ED.

Keywords: Chest pain, Emergency department, Manchester triage system, HEART score, Acute coronary syndrome, Angina pectoris

Background

Chest pain management is one of the biggest challenges in the emergency department (ED). This symptom accounts for 5 to 20 % of all ED admissions [1], being the second most common reason to present to the ED in the United States of America [2]. Causes of chest pain range from musculoskeletal chest pain to potentially life-threatening emergencies as acute coronary syndrome (ACS), aortic dissection or pulmonary embolism. Therefore, accurate and fast risk stratification is paramount in the acute management of these patients, mainly to identify those patients with immediate risk of complications, as those with an ACS. This group of patients is challenging to discriminate, as there is a variety of clinical manifestations.

To minimize this problem, several risk stratifying tools have been developed in the last years. Some of these tools are applicable to all clinical situations presenting to the ED, as the Manchester triage system. This validated system is performed by specifically trained nurses and prioritize patients according to illness severity and is based on the main complaint and in the presence of certain

*Correspondence: luispcleite@gmail.com
[1]Departament of Cardiology, Centro Hospitalar e Universitário de Coimbra, Praceta Prof. Mota Pinto, Coimbra 3000-075, Portugal
Full list of author information is available at the end of the article

discriminators, according to a structured questionnaire [3]. A colour is assigned to each level of urgency, specifying a target time to first medical observation: red (immediate); orange (<10 min); yellow (<60 min); green (<120 min) and blue (<240 min).

Other systems, more selective, are devoted to the risk stratification of suspected ACS in the ED. One is the HEART score, designed to be performed by the ED physician, predicting the short-term occurrence of major adverse cardiac events (MACE) - all-cause death, myocardial infarction or revascularization – in the ED population of chest pain patients [4].

We aimed (1) to describe an unselected population of chest pain patients presenting to the ED; (2) to characterize the subgroup of patients diagnosed with an ACS and (3) to determine the value of Manchester triage system and HEART score for risk stratification in acute chest pain.

Methods

Study design

We conducted a retrospective cohort study, which included all patients admitted to the ED of a tertiary referral hospital, with non-traumatic chest pain as the chief complaint. This ED receives around 400 to 500 patients daily, having no dedicated chest pain unit. There was no exclusion criterion in the selection of patients.

All clinical, laboratory and imaging data were recorded in a proprietary software specially developed for ED environments (ALERT®, ALERT systems, Vila Nova de Gaia, Portugal). In our ED, all patients are stratified by priority using a risk stratification protocol - the Manchester triage system - performed by specifically trained nurses. From the data introduced in ALERT®, we collected clinical information from the ED patients, analysed the level of priority given, prior medical history, diagnostic tests results and the final diagnosis. According to the diagnosis made by the ED cardiologist, using the current definition [5], patients were divided into two groups: group 1 – established ACS diagnosis; group 2 – no ACS. Nevertheless, every patient admitted to in-hospital care was reviewed by the authors to confirm the diagnosis. The research protocol was approved by the local ethics committee (*Comissão de Ética para a Saúde do Centro Hospitalar e Universitário de Coimbra*).

ACS risk-stratifying systems

The HEART score was retrospectively applied to the population according to the information available in the ALERT® system and in the electronic health records of the hospital. The acronym HEART is an abbreviation of the five parameters evaluated [6]:

- History (highly suspicious – 2 points; moderately suspicious – 1 point; slightly suspicious – 0 points)
- ECG (significant ST-depression – 2 points; non-specific repolarization disturbance – 1 point; normal – 0 points)
- Age (≥65 years – 2 points; 45–65 years – 1 point; ≤ 45 years – 0 points)
- Risk factors for coronary heart disease (≥3 risk factors – 2 points; 1 or 2 risk factors – 1 point; no risk factors – 0 points)
- Troponin (≥3 times the threshold for positivity – 2 points; 1 to 3 times the threshold for positivity – 1 point; normal limit – 0 points)

Two independent authors, blinded to the final diagnosis, performed the classification of the degree of suspicion in the 'history' parameter. In the cases with two different scores, the mean value was considered. The ECG's were interpreted by the attending physician in the ED, specialist in internal medicine or in cardiology.

According to the total score received, patients are divided into low (0–3), intermediate (4–6) or high (7–10) risk of a MACE, within 6 weeks after presentation at the ED. Lower scores lead to a recommendation of early discharge, intermediate scores suggest clinical observation or performance of non-invasive investigations and high scores admission for more invasive strategies [4]. In the analysis of HEART score data, we only used patients with available records to complete all the five parameters of the score, excluding patients without ECG or troponin measurement. This has led to a dropout of 59 patients (25.3 %).

A 6-week follow-up of all patients was conducted through the electronic health records information of the hospital and through direct phone calls to the patients involved. The follow-up focused on the composite endpoint of MACE, comprising all-cause death, myocardial infarction or unscheduled revascularization. No patient was lost to follow-up.

Statistical analysis

We aimed to find a difference in 6-week MACE between low, intermediate and high risk categories of HEART score. Based on the proportions of the multicentre study of Backus et al. [4] and assuming an alpha of 0.05, we would need a sample of 168 patients to detect differences with 80 % power. Since we anticipate that 20–25 % of patients could not have records to complete all the parameters of the score, we aimed for a sample size of 220 patients. The period of time analysed included 1 week from winter (23rd to 29th January 2012) and 1 week from summer (23rd to 29th July 2012), randomly selected, in order to balance the list of final diagnosis. Statistical analysis was carried out using IBM SPSS Statistics for Windows software version 20.0® (Armonk, New York). Normality of continuous variables was tested by histogram observation and Kolmogorov-Smirnov test. Continuous variables are presented by mean ± standard deviation and categorical variables as percentage. We used Student's *T* test and Mann–Whitney test for comparison of means for continuous variables, Chi-square and Fisher's exact test for comparison of categorical variables. Multiple logistic regression adjusted for confounding factors was performed considering any variable with $p < 0.25$ in univariate analysis. A received operator characteristics (ROC) curve was used to determine the discriminatory power of HEART score. Results with $p < 0.05$ were considered as statistically significant.

Results

Characterization of the chest pain population in the ED

We evaluated 233 patients presenting with non-traumatic chest pain, which accounted for 4.2 % of all ED admissions. The demographic characteristics and the priority stratification according to Manchester triage system are shown on Table 1. Age ranged from 19 to 98 years and women were significantly older than men (60.7 ± 20 vs. 55.4 ± 13, $p = 0.012$).

The most frequently requested diagnostic tests were chest X-ray (85.4 %), ECG (81.5 %) and cardiac biomarkers (74.2 %). The median time from patient ED arrival to ECG acquisition was 20 (IQR 12–41) minutes. According to Manchester triage system, patients stratified with a red or orange priority performed the ECG significantly faster than those with yellow or green priority (median 15 vs. 28 min, $p < 0.001$)

Table 1 Demographic characteristics and Manchester triage system

Variable	
Age, mean ± SD	57.7 ± 19
Male gender, n (%)	129 (55.4)
Manchester triage system, n (%)	
- Red	1 (0.4)
- Orange	102 (43.8)
- Yellow	99 (42.5)
- Green	31 (13.3)
Past medical history, n (%)	
- Hypertension	125 (53.6)
- Dyslipidemia	90 (38.6)
- Type 2 diabetes	33 (14.2)
- Active smoker	31 (13.3)
- Coronary artery disease	36 (15.5)
- Atrial fibrillation	42 (18)
- Heart failure	38 (16.3)
- Chronic pulmonary obstructive disease	16 (6.9)
- Chronic kidney disease	11 (4.7)
- Others	31 (13.3)

SD standard deviation

As presented in Fig. 1, after clinical observation and interpretation of diagnostic tests, the most common diagnosis made by the attending physician was non-specific chest pain ($n = 86$, 36.9 %), followed by ACS ($n = 22$, 9.4 %), anxiety-depressive disorder ($n = 21$, 9.0 %) and respiratory infection ($n = 20$, 8.6 %). The group of the less frequent diagnosis (10.3 %) included: cardiovascular diseases, as aortic dissection or acute pericarditis; pulmonary diseases, as acute asthma; and gastrointestinal diseases, as gastro-oesophageal reflux disease or biliary colic.

Stratifying the final diagnosis by season of the year, we found a higher proportion of patients being diagnosed with respiratory infections in the winter than in summer (15.9 % vs. 1.7 %, $p < 0.001$), whereas the proportion of the other final diagnosis, like non-specific chest pain or ACS, were similar in both seasons.

The great majority of patients presenting in the ED with chest pain were discharged home ($n = 189$, 81.1 %), while the remaining were admitted to hospital ($n = 44$, 18.9 %). The incidence of the composite endpoint of MACE was 9.4 %.

The patient flow diagram is summarized in Fig. 2.

Subgroup of acute coronary syndrome patients

Among the group of patients with a final diagnosis of ACS (group 1, $n = 22$), the most common ACS subtype was unstable angina (10 patients - 46 %), followed by non-ST-elevation myocardial infarction (NSTEMI) (7 patients - 32 %) and ST-elevation myocardial infarction (STEMI) (5 patients - 23 %). Group 1 patients were older and had a higher proportion of males, compared with the group of patients without ACS. Moreover, they had a significantly higher prevalence of hypertension, type 2 diabetes, dyslipidaemia, smoking habits, previously known coronary artery disease and chronic kidney disease (Table 2).

The great majority of patients diagnosed with an ACS were given high priorities by the Manchester triage system, with only 1 patient given the colour green (4.5 %). Most patients were classified as orange ($n = 16$, 72.8 %), followed by yellow ($n = 4$, 18.2 %) and red ($n = 1$, 4.5 %). The five STEMI patients were triaged with orange ($n = 4$, 80 %) or red ($n = 1$, 20 %) priority, while the seven NSTEMI patients were triaged as orange ($n = 6$, 85.7 %) or green ($n = 1$, 14.3 %).

There was a correlation between Manchester's priority category in chest pain patients and the final diagnosis of ACS: 3.2 % in the green category, 4.0 % in the yellow category, 15.7 % in the orange category and 100.0 % in the red category. Patients stratified red or orange had a significantly higher incidence of ACS compared with those with yellow or green levels of priority (16.5 % vs. 3.8 %, $p = 0.006$).

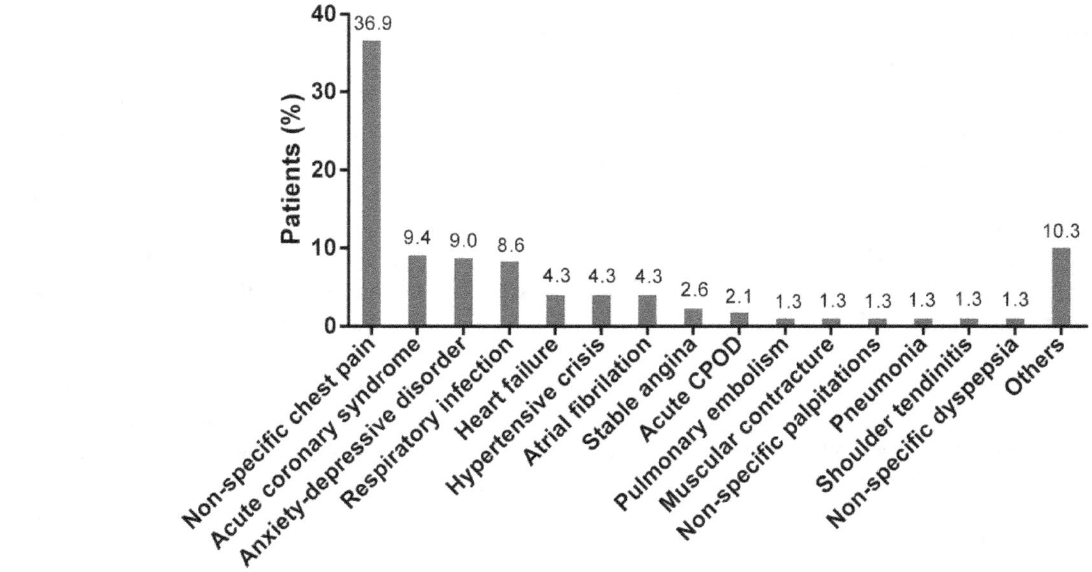

Figure 1 Final diagnosis of patients. COPD, chronic obstructive pulmonary disease

Using a multivariate analysis model controlling for age, gender, hypertension, dyslipidaemia, type 2 diabetes, smoking, coronary artery disease and chronic kidney disease, male gender (odds-ratio (OR) 4.48; 95 % confidence interval (CI), 1.12–17.40; $p = 0.030$), smoking (OR 4.22; 95 % CI, 1.21–14.74; $p = 0.024$) and chronic kidney disease (OR 8.21; 95 % CI, 1.76–38.16; $p = 0.007$) emerged as independent predictors of ACS in this population.

The use of HEART score in risk stratification

The determination of the HEART score in the population with complete datasets ($n = 174$) showed that most chest pain patients were low risk ($n = 98$, 56.3 %), followed by intermediate ($n = 64$, 36.7 %) and high risk ($n = 12$, 6.9 %).

Figure 3 illustrates the relationship between the HEART score and the incidence of the composite endpoint, with higher scores associated with higher incidence of 6-week MACE.

When the three externally validated categories of the HEART score were used (low risk 0–3; intermediate risk 4–6; high risk 7–10), a good discrimination of the incidence of 6-week MACE was obtained (2 %, 15.6 % and 76.9 %, $p < 0.001$), as showed in Fig. 4.

The HEART score had a good discriminatory power (c-statistic 0.880; 95 % CI, 0.807 – 0.950, $p < 0.001$) to predict the probability of the composite endpoint. The sensitivity, specificity, positive and negative predictive values for the established cut-off scores of 4 and 7 are shown in Table 3.

Discussion

In this study we described a population of patients presenting to an ED with chest pain as their main complaint. We demonstrated that less than 10 % have an ACS as the aetiology basis of this symptom and that the Manchester triage system correctly prioritized the patients with most severe causes of pain. Finally, we retrospectively tested the HEART score in our population, demonstrating that it has a good discriminatory power to identify the risk of MACE in a short term period.

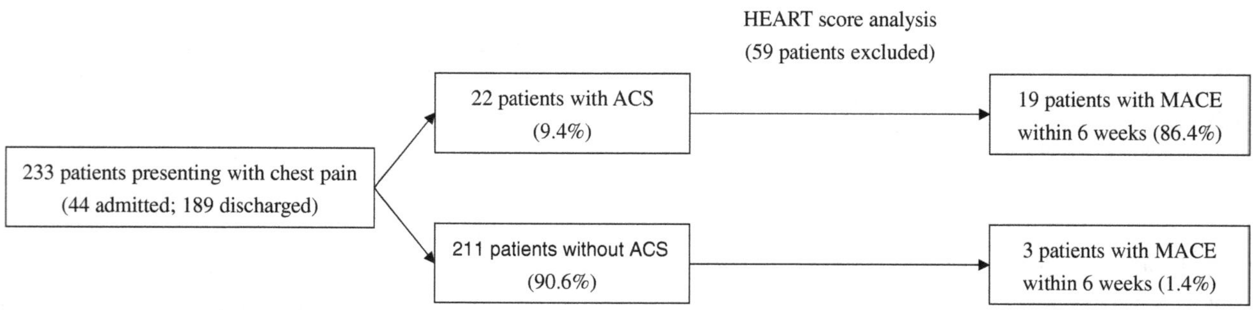

Figure 2 Flow diagram of patients presenting with chest pain. ED, emergency department; ACS, acute coronary syndrome; MACE, major adverse cardiovascular events

Table 2 Comparative of population characteristics ACS versus no ACS

	Group 1 – ACS (n = 22)	Group 2 – No ACS (n = 211)	p
Age, mean ± SD	65.6 ± 15	56.9 ± 19	0.043
Male gender, n (%)	18 (81.8)	111 (52.6)	0.012
Hypertension, n (%)	18 (81.8)	107 (50.7)	0.006
Dysl pidemia, n (%)	17 (73.9)	73 (34.6)	0.001
Type 2 diabetes, n (%)	8 (36.4)	25 (11.8)	0.005
Smcking, n (%)	8 (36.4)	23 (10.9)	0.003
Coronary artery disease, n (%)	9 (40.9)	27 (12.7)	0.002
Atrial fibrillation, n (%)	3 (13.6)	39 (18.5)	0.773
Heart failure, n (%)	3 (13.6)	35 (16.6)	0.957
Chronic pulmonary obstructive disease, n (%)	1 (4.5)	16 (7.6)	0.376
Chronic kidney disease, n (%)	5 (22.7)	6 (2.8)	0.002

ACS acute coronary syndrome, *SD* standard deviation

Our sample presented a male predominance, a wide range of age and a mean age similar to previous studies [7–9]. The analysis of the Manchester triage system in this population showed that more than a half of the patients were stratified with a green or a yellow level of severity, in accordance with the high incidence of potentially benign causes of chest pain. The most frequent comorbidities were similar to other studies [7, 9]; however we found a higher prevalence of hypertension and lower proportion of active smokers.

Considering the diagnostic tests, and in comparison with the results of the Spanish study of Martínez-Sellés et al. [7], our ED physicians requested more chest X-rays and cardiac biomarkers in this sample. The ECG is a first-line diagnostic tool in chest pain assessment and the time from ED arrival to ECG acquisition in this cohort was greater than the 10 min recommended in the current European Society of Cardiology guidelines [5]. Therefore, an effort must made to shorten this time, in order to identify life-threatening emergencies, namely to reduce time to revascularization therapy in STEMI.

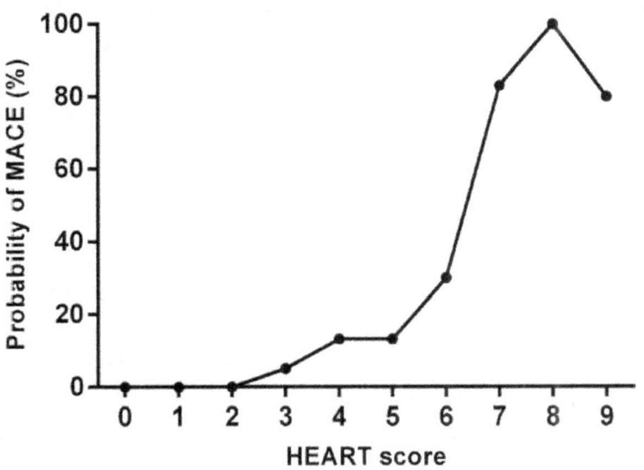

Figure 3 Incidence of 6-week MACE in each HEART score. MACE, major adverse cardiovascular events

The final diagnostic list of this population was extensive, with very different levels of severity, as in the literature [10]. Non-specific chest pain (mostly musculoskeletal pain) was the most frequent diagnosis, but with a proportion slightly lower than that reported in other studies, were it ranges from 43 to 59 % [7, 11]. This diagnosis is thus probably the most frequent one in an unselected population. ACS represented the second most common final diagnosis of chest pain in our population, albeit with a lower percentage than that reported in the literature (15.7 %) [7]. Stable angina had a relatively low proportion (2.6 %) on the list of the final diagnosis. Although this percentage is only slightly lower than in other studies [7], this clinical presentation of coronary artery disease may be underdiagnosed as non-specific chest pain.

Our study reports some traditional cardiovascular risk factors [12] that can increase significantly the odds of chest pain being of unstable coronary artery disease origin, as male gender, smoking and chronic kidney disease.

Considering the Manchester triage system, most of ACS patients were stratified with an orange or red level of priority, but this percentage was slightly lower than in previous studies [13, 14]. Although the proportion of patients stratified as yellow or green (n = 5, 22.7 %) could lead to an important delay in the management of ACS, namely in the time from arrival to ECG acquisition, none of these cases were STEMI, a reassuring finding that highlights the clinical value of the triage system. Taking in consideration all chest pain patients in the ED, the proportion of ACS is significantly higher in orange or red priority patients, in comparison to green or yellow, showing that the Manchester triage system has a reasonable discriminatory power. Our data are in line with another Portuguese cohort, where the sensitivity of this system in assigning red or orange priority to patients with ACS was 87.3 % [13].

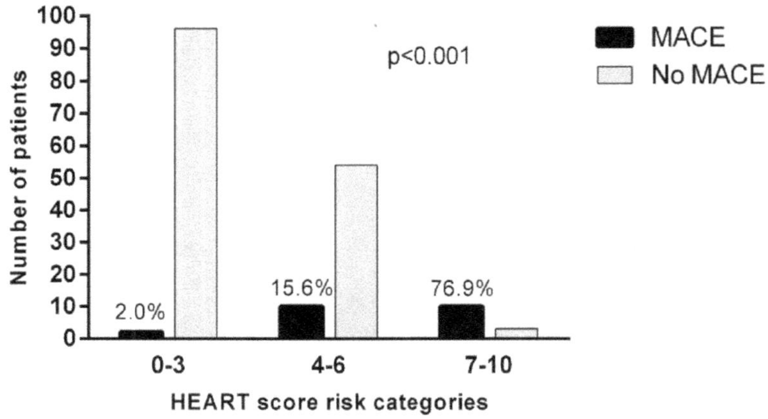

Figure 4 Incidence 6-week MACE in each HEART score risk category. MACE, major adverse cardiovascular events

In search for the optimal risk stratifying system for chest pain patients, we analysed the HEART score. This score was developed as an attempt to create an easy-to-use ACS risk quantification, incorporating well known markers of increased risk available on the ED, allowing a more firmly based decision, mainly in cases of atypical presentation or absence of ECG abnormalities [6]. The application of the HEART score to our population showed that the majority of patients are low risk, as it was reported in the first cohort where this score was applied [6]. The relationship between the HEART category and adverse outcomes, defined as the occurrence of MACE within 6 weeks, showed a curve with three different patterns, corresponding to the three risk categories defined by the literature [15]. The risk stratification using the three categories (0–3; 4–6; 7–10) identified MACE with similar proportions than in the multicentre study of Backus et al. [4], but with greater risk of MACE in the high risk category.

Our study confirmed the appropriate discriminatory power of the three risk categories of HEART score to predict short-term occurrence of MACE. A score <4, corresponding to low risk category, had a very high negative predictive value, identifying a small risk population. Moreover, the high risk category (score ≥7) showed a reasonable positive predictive value, allowing the identification of a high risk population, even in patients with more atypical presentations. This risk score may help in making accurate management choices in a setting that is frequently denoted by uncertainty, by being a strong predictor of event free survival and of potentially life threatening cardiac events.

Table 3 Sensitivity, specificity, positive and negative predictive values for six-week incidence of MACE using HEART score

	Cut-off = 4[a]	Cut-off = 7[b]
Sensitivity, % [95 % CI]	90.9 [70.8; 98.9]	45.5 [24.4; 67.79]
Specificity, % [95 % CI]	63.2 [55.0; 70.8]	98.7 [95.3; 99.8]
Positive predictive value, % [95 % CI]	26.3 [16.9; 37.7]	83.3 [51.59; 97.9]
Negative predictive value, % [95 % CI]	97.9 [92.8; 99.8]	92.6 [87.4; 96.1]

[a]98 patients with score <4 and 76 with score ≥4
[b]162 patients with score <7 and 12 with score ≥7

The limitations of this study are mainly those inherent to single-centre retrospective studies. The prevalence of obesity, an important cardiovascular risk factor, was not analysed because of lack of data about body mass index. In the analysis of HEART score, we only used patients with all the five parameters available to complete the score, which could lead to a selection bias. However, when comparing the characteristics of the patients with incomplete datasets with patients with complete datasets, no differences were found in the available variables. We are unaware of studies where the HEART score has been applied prospectively in real time, but such studies would be useful to confirm the prognostic value of the score. Furthermore, during the period of time analysed, the laboratory was using conventional troponin I assays, so we could not evaluate the potential impact of high-sensitivity troponin in chest pain management.

Conclusions

Chest pain is a common complaint in the ED and has an extensive differential diagnosis list with very different levels of severity. Age, gender, traditional cardiovascular risk factors and the priority attributed by the Manchester triage system should be considered in the assessment of patients. Moreover, the HEART score seems to be a useful tool for risk stratification and decision making in acute chest pain.

Abbreviations

ACS: Acute coronary syndrome; CI: Confidence interval; ED: Emergency department; MACE: Major adverse cardiac events; NSTEMI: Non-ST-elevation myocardial infarction; OR: Odds-ratio; SD: Standard deviation; STEMI: ST-elevation myocardial infarction.

Competing interests

The authors declare that they have no competing interests.

Authors' contributions

LL, conception and design, analysis and interpretation of data, manuscript writing. RB, substantial contribution to the design of the work, analysis of data, manuscript writing. JL, conception and design, analysis and interpretation of data, revising it critically for important intellectual content. JC and FB, acquisition and analysis of data, revising it critically for important intellectual content. LE, IF, AC and JNC, interpretation of data, revising it critically for important intellectual content. All authors read and approved the final manuscript.

Author details

[1]Departament of Cardiology, Centro Hospitalar e Universitário de Coimbra, Praceta Prof. Mota Pinto, Coimbra 3000-075, Portugal. [2]Department of Internal Medicine, Centro Hospitalar e Universitário de Coimbra, Praceta Prof. Mota Pinto, Coimbra 3000-075, Portugal. [3]Emergency Department, Centro Hospitalar e Universitário de Coimbra, Praceta Prof. Mota Pinto, Coimbra 3000-075, Portugal.

References

1 Fernández JB, Ezquerra EA, Genover XB, O'Callaghan AC, Gárriz I, Nácher J, et al. Chest pain units. Organization and protocol for the diagnosis of acute coronary syndromes. Rev Esp Cardiol. 2002;55:143–54.
2 Pitts SR, Niska RW, Xu J, Burt CW. National Hospital Ambulatory Medical Care Survey: 2006 emergency department summary. Natl Health Stat Report. 2008;7:1–38.
3 Cooke MW, Jinks S. Does the Manchester triage system detect the critically ill? J Accid Emerg Med. 1999;16:179–81.
4 Backus BE, Six AJ, Kelder JC, Mast TP, van den Akker F, Gijis Mast EG, et al. Chest pain in the emergency room: a multicenter validation of the HEART Score. Crit Pathw Cardiol. 2010;9:164–9.
5 Hamm CW, Bassand J-P, Agewall S, Bax J, Boersma E, Bueno H, et al. ESC Guidelines for the management of acute coronary syndromes in patients presenting without persistent ST-segment elevation: The Task Force for the management of acute coronary syndromes (ACS) in patients presenting without persistent ST-segment elevation. Eur Heart J. 2011;32:2999–3054.
6 Six AJ, Backus BE, Kelder JC. Chest pain in the emergency room: value of the HEART score. Neth Heart J. 2008;16:191–6.
7 Martínez-Sellés M, Bueno H, Sacristán A, Estévez A, Ortiz J, Gallego L, et al. Chest pain in the emergency department: incidence, clinical characteristics and risk stratification. Rev Esp Cardiol. 2008;61:953–9.
8 Burman RA, Zakariassen E, Hunskaar S. Acute chest pain - a prospective population based study of contacts to Norwegian emergency medical communication centres. BMC Emerg Med. 2011;11:9.
9 Hess EP, Perry JJ, Calder LA, Thiruganasambandamoorthy V, Roger VL, Wells GA, et al. Sex differences in clinical presentation, management and outcome in emergency department patients with chest pain. CJEM. 2010;12:405–13.
10. Erhardt L, Herlitz J, Bossaert L, Halinen M, Keltai M, Koster R, et al. Task force on the management of chest pain. Eur Heart J. 2002;23:1153–76.
11. Groarke J, O'Brien J, Go G, Susanto M, Owens P, Maree AO. Cost burden of non-specific chest pain admissions. Ir J Med Sci. 2013;182(1):57–61.
12. Perk J, De Backer G, Gohlke H, Graham I, Reiner Z, Verschuren M, et al. European Guidelines on cardiovascular disease prevention in clinical practice (version 2012). The Fifth Joint Task Force of the European Society of Cardiology and Other Societies on Cardiovascular Disease Prevention in Clinical Practice. Eur Heart J. 2012;2012(33):1635–701.
13. Pinto D, Lunet N, Azevedo A. Sensitivity and specificity of the Manchester Triage System for patients with acute coronary syndrome. Rev Port Cardiol. 2010;29:961–87.
14. Providência R, Gomes PL, Barra S, Silva J, Seca L, Antunes A, et al. Importance of Manchester Triage in acute myocardial infarction: impact on prognosis. Emerg Med J. 2011;28:212–6.
15. Backus BE, Six AJ, Kelder JH, Gibler WB, Moll FL, Doevendans PA. Risk scores for patients with chest pain: evaluation in the emergency department. Curr Cardiol Rev. 2011;7:2–8.

Correlations of serum cystatin C and glomerular filtration rate with vascular lesions and severity in acute coronary syndrome

Jinjin Zhang[1†], Xianhao Wu[2†], Peizhen Gao[3] and Pingping Yan[1*]

Abstract

Background: The aim of this study was to evaluate the predictive value of cystatin C (CysC) and estimated glomerular filtration rate (eGFR) regarding vascular lesions and their severity in patients with acute coronary syndrome (ACS).

Methods: According to the results of coronary angiography, 195 ACS patients were divided into a single-vascular-lesion group (91 cases), a dual-vascular-lesion group (67 cases), and a multiple-vascular-lesion group (37 cases) to assess the severity of coronary artery disease according to Gensini scores and to analyze the correlations of CysC and eGFR level with vascular lesions and severity in ACS patients.

Results: Intergroup comparisons of univariate and multivariate regression analyses showed that CysC was positively correlated with vascular lesions ($P < 0.05$), but eGFR showed no correlation. Regarding the severity of vascular lesions, CysC was positively correlated with Gensini score (Pearson's correlation coefficient $r = 0.1811$, $P < 0.05$), but eGFR was not correlated ($P > 0.05$).

Conclusions: Serum CysC levels could reflect the severity of vascular lesions in ACS patients, and a high CysC level had predictive value regarding the severity of vascular lesions in ACS.

Keywords: Acute coronary syndrome, Serum cystatin C, Glomerular filtration rate, Correlation study

Background

With changes in lifestyles and diet structures in China, current heart disease spectra have changed, and coronary heart disease (CHD) has become the most common cardiac disease. Meanwhile, with the acceleration of the aging process, the morbidity and mortality of CHD are exhibiting a rapidly increasing trend, and it has become a major chronic noncommunicable disease severely harming public health. Acute coronary syndrome (ACS), characterized by high incidence, high mortality, and high recurrence, is currently one of the diseases that is a serious hazard to human health. ACS includes ST segment-elevated myocardial infarction (STEMI), non-ST segment-elevated myocardial infarction (NSTEMI), and unstable angina. Different forms of ACS share a common pathophysiological basis, namely coronary atherosclerosis-based atheromatous plaque loosening, cracks, or rupture, so the intra-plaque substances that might result in thrombosis would be exposed in the blood, causing adhesion, activation, and aggregation of platelets on the damaged surface, followed by thrombosis as well as complete or incomplete occlusion of the diseased vessels. Cystatin C (CysC) and glomerular filtration rate (GFR) are indicators that could reflect renal dysfunction; the former is one of the sensitive indexes used to evaluate GFR [1] and could detect early renal damage. The important function of CysC is to regulate the hydrolysis of cysteine proteases; by inhibiting the activity of endogenous cysteine proteases, cell damage can

* Correspondence: pingpingyandoc@163.com
†Equal contributors
[1]Department of Cardiology, North Huashan Hospital of Fudan University, Shanghai 201907, People's Republic of China
Full list of author information is available at the end of the article

be avoided. Recent studies showed that CysC participates in inflammatory reactions, production of vascular wall matrix, and homeostasis of degradation as well as the pathological processes of vascular injuries; it might also participate in regulating the formation, stabilization, and regression of atherosclerotic plaques [2]. Therefore, it would have predictive value regarding the prognosis of coronary artery disease (CAD) [3–5]. Meanwhile, CysC also exhibited predictive value regarding the morbidity and mortality of cardiovascular disease in people with normal renal function [6–8]. GFR equations based on CysC or a combination of CysC with creatinine may be superior to GFR equations based on creatinine alone in patients with CAD [9]. However, because the correlations of these two factors with ACS are rare, further study is still needed to determine whether CysC could be used to predict the severity of vascular disease. A number of studies about the correlations of CysC and CHD reported inconsistent conclusions. Therefore, this study aimed to further clarify the correlations of these two factors with vascular lesions and their severity in ACS.

Methods

Clinical data

Inclusion criteria: A total of 195 patients with ACS diagnosed and hospitalized in our hospital from July 2012 to June 2013 were enrolled. All the patients met the diagnostic criteria of ACS defined by the ACC/AHA in 2014 [10] and were confirmed by coronary angiography (CAG) to have stenosis ≥50% in at least one coronary artery. Another 39 patients with negative CAG results were selected during the same period for a total enrollment of 234 patients. This study was conducted in accordance with the declaration of Helsinki. This study was conducted with approval from the Ethics Committee of the North Huashan Hospital. Written informed consent was obtained from all participants.

Exclusion criteria: Patients were excluded if they had severe liver dysfunction (combined with jaundice, portal hypertension, ascites, and hepatic encephalopathy), severe renal dysfunction (estimated GFR [eGFR] < 30 mL/min/1.73 m^2), acute cerebrovascular accident, acute infection, advanced cancer, a history of old myocardial infarction or structural heart diseases including cardiomyopathy or valvular disease, or a history of coronary stenting or coronary bypass surgery.

Grouping

According to the results of CAG, the patients were divided into a single-vascular-lesion group (group S, 91 cases), a dual-vascular-lesion group (group D, 67 cases), and a multiple-vascular-lesion group (group M, 37 cases).

Count of CAS lesions: Stenosis ≥50% in any one of the three main coronary arteries (LAD, LCX, or RCA) was considered a significant lesion. Stenosis ≥50% of the left main stem was considered a dual-vascular lesion. Stenosis ≥50% of the intermediate branch was considered a single vascular lesion. Stenosis of a branch was considered a main vascular lesion. The sum of the diseased vessels with meaningful stenosis was then calculated.

Baseline information

In addition to the baseline data, all the patients underwent electrocardiography (ECG) to calculate the left ventricular ejection fraction (LVEF) before and after admission (outpatient). The patients with STEMI and NSTEMI in each ACS subgroup were then categorized according to the Killip classification.

ECG evaluation

A total of 187 patients completed ECG, with 152 completed within 48 h of admission using the Philips IE 33 ultrasound system. Thirty-five patients underwent ECG within 1 month of admission using the Philips HD 11 ultrasound system. LVEF was checked using M-mode ultrasonography and obtained using Simpson's principle.

Assessment of CAD severity

Assessment of CAD was performed according to the modified Gensini score [11].

Killip classification

The Killip classification is a clinical classification of acute myocardial infarction-induced heart failure, and its classification standards were in accordance with the diagnostic criteria of ACS defined by the ACC/AHA in 2014 [10].

Detection and grouping of serum CysC levels

A 4-mL sample of serum from each patient was subjected to a turbidimetric immunoassay to measure the concentration of serum CysC using was the Hitachi 7600-120 automatic biochemical analyzer; the kit was provided by Kyokuto (Tokyo, Japan). The normal reference value of CysC is ≤1.0 mg/L. The serum CysC concentration for all patients was measured within 24 h after admission.

CysC grouping: The CysC levels of all the hospitalized patients (234 cases) were divided into four subgroups according to the interquartile method: subgroup Q1, CysC < 1.1 mg/L (45 cases); subgroup Q2, 1.1 mg/L ≤ CysC < 1.2 mg/L (35 cases); subgroup Q3, 1.2 mg/L ≤ CysC < 1.5 mg/L (88 cases); and subgroup Q4, CysC ≥ 1.5 mg/L (66 cases).

eGFR and grouping

The level of serum creatinine (Scr) was determined using a Hitachi automatic biochemical analyzer, and eGFR was calculated using the Cockcroft–Gault formula: Ccr (mL/min) = [(140 - age) × body weight (kg) × (0.85 (female)]/(72 × Scr [mg/dL]).

The eGFR levels of all the hospitalized patients (234 cases) were divided into three subgroups according to the degree of renal dysfunction: subgroup q1, moderate to severe renal dysfunction (30 mL/min ≤ eGFR < 60 mL/min) (44 cases); subgroup q2, mild to moderate renal dysfunction (60 mL/min ≤ eGFR < 90 mL/min) (94 cases); and subgroup q3, normal renal function (96 cases).

Statistical analysis

The quantitative data are expressed as mean ± standard deviation. When homogeneity of variance existed among the groups, a t test was used to compare count data; otherwise, the t' test was used. The CysC classification data are described as median (interquartile range), and the intergroup comparisons were made using the Wilcoxon rank sum test. Qualitative data are described as frequency (percentage), and the differences in CysC and eGFR in different vascular lesion subgroups were analyzed used the χ^2 test. Correlations of CysC and eGFR with the Gensini score were analyzed using Pearson's correlation coefficient. The relationship of each individual variable with ACS was then observed, and a single logistic regression model was established. To eliminate interference of confounding factors, a multivariate logistic regression model containing the main effects was established, and the predictive values of the variables with respect to the results were then analyzed. A multivariate logistic prediction model was established, with the inclusion criterion of $P \leq 0.05$ and the exclusion criterion of $P > 0.05$. When the outcome variables were dichotomous, a nonconditional logistic regression model was established; when the outcome variables were ordered and categorical, an ordinal logistic regression model was established. Bilateral levels were set for the P values of all hypothetical tests, with the significance level set at 5% and the homogeneity of variance level was set at 10%. Statistical analysis was performed using STATA version 12.0 software.

Results

Index comparison

Compared with the control group, the proportion of male patients was significantly higher ($P < 0.01$), age was lower ($P < 0.05$), and the low-density lipoprotein cholesterol (LDL-C) level was higher ($P < 0.01$) in the STEMI group. Compared with the control group, the proportion of male patients was significantly higher ($P < 0.01$), the percentage of patients with diabetes was higher ($P < 0.05$), and the LDL-C level was higher ($P < 0.05$) in the NSTEMI group (Table 1).

The comparison of different variables among different ACS subgroups (group S, D, and M) and the control group showed that the proportion of male patients in each ACS subgroup was higher than that of the control group, and the comparison among different ACS subgroups showed the results as group M > group S > group D ($P < 0.05$); the LDL-C level in each ACS subgroup was higher than that of the control group, and the comparison among different ACS subgroups showed the results as group D > group M > group S ($P < 0.05$); the CysC levels in groups D and M were higher than that of the control group, and the comparison among different ACS subgroups showed the results as group M > group D > group S ($P < 0.05$). Differences in age, proportion of patients with hypertension, proportion of patients with diabetes, LVEF, Killip grades, Scr level, and eGFR among the groups were not statistically significant ($P > 0.05$, Table 2).

Table 1 Baseline clinical baseline characteristic of all patients

		STEMI group ($n = 77$)	NSTEMI group ($n = 35$)	UAP group ($n = 83$)	Control group ($n = 39$)
Sex	Male	165 (84.42%)**	29 (82.86%)**	57 (68.67%)	20 (51.28%)
	Female	412 (15.58%)	6 (17.14%)	26 (31.33%)	19 (48.72%)
Age		59.19 ± 11.76*	67.14 ± 10.74	64.12 ± 10.36	64.59 ± 8.14
Hypertension		42 (54.55%)	25 (71.43%)	56 (67.47%)	23 (58.97%)
Diabetes		20 (25.97%)	14 (40.00%)*	25 (30.12%)	6 (15.38%)
LDL-C		3.11 ± 1.02**	3.07 ± 0.91*	2.65 ± 0.98	2.60 ± 0.77
Serum creatinine		74.78 ± 19.63	82.05 ± 24.91	75.55 ± 18.82	75.87 ± 19.73
Cys C		1.34 ± 0.48	1.46 ± 0.58	1.26 ± 0.27	1.30 ± 0.35
eGFR		99.47 ± 35.44	84.72 ± 35.42	83.03 ± 25.02	81.44 ± 23.95

Note: compared with control group
*$P < 0.05$
**$P < 0.01$

Table 2 Variable comparison among different lesion groups

Index	Control ($n = 39$)	S ($n = 91$)	D ($n = 67$)	M ($n = 37$)	P
Gender					0.0153
F	19 (48.72%)	20 (21.98%)	16 (23.88%)	8 (21.62%)	
M	20 (51.28%)	71 (78.02%)	51 (76.12%)	29 (78.38%)	
Age	63.59 ± 9.14	62.40 ± 10.56	61.67 ± 12.12	66.49 ± 10.70	0.1591
Hypertension	23 (58.97%)	53 (58.24%)	40 (59.70%)	30 (81.08%)	0.0670
LDL-C	2.60 ± 0.77	2.74 ± 1.07	3.10 ± 0.91	2.97 ± 1.03	0.0449
Diabetics	6 (15.38%)	27 (29.67%)	21 (31.34%)	11 (29.73%)	0.2608
LVEF	-	59.16 ± 5.17[a]	60.60 ± 5.67[b]	58.05 ± 8.00	0.0644
Killip classification					0.1090
Grade I	-	31 (77.50%)[c]	32 (86.49%)[d]	15 (68.18%)[e]	
Grade II	-	8 (20.00%)[c]	3 (8.11%)[d]	2 (9.09%)[e]	
Grade III	-	1 (2.50%)[c]	2 (5.41%)[d]	4 (18.18%)[e]	
Grade IV	-	0 (0.00%)[c]	0 (0.00%)[d]	1 (4.55%)[e]	
Cys C	1.30 ± 0.35	1.27 ± 0.30	1.34 ± 0.44	1.51 ± 0.59	0.0296
Scr	75.87 ± 19.73	73.29 ± 14.82	77.87 ± 21.31	80.84 ± 29.00	0.2370
eGFR	81.44 ± 23.95	92.31 ± 31.02	90.05 ± 32.50	83.56 ± 34.39	0.2146

Note:
[a]the cases with valid LVEF data in group S were 88 cases
[b]the cases with valid LVEF data in group D were 62 cases
[c]the cases with valid Killip classification data in group S were 40 cases
[d]the cases with valid Killip classification data in group D were 37 cases
[e]the cases with valid Killip classification data in group M were 22 cases

Relationships between different variables and vascular lesions

Using a univariate logistic regression model while not controlling other factors, each variable was evaluated regarding correlation with vascular lesions. The results showed that the gender composition (male) and LDL-C and CysC levels were positively correlated with vascular lesions ($P < 0.05$), but the correlations of eGFR and other variables did not reach statistical significance ($P > 0.05$) (Table 3).

Using a multivariate logistic regression model while controlling other factors, each variable was analyzed regarding correlation with vascular lesions. The results showed that CysC level, gender composition (male), LDL-C level, and hypertension were positively correlated with vascular lesions ($P < 0.05$). For the CysC level, the odds ratio was 2.09, indicating that when CysC was increased by 1 mg/L, the risk of an additional vascular lesion increased by 2.09 times. Because the P value of eGFR in the univariate regression analysis was too high (0.937), it was not included in the multivariate statistical regression model (Table 4).

Linear relation of CysC and eGFR with Scr values

CysC and Scr levels were measured in 234 patients after they were hospitalized, and eGFR values were calculated. A positive correlation was detected between CysC and Scr values based on Pearson's correlation coefficient ($r = 0.6158$, $P < 0.0001$), and a negative correlation was detected between eGFR and CysC level ($r = -0.5115$, $P < 0.0001$) and between eGFR and Scr level ($r = -0.5545$, $P < 0.0001$) (Fig. 1).

Relationships of CysC level and kidney function with vascular lesions

By comparing the constitute ratio differences of different CysC levels (four subgroups) and different eGFR levels (three subgroups) in different vascular lesion groups, the correlations of different CysC levels and kidney dysfunction with vascular lesions were determined. Among the CysC subgroups, the constitute ratios in subgroup Q1 (low CysC concentration) were group S > group D > group M and those in subgroup Q4 (high CysC concentration) were group M > group D > group S; these differences were statistically significant ($P < 0.05$). Among the different eGFR subgroups, the constitute ratios in subgroup q1 (moderate to severe renal dysfunction) were group M > group D > group S, those in subgroup q2 (mild to moderate renal dysfunction), and those in subgroup q3 (normal renal function) were group S > group D > group M, but the differences were not statistically significant ($P > 0.05$) (Table 5).

Comparison of CysC medians

According to the CysC ranges and medians in different vascular lesion subgroups, a box plot could be drawn

Table 3 Univariate logistic regression analysis of different variables with vascular lesions

Factor	Coefficient	SD	Statistic	P	OR (95%CI)
M	0.6362047	0.2794	2.28	0.0230	1.8893 (1.0927–3.2667)
Age	0.0080341	0.0108	0.75	0.4560	1.0081 (0.9870–1.0296)
Hypertension	0.4309775	0.2446	1.76	0.0780	1.5388 (0.9528–2.4851)
LDL-C	0.3062137	0.1254	2.44	0.0150	1.3583 (1.0623–1.7367)
Diabetics	0.3487115	0.2616	1.33	0.1830	1.4172 (0.8487–2.3666)
Cys C	0.7297879	0.3015	2.42	0.0150	2.0746 (1.1490–3.7459)
Scr	0.0103784	0.0061	1.70	0.0890	1.0104 (0.9984–1.0226)
eGFR	0.0002985	0.0038	0.08	0.9370	1.0003 (0.9929–1.0078)

(Fig. 2a). As seen from the box plot, with an increase in vascular lesions, the median CysC level showed an increasing trend. The Spearman rank correlation coefficient between these two was 0.1576, which reached statistical significance ($P = 0.0278$). Quantile regression analysis showed that the median CysC level was increased on average by 0.1 mg/L for each additional vascular lesion ($P = 0.513$) (Fig. 2a).

Comparison of eGFR medians

According to the eGFR ranges and medians in different vascular lesion subgroups, a box plot could be drawn (Fig. 2b). As seen from the box plot, with an increase in vascular lesions, the median eGFR showed a decreasing trend. The Spearman rank correlation coefficient between these two was -0.0993, which did not reach statistical significance ($P = 0.1671$). Quantile regression analysis showed that the median eGFR was decreased on average by 2.0 for each additional vascular lesion ($P = 0.086$) (Fig. 2b).

Correlation comparison of different vascular lesions and severity

By comparing the differences in Gensini scores among the different vascular lesion subgroups, the correlations of vascular lesions with Gensini scores were determined. Gensini scores showed differences among different subgroups, with group M > group D > group S, and the differences were statistically significant (67.32 ± 40.04 vs. 43.78 ± 25.50 vs. 30.20 ± 22.92, $P < 0.0001$).

Table 4 Multivariate logistic regression analysis of different variables with vascular lesions

Factor	Coefficient	SD	Statistic	P	OR (95%CI)
Cys C	0.736095	0.3095	2.38	0.0170	2.0878 (1.1382–3.8295)
Male	0.776684	0.2928	2.65	0.0080	2.1743 (1.2250–3.85920)
LDL-C	0.329243	0.1270	2.59	0.0100	1.3899 (1.08360–1.7828)
Hypertension	0.514262	0.2565	2.00	0.0450	1.6724 (1.0115–2.7650)

Correlations of different CysC levels with vascular lesion severity

By comparing the differences of Gensini scores among different CysC subgroups, the correlations of CysC levels with Gensini scores were then determined. The results showed that the Gensini scores showed differences among different CysC subgroups, subgroup Q4 > subgroup Q 3 > subgroup Q2 > subgroup Q1, and the differences were statistically significant (50.00 ± 37.37 vs. 42.67 ± 30.40 vs. 39.13 ± 22.58 vs. 30.24 ± 22.25 mg/L, $P < 0.05$).

Correlations of different renal functions with vascular lesion severity

By comparing the differences of Gensini scores among different eGFR subgroups, the correlations of different renal functions with Gensini scores were then determined. The results showed that the Gensini scores showed differences among different eGFR subgroups, subgroup q3 > subgroup q1 > subgroup q2, but the differences were not statistically significant (43.2 ± 29.84 vs. 41.54 ± 35.65 vs. 40.91 ± 30.97 mL/min/1.73 m^2, $P > 0.05$).

Linear relationships of serum CysC level, eGFR, and Gensini score

Pearson's correlation coefficient was used to calculate the paired linear relationships among CysC level, eGFR, and Gensini score. CysC was negatively correlated with eGFR ($r = -0.5073$, $P < 0.0001$) but positively correlated with Gensini score ($r = 0.1811$, $P < 0.05$); eGFR and Gensini score were positively correlated ($r = 0.0738$, $P > 0.05$) (Fig. 3).

Correlations of different Killip grades with vascular lesion severity

By comparing the differences in Gensini scores among the different Killip classification subgroups, the correlations of

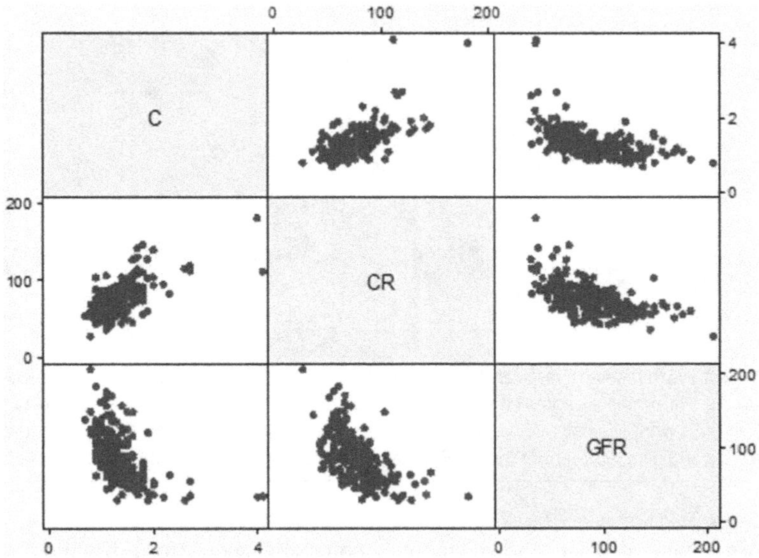

Fig. 1 Scatterplots showed linear relationships between serum cystatin C, eGFR and Scr

Killip grades with Gensini scores were then determined. Gensini scores showed differences among different Killip classification subgroups, with Killip grade IV (one case) > Killip grade II > Killip grade III > Killip grade I, but the differences were not statistically significant (168.00 ± 0.00 vs. 67.15 ± 39.32 vs. 51.57 ± 16.78 vs. 46.36 ± 26.53, $P > 0.05$).

Discussion

The purpose of this study was to investigate the correlations of serum CysC level and eGFR with vascular lesions and their severity in patients with ACS. In recent years, some scholars suggested that inflammation and immune responses were the intermediary and key factors of cardiovascular remodeling and onset [12]. Cardiovascular events such as acute myocardial infarction are related to the inflammatory activities of lesions and matrix remodeling induced by plaque rupture. Optical coherence tomography is a feasible and safe imaging modality for patients with CAD and allows identification of the various microstructures of the atherosclerotic plaque such as plaque rupture, thin-cap fibroatheroma, lipid core, and intracoronary thrombus [13]. Many studies observed that the weakening process of fibrous caps mainly resulted from extracellular matrix degradation, which was caused by activated proteases such as matrix metalloproteinases and serine proteases released by the activated macrophages and smooth muscle cells in the plaques [14, 15]. Recently, two cysteine proteases that could promote the dissolving of elastic tissues, cathepsin S and cathepsin K, were found to be overexpressed in atherosclerotic lesions [16]. The main functions of serum CysC are to inhibit the activity of endogenous cysteine proteases, to regulate the intracellular metabolism of proteins [17], and to play the role of inflammatory mediators through activating neutrophils [18]; its mechanisms are involved in inhibiting inflammatory factors, confronting plasminogens, regulating the activity of pre-hormones, and regulating proteinases inside and outside cells [19–21]. Studies have shown that the serum CysC level was related to the severity of ACS [22]. Tebaldi [23] found that a reduced CrCl value (45 mL/min) was independently associated with a significantly lower incidence of positive FFR (0.80 or less). Regarding correlations between coronary vascular lesions and the severity of coronary vascular diseases, Corpus [24] found that the incidence of major adverse cardiac events such as death, repeated myocardial infarction, or repeated revascularization in patients with acute myocardial infarction plus multiple vascular lesions during the 1-year follow-up period was significantly higher than in patients with a single vascular lesion. Their results suggested that the ACS patients with multiple

Table 5 Comparison of constitute ratio differences of different Cys C subgroups and different eGFR subgroups in different vascular lesion groups

Index		S	D	M	Statistic	*P*
Cys C	Q1	23 (25.27%)	10 (14.93%)	4 (10.81%)	Z = 7.25	0.0267
	Q2	12 (13.19%)	13 (19.40%)	5 (13.51%)		
	Q3	35 (38.46%)	26 (38.81%)	10 (27.03%)		
	Q4	21 (23.08%)	18 (26.87%)	18 (48.65%)		
eGFR	q1	13 (14.29%)	12 (17.91%)	10 (29.73%)	Z = 2.90	0.2342
	q2	36 (39.56%)	26 (38.81%)	13 (35.14%)		
	q3	42 (46.15%)	29 (43.28%)	13 (35.14%)		

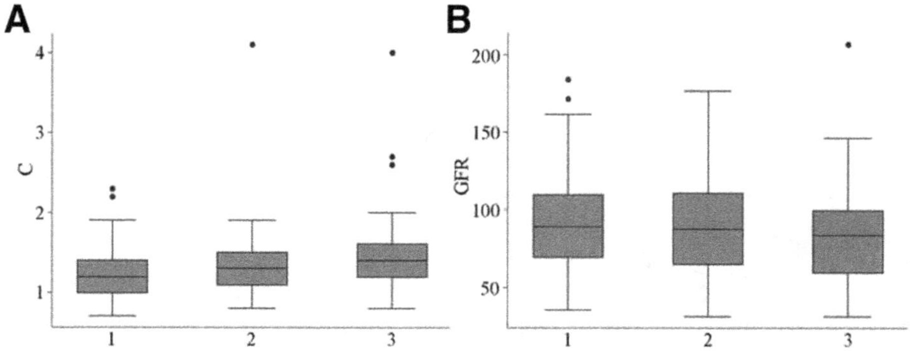

Fig. 2 **a** Correlation of Cys C median with different vascular disease variables by box-plot; Note: Abscissa 1 represented group S, 2 represented group D, 3 represented group M, the ordinate represented the Cys C value, and the transverse lines in the blocks represented the medians. **b** Correlation of eGFR median with different vascular disease variables by box-plot. Note: Abscissa 1 represented group S, 2 represented group D, 3 represented group M, the ordinate represented the eGFR value, and the transverse lines in the blocks represented the medians

vascular lesions had more severe disease and a worse prognosis.

The analysis of correlations between CysC level and vascular lesions in the ACS patients showed the CysC levels in group D and M were higher than those in the control group, and the comparison among different ACS subgroups showed group M > group D > group S (group M 1.51 ± 0.59 mg/L vs. group D 1.34 ± 0.44 mg/L vs. group S 1.27 ± 0.30 mg/L vs. control group 1.30 ± 0.35 mg/L, $P = 0.0296$). The single-factor regression analysis of the vascular lesions in these ACS patients suggested that the CysC level was positively correlated with the vascular lesions ($P = 0.0150$), and the multifactor regression analysis showed the same result ($P = 0.017$); among different CysC subgroups, the constitute ratios in the lower-quartile groups were group S > group D > group M, and those in the high-quartile groups were group M > group D > group S, and the differences were statistically significant ($P < 0.0267$). It could be seen from the box plot (Fig. 2a) that with increasing vascular lesions, the median CysC level also showed an increasing trend. The Spearman rank correlation coefficient of these two was 0.1576 ($P = 0.0278$).

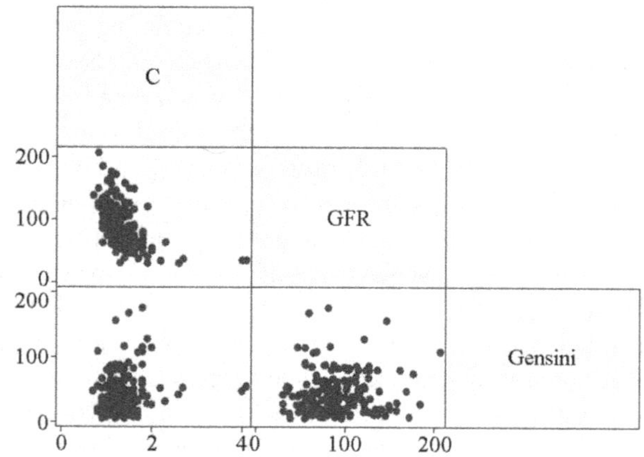

Fig. 3 Scatterplot matrix among Cys C, eGFR, and Gensini score in patients with ACS. The pair Pearson correlation coefficients among the above three indexes

The analysis of correlations between CysC level and vascular lesion severity in the ACS patients showed that the Gensini scores exhibited differences among different CysC subgroups, with subgroup Q4 (high-quartile group, 50.00 ± 37.37 mg/L) > subgroup Q3 (42.67 ± 30.40 mg/L) > subgroup Q2 (39.13 ± 22.58 mg/L) > subgroup Q (lower-quartile group) 30.24 ± 22.25 mg/L ($P = 0.0286$). Using the scatterplot matrix of CysC, eGFR, and Gensini scores, Pearson's correlation coefficient calculation showed that CysC was positively correlated with the Gensini score ($r = 0.1811$, $P < 0.05$).

The results of this study suggested that CysC level was positively correlated with the vascular lesions and their severity in these ACS patients, and the differences were statistically significant, consistent with the results of Jernberg [22]. Meanwhile, the comparison between the vascular lesions and Gensini scores in the ACS patients showed that group M (67.32 ± 40.04 mg/L) > group D (43.78 ± 25.50 mg/L) > group S (30.20 ± 22.92 mg/L) ($P < 0.0001$), fully consistent with the results of Corpus [24].

The inconsistent results regarding CysC mainly derives from the fact that CysC is just one member of the cysteine protease inhibitors, and CysC and its fragment can regulate inflammatory processes and participate in the pathological physiological process of atherosclerotic plaque formation. CysC may inhibit the activity of cathepsin S and K, reduce degradation of blood vessels and vascular remodeling, and postpone the occurrence and development of atherosclerosis. Patients with increased CysC levels may have higher cardiac mortality, and the mortality of patients with higher CysC levels was 3.87-fold higher than that in patients with lower CysC levels. Sai E et al. [25] found that increased CysC levels can be a predictive factor of recurrence of cardiovascular events, which may be derived from the fact that CysC contributes to the pathological physiological process of atherosclerosis and inflammation. However, there are still multiple contradictions with respect to the relationship between CysC and CHD. For these contradictions, Noto et al. [26] believed that the difference is mainly caused by a negative acute-phase reaction during acute myocardial infarction. The case of a patient with acute myocardial infarction who had normal expression levels of CysC after 7 days in the hospital also supports this hypothesis. However, another hypothesis indicated that the expression of CysC is reduced before acute cardiovascular events, which further activates inflammatory factors and cell factors and induces a lower level of CysC. One study showed that transforming growth factor β1 (TGF-β1) is an important factor inducing CysC [27]; serum TGF-β1 levels are significantly reduced in atherosclerosis, and increased TGF-β1 can inhibit the process of lesion formation. CysC levels are near normal in the recovery phase, and may even be increased, which is also caused by regulation of inflammatory and cell factors, body compensatory mechanisms, and the gradual repair and conserved result of inflammatory patches. Luc et al. [28] found that ischemic events may be caused by a relative shortage of proteinase inhibitors (such as CysC). Although the inflammatory process increased the expression of CysC, CysC is still not enough than increased protease in inflammatory atheromatous plaques.

Collectively, many clinical studies have shown that CysC is related to CHD. Patients with ACS with vascular lesions should be further studied owing to the limited number of samples in this study. Simultaneously, determining whether CysC can be used as a potential biomarker for prognostic evaluation and prediction of major adverse cardiac events and has potential guiding significance and value for revascularization will be the next research direction.

Conclusions

Serum CysC levels might reflect the severity of vascular lesions in patients with ACS, and high CysC levels had a predictive value regarding the severity of vascular lesions in ACS.

Abbreviations

ACS: Acute coronary syndrome; CAD: Coronary artery disease; CAG: Coronary angiography; CHD: Coronary heart disease; CysC: Cystatin C; GFR: Glomerular filtration rate; LVEF: Left ventricular ejection fraction; NSTEMI: Non-ST segment-elevated myocardial infarction; STEMI: ST segment-elevated myocardial infarction

Acknowledgements

We appreciate all the colleagues provide help in North Huashan Hospital of Fudan University.

Funding

No funding was received for this study.

Authors' contributions

PY designed the study; XW collected data and performed statistical analysis; JZ and PG performed the study and wrote the paper. All authors read and approved the final manuscript.

Competing interests

The authors declare that they have no competing interests.

Author details

[1]Department of Cardiology, North Huashan Hospital of Fudan University, Shanghai 201907, People's Republic of China. [2]Department of Cardiology, Tongren Hospital, Shanghai 200050, People's Republic of China. [3]Department of Beixinjing Community Health Center, Shanghai 200335, People's Republic of China.

References

1. Yang XH, Wang QX. Cystain C and research progess of cardiovescular disease. Clin Med. 2012;32:125–8.
2. Royakkers AA, Korevaar JC, van Suijlen JD, Hofstra LS, Kuiper MA, Spronk PE, et al. Serum and urine cystatin Care poor biomarkers for acute kidney injury and renal replacement therapy. Intensive Care Med. 2011;37:493–501.
3. Ix JH, Shlipak MG, Chertow GM, Whooley MA. Association of cystatinC with mortality, cardiovascular events and incident heart failure among persons with coronary heart disease: data from the Heart and Soul Study. Circulation. 2007;115:173–9.
4. Keler T, Messow CM, Lubos E, Nicaud V, Wild PS, Rupprecht HJ, et al. Cystatin C and cardiovascular mortality in patients with coronary artery disease and normal or mildly reduced kidney function: results from the AtheroGene study. Eur Heart J. 2009;30:314–20.
5. Dupont M, Wu Y, Hazen SL, Tang WH. Cystatin C identifies patients with stable chronic heart failure at increased risk for adverse cardiovascular events. Circ Heart Fail. 2012;5:602–9.
6. Meng L, Yang Y, Qi LT, Wang XJ, Xu GB, Zhang BW. Eletated serum cyctatin C is an independent predictor of cardiovascular events in people with relatively nomal renal function. J Nephrol. 2012;25:426–30.
7. He F, Zhang J, Lu ZQ, Gao QL, Sha DJ, Pei LG, et al. Risk factors and outcomes of acute kidney injury after intracoronary stent implantation. World J Emerg Med. 2012;3:197–201.
8. Doganer YC, Aydogan U, Aydogdu A, Aparci M, Akbulut H, Nerkiz P, et al. Relationship of cystatin C with coronary artery disease and its severity. Coron Artery Dis. 2013;24:119–26.
9. Doğaner YÇ, Aydoğan Ü, Rohrer JE, Aydoğdu A, Çaycı T, Barçın C, et al. Comparison of estimated GFR equations based on serum cystatin C alone and in combination with serum creatinine in patients with coronary aaery disease. Anatol J Cardiol. 2015;15:571–6.
10. Amsterdam EA, Wenger NK, Brindis RG, Casey Jr DE, Ganiats TG, Holmes Jr DR, et al. 2014 AHA/ACC Guideline for the Management of Patients with Non-ST-Elevation Acute Coronary Syndromes: a report of the American College of Cardiology/American Heart Association Task Force on Practice Guidelines. J Am Coll Cardiol. 2014;64:e139–228.
11. Yu JH, Hu JZ, Zhou H, Liu X, Cao Q, Shen Y, et al. SCN5A mutation in patients with Brugada electrocardiographic pattern induced by fever. ZhonghuaXinXue Guan Bing ZaZhi. 2013;41:1010–4.
12. Libby P, Ridker PM, Maseri A. Inflammation and atherosclerosis. Ciculation. 2002;105:1135–43.
13. Iannaccone M, Quadri G, Taha S, D'Ascenzo F, Montefusco A, Omede' P, et al. Prevalence and predictors of culprit plaque rupture at OCT in patients

with coronary artery disease: a meta-analysis. Eur Heart J Cardiovasc Imaging. 2016;17:1128–37.
14. Galis ZS, Khatri JJ. Matrix metalloproteinases in vascular remodeling and atherogesis: the good, the bad, and the ugly. Circ Res. 2002;90:251–62.
15. Rao SK, Reddy KV, Cohen JR. Role of serine proteases in aneurysm development. Ann N Y Acad Sci. 1996;800:131–7.
16. Sukhova GK, Shi GP, Simon DI, Chapman HA, Libby P. Expression of elastolyticcathepsins S and K in human atheroma and regulation of their production in smooth muscles cells. J Chin Invest. 1998;102:576–83.
17. Abdallah E, Waked E, Al-Helal B, Asad R, Nabil M, Harba T. Novel troponin-like biomarkers of acute kidney injury. Saudi J Kidney Dis Transpl. 2013;24: 1111–24.
18. Longenecker CT, Hileman CO, Funderburg NT, McComsey GA. Rosuvastatin preserves renal function and lowers cystatin C in HIV-infected subjects on antiretroviral therapy: the SATURN-HIV trial. Clin Infect Dis. 2014;59:1148–56.
19. Ganda A, Magnusson M, Yvan-Charvet L, Hedblad B, Engström G, Ai D, et al. Mildrenal dysfunction and metabolites tied to low HDL cholesterol are associated with monocytosis and atherosclerosis. Circulation. 2013;127: 988–96.
20. Ge C, Ren F, Lu S, Ji F, Chen X, Wu X. Clinical prognostic significance of plasma cystatin C levels among patients with acute coronary syndrome. Clin Cardiol. 2009;32:644–8.
21. Negrusz-Kawecka M, Poręba R, Hulok A, Sciborski K, Marczak J, Bańkowski T. Evaluation of the significance of cystatin C levels in patients suffering from coronary artery disease. Adv Clin Exp Med. 2014;23:551–8.
22. Jernberg T, Lindahl B, James S, Larsson A, Hansson LO, Wallentin L. Cystatin C: a novel predictor of outcome in suspected or confirmed non-ST-elevation acute coronary syndrome. Circulation. 2004;110:2342–8.
23. Tebaldi M, Biscaglia S, Fineschi M, Manari A, Menozzi M, Secco GG, et al. Flow reserve evaluation and chronic kidney disease: analysis from a multicenter Italian registry (the FREAK Study). Catheter Cardiovasc Interv. 2016;88:555–62.
24. Corpus RA, House JA, Marso SP, Grantham JA, Huber Jr KC, Laster SB, et al. Multivessel percutaneous coronary intervention in patients with multivessel disease and acute myocardial infarction. Am Heart J. 2004;148:493–500.
25. Sai E, Miyauchi K, Kojima T, Masaki Y, Kojima T, Miyazaki T, et al. Increased cystatin C levels as a risk factor of cardiovascular events in patients with preserved estimated glomerular filtration rate after elective percutaneous coronary intervention with drug-eluting stents. Heart Vessels. 2016;31:694–701.
26. Noto D, Cefalu AB, Barbagallo CM, Pace A, Rizzo M, Marino G, et al. Cystatin C levels are decreased in acutemyocardial infarction, effect of cystatin C G73A gene polymorphism on plasma levels. Int J Cardiol. 2005;101:213–7.
27. Shi GP, Sukhova GK, Grubb A, Ducharme A, Rhode LH, Lee RT, et al. Cystatin C deficiency in human atheroscler-osis and aortic aneurysms. J Chin Invest. 1999;104:1191–7.
28. Luc G, Bard JM, Lesueur C. Plasmacystatin-C and development of coronary heartdisease: The PRIME Study. Atherosclerosis. 2006;85:375–80.

18

Predictors of high-cost hospitalization in the treatment of acute coronary syndrome in Asia: findings from EPICOR Asia

Stephen Jan[1*], Stephen W-L. Lee[2], Jitendra P. S. Sawhney[3], Tiong K. Ong[4], Chee Tang Chin[5], Hyo-Soo Kim[6], Rungroj Krittayaphong[7], Vo T. Nhan[8], Stuart J. Pocock[9], Ana M. Vega[10], Nobuya Hayashi[11] and Yong Huo[12]

Abstract

Background: The EPICOR Asia (long-tErm follow-uP of antithrombotic management patterns In acute CORonary syndrome patients in Asia) study (NCT01361386) was an observational study of patients hospitalized for acute coronary syndromes (ACS) enrolled in 218 hospitals in eight countries/regions in Asia. This study examined costs, length of stay and the predictors of high costs during an ACS hospitalization.

Methods and results: Data for patients hospitalized for an ACS ($n = 12{,}922$) were collected on demographics, medical history, event characteristics, socioeconomic and insurance status at discharge. Patients were followed up at 6 weeks' post-hospitalization for an ACS event to assess associated treatment costs from a health sector perspective. Primary outcome was the incurring of costs in the highest quintile by country and index event diagnosis, and identification of associated predictors. Cost data were available for 10,819 patients. Mean length of stay was 10.1 days. The highest-cost countries were China, Singapore, and South Korea. Significant predictors of high-cost care were age, male sex, income, country, prior disease history, hospitalization in 3 months before index event, no dependency before index event, having an invasive procedure, hospital type and length of stay.

Conclusions: Substantial variability exists in healthcare costs for hospitalized ACS patients across Asia. Of concern is the observation that the highest costs were reported in China, given the rapidly increasing numbers of procedures in recent years.

Keywords: Acute coronary syndrome, Asia, Health insurance, Costs, Hospitalization

Background

Ischemic heart disease is associated with a substantial healthcare burden worldwide, in terms of both deaths and disability-adjusted life years [1], while the costs of treating acute coronary syndromes (ACS) also represent a major burden for healthcare systems globally [2–6]. With the increasing prevalence of lifestyle-related chronic-disease risk factors, increasing healthcare costs, technological innovation, and growing consumer and patient expectations regarding access to twenty-first century healthcare, it is expected this burden will likely continue to increase [5]. This will have implications for the future financial sustainability of healthcare systems globally. These pressures are particularly pronounced in low- and middle-income countries in Asia where large-scale policies are underway or in planning; notably, in India and China to achieve universal coverage through the expansion of financial coverage for treatments to previously under-served populations. Such reforms, while critical in promoting social protection and equity of access to healthcare, come with significant resource requirements and will inevitably magnify future health sector financing challenges.

In addressing issues of cost and financial sustainability, understanding of the factors that drive variation in resource

* Correspondence: sjan@georgeinstitute.org
[1]The George Institute for Global Health, Sydney Medical School, University of Sydney, King George V Building, 83–117 Missenden Rd, Camperdown, NSW 2050, Australia
Full list of author information is available at the end of the article

use is important, particularly those factors that contribute to higher treatment costs. Notably, only very few studies have examined the factors associated with variation in treatment costs for ACS. Evidence from the US, comparing inpatient resource use for ACS in patients who died in hospital with that for a surviving ACS cohort, indicated that inpatient mortality for ACS is associated with a 47% greater duration of hospital stay along with an incremental cost of around US$43,000 [7]. Similarly, in a study conducted in Italy, which followed up patients for 12 months' post-hospitalization for ACS, patients who died of a cardiovascular event had an average cost of around €16,000 compared with an average cost of around €11,000 for the entire ACS cohort [8]. In China, a small study in a single hospital in Shandong found that increased age was associated with increased treatment costs and poorer clinical outcomes [9]. In a study in the US of over 12,000 patients with ACS, which compared those with and without diabetes, the presence of diabetes was reported to incur significant additional hospitalization costs of $32,577 versus no diabetes $29,150 [10]. Although evidence from such studies helps to clarify how resource use varies for patients with differing clinical presentations, the implications for policy are limited insofar as they reinforce the well-acknowledged relationship between more severe and complex illness and higher healthcare costs.

Investigation into the broader socioeconomic and regional health systems factors that influence costs is generally limited. Notably, however, a study in India using national administrative and household survey data reported that costs of hospitalization for cardiovascular disease were significantly higher in private health centers, in patients of high-fertility status, and in those of high socioeconomic status [11]. Studies of this kind, which examine broader healthcare systems and socioeconomic drivers of healthcare costs, provide potential policy lessons by addressing disparities in costs that reflect possible inefficiencies in healthcare systems, and are thus amenable to policy intervention.

In this study we assessed hospitalization costs associated with treating ACS patients across eight countries/regions in Asia: China, Hong Kong, India, Malaysia, Singapore, South Korea, Thailand, and Vietnam. The aim was to highlight variations in care costs across different healthcare settings and by different categories of ACS (ST-elevation myocardial infarction [STEMI], non-STEMI [NSTEMI] and unstable angina [UA]), and to determine the clinical, socioeconomic, and healthcare system factors that predict whether patients incur a level of treatment cost equivalent to the highest quintile by country and type of ACS.

Methods

The EPICOR Asia (long-tErm follow-uP of antithrombotic management patterns In acute CORonary syndrome patients in Asia) study (NCT01361386; registration, May 26, 2011), was a prospective, multinational, observational, cohort study of patients hospitalized for ACS enrolled in 218 hospitals in eight countries/regions in Asia [12]. These countries represent a combination of high- (Singapore, Hong Kong, Republic of Korea), upper-middle (China, India, Malaysia), and lower-middle (India, Vietnam) income settings. EPICOR Asia recruited consecutive patients hospitalized for ACS within 48 h of symptom onset and who were discharged with a final diagnosis of STEMI, NSTEMI, or UA, with 2-yearfollow-up. Data collection occurred between 2011 and 2014.

The study was conducted in compliance with the principles of the Declaration of Helsinki, International Conference on Harmonization Good Clinical Practice guidelines and applicable legislation on non-interventional studies in participating countries and regions. The protocol, including the informed consent form, was approved in writing by the applicable ethics committee of the participating centers in accordance with local regulations in each country. The ethics committee also approved any other non-interventional study documents in accordance with local regulations. A list of participating centers is provided in Additional file 1: Table S1. Patients provided written informed consent at discharge and completed a contact order form agreeing to be contacted for regular follow-up interviews post-discharge.

Data were collected from 12,922 patients on demographics, medical history, event characteristics, and socioeconomic and insurance status at discharge. Patients were followed up at 6 weeks following hospitalization for the index event in regard to treatment course. Costs associated with hospitalization were estimated from a health sector perspective based on health system payments for individual items at each specific hospital. Such payments reflect the outlay required of payers and are therefore of primary relevance from a policy standpoint. Costs were converted into US dollars at the prevailing exchange rates (see footnote to Table 2). These have not been converted into international dollars although prevailing purchasing power parities (PPPs) are presented to enable the reader to make such a conversion. In spite of potentially skewed distributions, mean costs were reported in accordance with economic theory which deems that the arithmetic mean (unlike the median) best informs resource allocation given a budgetary constraint [13–17].

The primary outcome was whether a patient incurred costs in the highest quintile for their specific country and index event diagnosis. This type of binary outcome, standardized against country and condition-specific norms, facilitated the pooling of data from multiple countries with differences in living standards and cost structures.

We assessed the association between the outcomes variable and several demographic, socioeconomic, health and clinical systems variables through univariate analyses. These variables included age, sex, smoking status, income (defined by country-specific quintiles based on country-specific income distributions, with quintile 1 representing the lowest income group, and quintile 5 the highest), country, place of residence (rural versus metropolitan), insurance status, cardiovascular disease history, hospitalization in the 3 months prior to the index event, dependence before the index event, index event medical management (invasive, non-invasive or unknown), type of hospital (regional/community/rural, non-university general hospital, university general hospital, other type of hospital/clinic), number of beds within the facility, and length of stay. A multivariable logistic regression model was constructed using stepwise selection, forcing in a variable of interest – health insurance status. A conditional binary regression model [18] to conduct a matched analysis was not used because the objective in this study was not to estimate a treatment effect.

Analyses were undertaken using SAS® v8.2 or later (SAS Institute, Cary, USA).

Results

Cost data were available for 10,819 participants; data from Malaysia ($n = 42$ patients) were excluded as costs were incorrectly recorded. Overall, 71% of participants were from China and 21% from India. Hong Kong, South Korea, Thailand, and Vietnam comprised between 1.2–2.3% of participants, with Singapore representing the fewest participants (0.6%).

Participant mean age was 60 years, 77% were males and 33% were current smokers compared with 20% former smokers, and 40% who had never smoked. Most participants were concentrated in the second (42%) and third (25%) income quintiles. Quintile 1 comprised less than 1% of participants, quintile 4 had 2% and quintile 5 had 24% (Table 1).

The majority (65%) of participants were resident in metropolitan areas compared with 35% in rural areas; 83% of participants had health insurance; 28% had some cardiovascular disease history; 7% had been hospitalized in the 3 months before the index event; 13% had some degree of dependence before the index event; and 83% underwent an invasive procedure during hospitalization. In terms of hospital type, 5% were admitted to a regional/community/rural hospital, 23% to a non-university general hospital, 56% to a university general hospital, and 17% to a 'other' type of hospital or clinic. The mean number of beds was 1312, and mean length of stay was 10.1 days, with little difference between STEMI (10.3 days), NSTEMI (10.2 days) and UA (9.8 days) (Table 1).

When compared in US dollars, the highest-cost countries were China (STEMI mean cost = \$7790; NSTEMI = \$7450; UA = \$6585), Singapore (\$6978; \$4910; \$3394), the Republic of Korea (\$4300; \$4621; \$3552), and Thailand (\$4427; \$3321; \$2008); across the three index-event types, UA generally represented the lowest-cost category except in India where it was the highest, albeit modestly (Fig. 1). In Hong Kong, all emergency admissions for ACS are subsidised by the Government and although the real cost incurred is not clear, health system payments to the patient are generally low. In terms of invasive interventional procedures, the highest costs were associated with (in descending order) coronary artery bypass graft, percutaneous coronary intervention (PCI) with one drug-eluting stent, PCI with one bare metal stent, and angiography; the costs for these procedures being highest in China, Hong Kong, Singapore, and Thailand (Table 2; also, conversion of these costs based on purchasing power parities (PPP) into international dollars is provided in Additional file 1: Table S2). Univariate analyses indicated that high-cost utilization was significantly associated with income, hospitalization in the 3 months prior to the index event, degree of dependence before the index event, index-event medical management, length of stay, sex, type of hospital and disease history (Table 3).

In controlling for all these variables at once, a multivariate analysis indicates the significant predictors of high-cost care were age (odds ratio [OR] = 1.10 per 10-year increment), being male (OR = 1.17), income (quintile 2 versus 5: OR = 0.76), prior disease history (OR = 1.25), hospitalization in the 3 months prior to index event (OR = 1.48), no dependency prior to index event (OR = 1.96), having an invasive procedure (OR = 5.48), hospital type (community versus university general: OR = 1.74), country (Hong Kong versus China: OR = 1.92; India versus China: OR = 2.54; Thailand versus China: OR = 1.52) and length of stay (OR = 1.06 per day) (Table 4).

Discussion

This study in more than 10,000 participants represents one of the largest prospective cost analyses of ACS and one of only few such analyses to provide cross-country comparisons. We found substantial variations across countries/regions and index diagnosis in healthcare costs incurred by patients during hospitalization for treatment of an ACS event. This is perhaps to be expected given the milieu of high, upper-middle and lower-middle income countries included in EPICOR Asia. What seems surprising is that the cost of treating ACS appeared relatively high in China across all three index-event types, exceeding those recorded for high-income countries/regions such as Singapore, the Republic of Korea, and Hong Kong. Interestingly, in contrast to Hong Kong and Singapore, costs in China were generally similar across all three index-event types. This suggests stratification of patients may not

Table 1 Baseline characteristics by final diagnosis of index event – all patients with cost data

	STEMI (*n* = 5478)	NSTEMI (*n* = 2030)	UA (*n* = 3311)	Total (*n* = 10,819)
Age, mean (SD)	58.5 (11.7)	61.9 (11.95)	61.4 (10.44)	60.0 (11.48)
Male, n (%)	4532 (82.7)	1520 (74.9)	2247 (67.9)	8299 (76.7)
Smoker, n (%)				
Current	2197 (40.1)	649 (32.0)	742 (22.4)	3588 (33.2)
Former	964 (17.6)	398 (19.6)	775 (23.4)	2137 (19.8)
Never	1896 (34.6)	855 (42.1)	1602 (48.4)	4353 (40.2)
Unknown	421 (7.7)	128 (6.3)	192 (5.8)	741 (6.8)
Income, n (%)				
Quintile 1	14 (0.3)	21 (1.0)	18 (0.5)	53 (0.5)
Quintile 2	2352 (42.9)	849 (41.8)	1342 (40.5)	4543 (42.0)
Quintile 3	1253 (22.9)	471 (23.2)	965 (29.1)	2689 (24.9)
Quintile 4	70 (1.3)	61 (3.0)	31 (0.9)	162 (1.5)
Quintile 5	1271 (23.2)	463 (22.8)	805 (24.3)	2539 (23.5)
Country, n (%)				
China	3716 (67.8)	1234 (60.8)	2754 (83.2)	7704 (71.2)
Hong Kong	75 (1.4)	45 (2.2)	5 (0.2)	125 (1.2)
India	1341 (24.5)	527 (26.0)	415 (12.5)	2283 (21.1)
Singapore	25 (0.5)	36 (1.8)	4 (0.1)	65 (0.6)
South Korea	101 (1.8)	70 (3.4)	76 (2.3)	247 (2.3)
Thailand	124 (2.3)	81 (4.0)	30 (0.9)	235 (2.2)
Vietnam	96 (1.8)	37 (1.8)	27 (0.8)	160 (1.5)
Place of residence, n (%)				
Rural	2088 (38.1)	624 (30.7)	1067 (32.2)	3779 (34.9)
Metropolitan	3390 (61.9)	1406 (69.3)	2244 (67.8)	7040 (65.1)
Insurance status, n (%)				
Yes	4396 (80.2)	1620 (79.8)	2950 (89.1)	8966 (82.9)
No	1082 (19.8)	410 (20.2)	361 (10.9)	1853 (17.1)
Disease history, n (%)	1008 (18.4)	630 (31.0)	1437 (43.4)	3075 (28.4)
Myocardial infarction	354 (6.5)	247 (12.2)	421 (12.7)	1022 (9.4)
Prior PCI	201 (3.7)	173 (8.5)	455 (13.7)	829 (7.7)
Prior CABG	43 (0.8)	39 (1.9)	70 (2.1)	152 (1.4)
CAG diagnostic for CAD	233 (4.3)	216 (10.6)	606 (18.3)	1055 (9.8)
Chronic angina	484 (8.8)	299 (14.7)	1018 (30.7)	1801 (16.6)
Heart failure	63 (1.2)	71 (3.5)	135 (4.1)	269 (2.5)
Atrial fibrillation	47 (0.9)	45 (2.2)	62 (1.9)	154 (1.4)
TIA/stroke	212 (3.9)	101 (5.0)	166 (5.0)	479 (4.4)
Peripheral vascular disease	24 (0.4)	24 (1.2)	41 (1.2)	89 (0.8)
Chronic renal failure	59 (1.1)	70 (3.4)	38 (1.1)	166 (1.5)
Hospitalization in 3 months prior to index event, n (%)	206 (3.8)	126 (6.2)	458 (13.8)	790 (7.3)
Dependence degree (need of help for daily activities) prior to index event, n (%)				
Some dependence	715 (13.1)	318 (15.7)	367 (11.1)	1400 (12.9)
No dependence	4601 (84.0)	1659 (81.7)	2826 (85.4)	9086 (84.0)
Unknown	162 (3.0)	53 (2.6)	118 (3.6)	333 (3.1)

Table 1 Baseline characteristics by final diagnosis of index event – all patients with cost data *(Continued)*

	STEMI (*n* = 5478)	NSTEMI (*n* = 2030)	UA (*n* = 3311)	Total (*n* = 10,819)
Index event medical management, n (%)				
Invasive	4713 (86.0)	1598 (78.7)	2612 (78.9)	8923 (82.5)
Non-invasive	724 (13.2)	422 (20.8)	617 (18.6)	1763 (16.3)
Unknown	41 (0.7)	10 (0.5)	82 (2.5)	133 (1.2)
Type of hospital, n (%)				
Regional/community/rural hospital	296 (5.4)	111 (5.5)	76 (2.3)	483 (4.5)
Non-university general hospital	1269 (23.2)	368 (18.1)	792 (23.9)	2429 (22.5)
University general hospital	2931 (53.5)	1074 (52.9)	2092 (63.2)	6097 (56.4)
Other type of hospital/clinic	982 (17.9)	477 (23.5)	351 (10.6)	1810 (16.7)
Number of beds, mean (95% CI)	1307.1 (1280.0, 1334.2)	1223.1 (1181.9, 1264.3)	1374.5 (1338.6, 1410.5)	1311.9 (1292.7, 1331.2)
Length of stay, mean (95% CI)	10.3 (10.2, 10.5)	10.2 (9.9, 10.6)	9.8 (9.6, 10.0)	10.1 (10.0, 10.3)

CABG Coronary artery bypass graft, *CAD* Coronary artery disease, *CAG* Coronary angiogram, *CI* Confidence interval, *NSTEMI* Non-ST-elevation myocardial infarction, *PCI* Percutaneous coronary intervention, *STEMI* ST-elevation myocardial infarction, *TIA* Transient ischemic attack, *UA* Unstable angina

have been optimal, with patients at high- and lower-risk variably receiving high-level interventional therapy, and of variable cost. This may be compounded by inaccurate recording as to whether percutaneous transluminal coronary angioplasty was provided with or without stenting. Further detailed study is required to establish the multifarious factors underlying the apparent high costs of treatment in China and alleviate any concerns to decision makers given the increasing burden of ACS and growing proliferation of treatment. For example, between 2007 and 2011, there was a virtual doubling in the number of PCI procedures performed from 180,000 to 330,000 [19].

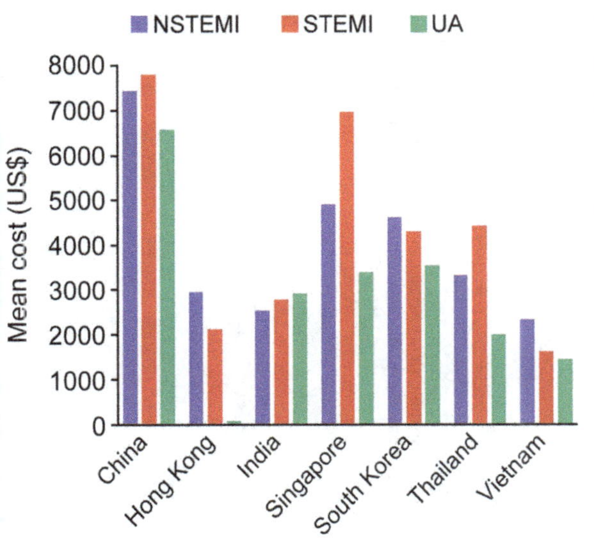

Fig. 1 Mean cost (US$) by country and index event. *NSTEMI* non-ST-elevation myocardial infarction, *STEMI* ST-elevation myocardial infarction, *UA* unstable angina

The finding that age is a positive predictor of high cost is consistent with potentially greater complexity and severity of illness, some of which may not have been captured and thus controlled for in the model. This is perhaps further evidenced by the positive association between hospitalization in the 3 months prior to the index event and high costs. Similar findings for male sex are consistent with a study in Italy where costs incurred by men were significantly greater than that for women, irrespective of index-event type [8]. Reports that women who present with ACS may be evaluated less intensively than men, may go some way towards explaining this [20].

The findings reported here also provide evidence of a potential income effect in that patients on relatively high income appear more likely to be categorized as highest cost. Odds ratios relative to income quintile 5 of 0.45 for quintile 1; 0.76 for quintile 2; 0.97 for quintile 3; 0.80 for quintile 4 (although only statistically significant in relation to quintile 2), ostensibly indicate a pattern in which the odds of incurring high costs increase with income. Such a finding, again, accords with expectations that wealthier patients will seek and have access to higher-cost treatments.

The findings that longer length of stay and having an invasive procedure (versus non-invasive medical management) were both positively associated with odds of incurring high costs is consistent with expectations and reflects, perhaps obviously, resource needs associated with longer treatment duration and need for an invasive procedure. Less intuitive is the finding that those patients who required no help with daily activities prior to hospitalization for their index condition ("no dependence") had significantly higher odds of being in the highest-cost category. Here, it is possible that patients with dependency at

Table 2 Mean (95% confidence interval [CI]) individual center-specific cost ($) per procedure by country[a]

	Country/Region							
	China ($n = 7704$)	Hong Kong ($n = 125$)	India ($n = 2283$)	Singapore ($n = 65$)	South Korea ($n = 247$)	Thailand ($n = 235$)	Vietnam ($n = 160$)	All ($n = 10,819$)
ECG	4.2 (3.9, 4.4)	43.7 (38.1, 49.3)	3.2 (2.8, 3.6)	35.0 (NA)	7.6 (5.5, 9.7)	8.8 (6.6, 11.0)	1.2 (0.7, 1.7)	5.9 (4.9, 6.8)
Cardiac markers	32.9 (30.2, 35.5)	51.5 (41.8, 61.1)	26.7 (23.0, 30.4)	84.0 (NA)	30.3 (22.6, 38.0)	15.5 (11.9, 19.0)	7.8 (0.9, 14.6)	35.8 (22.5, 49.1)
Echocardiography	53.9 (42.5, 65.3)	261.6 (226.9, 296.3)	25.2 (22.1, 28.3)	443.0 (NA)	184.9 (167.5, 202.3)	72.4 (65.7, 79.0)	9.3 (5.7, 12.9)	69.5 (59.3, 79.6)
Angiography	666.4 (613.1, 719.6)	1536.0 (816.9, 2255.1)	343.8 (203.6, 484.0)	4674.0 (NA)	667.0 (376.0, 958.0)	645.2 (539.3, 751.1)	284.2 (209.8, 358.6)	621.4 (549.6, 693.3)
PCI with 1 drug eluting stent	3072.8 (2820.6, 3325.1)	4359.2 (2615.1, 6103.3)	3696.7 (2251.7, 5141.8)	17,590.0 (NA)	1980.9 (1464.5, 2497.4)	4261.4 (3456.8, 5066.1)	3233.3 (2729.3, 2737.4)	3308.1 (2918.5, 3697.7)
PCI with 1 bare metal stent	2174.9 (1924.9, 2425.0)	1942.4 (617.2, 3715.6)	2192.2 (1858.5, 2525.9)	7995.0 (NA)	1752.4 (1291.4, 2213.4)	3247.6 (2609.0, 3886.1)	1900.0 (1542.6, 2257.4)	2251.1 (2067.0, 2435.3)
CABG	8864.1 (8173.1, 9555.1)	7561.0 (4368.2, 10,753.8)	3265.1 (2918.4, 3611.7)	29,520.0 (NA)	4458.6 (2879.3, 6038.0)	7240.7 (4485.7, 9995.7)	4160.0 (2980.1, 5339.9)	6906.7 (6284.3, 7529.0)
Stay in CCU per day	164.5 (119.7, 209.2)	1482.0 (1233.7, 1730.3)	90.7 (72.5, 108.8)	861.0 (NA)	123.2 (73.4, 173.0)	109.7 (59.3, 160.0)	35.3 (4.4, 72.3)	231.3 (102.1, 360.5)

CABG Coronary artery bypass graft, *CCU* Critical care unit, *ECG* Electrocardiogram, *NA* Not available, *PCI* Percutaneous coronary intervention

[a]Exchange rate conversion based on (March 2013): 1 USD = 6.2943 CNY; 7.7681 HKD; 53.060 INR; 3.1690 SGD; 1158.1 KRW; 31.545 THB; 21,030 VND

Table 3 Model-based point estimates for high-cost healthcare expenditure[a] using logistic models – univariate analysis (excluding Malaysia)

Factor	Odds ratio	95% CI	*P* value
Age, per 10-year increment	1.04	0.99, 1.08	0.0925
Sex, male versus female	1.18	1.06, 1.33	0.0038
Income (versus quintile 5)			< 0.0001
Quintile 1	0.45	0.19, 1.06	
Quintile 2	0.76	0.67, 0.85	
Quintile 3	0.97	0.85, 1.11	
Quintile 4	0.80	0.53, 1.20	
Health insurance, yes versus no	1.02	0.90, 1.16	0.7074
Residence, rural versus non-rural	1.02	0.92, 1.12	0.7516
Smoker (versus never)			0.2418
Current	0.92	0.83, 1.03	
Former	1.02	0.89, 1.15	
Disease history, yes versus no	1.15	1.04, 1.28	0.0068
Hospitalization in the 3 months prior to index event, yes versus no	1.37	1.16, 1.62	0.0002
Dependence degree before index event, none versus some	1.74	1.48, 2.05	< 0.0001
Index event medical management, invasive versus non-invasive	4.62	3.78, 5.64	< 0.0001
Type of hospital (versus UGH)			0.0030
Regional/community/rural hospital	0.92	0.72, 1.17	
Non-UGH	1.13	1.01, 1.27	
Other type of hospital/clinic	1.24	1.09, 1.40	
Number of beds	1.00	1.00, 1.00	0.5995
Length of stay	1.04	1.03, 1.05	< 0.0001
Country (versus China)			0.8569
Hong Kong	1.00	0.64, 1.56	
India	1.09	0.97, 1.23	
Singapore	0.91	0.48, 1.70	
South Korea	1.00	0.72, 1.36	
Thailand	1.00	0.72, 1.38	
Vietnam	0.96	0.65, 1.43	

UGH University general hospital, CI Confidence interval
[a]high cost defined as the top quintile within a country

baseline would have the ongoing support of a "carer" to rely on. The potential lack of such support for patients without dependency at baseline may have led to greater costs due to a greater need for in-hospital rehabilitation and extensive discharge planning.

Another ostensibly unexpected observation was that the odds of incurring high-cost treatment, relative to those encountered in patients admitted to a university general hospital, were higher for those patients admitted to all "other" categories of hospital, e.g. regional/community/rural hospitals, non-university general hospitals and other type of clinics. Here, it is possible that the multivariable analysis used in this study effectively controlled for factors implicated in higher costs seen in teaching (university) hospitals, such as size of facility, treatment mode, disease history and length of stay. Our findings suggest, therefore, that the independent effect of university status of a hospital was to lower costs, very likely associated with efficiency and an established degree of expertise in such centers.

The lack of significant association between insurance status and high-cost care may allay potential concerns about the inflationary effects of national programs to expand insurance coverage, e.g. due for instance to incentives created by a third-party payer for providers to overcharge/over-service (provider moral hazard) and patients to overuse (patient moral hazard) [21]. Although this study focuses only on ACS patients, the findings of

Table 4 Model-based point estimates for high-cost healthcare expenditure[a] using logistic models – multivariate analysis (excluding Malaysia)

Factor	Odds ratio	95% CI	*P* value
Age, per 10-year increment	1.10	1.05, 1.16	< 0.0001
Sex, male versus female	1.17	1.02, 1.33	0.0224
Income (versus quintile 5)			< 0.0001
Quintile 1	0.43	0.15, 1.19	
Quintile 2	0.76	0.67, 0.86	
Quintile 3	0.96	0.83, 1.11	
Quintile 4	0.74	0.45, 1.23	
Health insurance, yes versus no	1.11	0.89, 1.38	0.3686
Disease history, yes versus no	1.25	1.11, 1.41	0.0002
Hospitalization in the 3 months prior to index event, yes versus no	1.48	1.23, 1.77	< 0.0001
Dependence degree before index event, none versus some	1.96	1.60, 2.40	< 0.0001
Index event medical management, invasive versus non-invasive	5.48	4.34, 6.92	< 0.0001
Type of hospital (versus UGH)			0.00[illegible]6
Regional/community/rural hospital	1.74	1.25, 2.41	
Non-UGH	1.13	0.99, 1.29	
Other type of hospital/clinic	0.97	0.79, 1.19	
Length of stay	1.06	1.04, 1.06	< 0.0001
Country (versus China)			< 0.0001
Hong Kong	1.92	1.04, 3.53	
India	2.54	1.98, 3.25	
Singapore	1.58	0.77, 3.24	
South Korea	1.21	0.76, 1.95	
Thailand	1.52	1.05, 2.20	
Vietnam	0.90	0.57, 1.42	

UGH University general hospital
[a]Defined as the top quintile within a country

this study found no evidence of an inflationary impact associated insurance coverage. Further country-specific research is needed to determine whether the roll out of social insurance programs will increase costs to any significant degree.

There were several limitations in the present study. First, inclusion only of patients alive and followed up at 6 weeks might suggest a possible survivor bias to the findings. As mentioned, earlier studies have reported in-hospital mortality to be associated with higher costs, suggesting our estimates of average costs may have been underestimated. In addition, the costs examined in this study reflect only health system cost whereas a broader societal perspective would have considered costs to households and the community associated with indirect loss of income and reduced productivity. Also, the costs included in this analysis were confined to hospitalization for the index condition and excluded costs of potential re-hospitalizations for ACS; in the US, such costs have been estimated at over 30% [22], suggesting there are significant costs associated with ACS outside of the scope of this analysis. Furthermore, the costs of sub-acute follow-up care were not included. These may vary across countries due to differences in treatment norms, funding models and other health system characteristics. Despite these potential limitations in capturing the high costs to health systems associated with ACS, the study highlights the major policy challenges associated with a high burden of illness in Asia. Some countries in this analysis were represented by a relatively small number of participants, thus precluding detailed country-specific analyses. Thus, the way in which the primary outcome for this study was specified (i.e. occurrence of cost in the highest quintile specific to each country and index condition) served as a standardized outcome that facilitated the pooling of data across all countries. An alternative approach would have been to adjust for differences in purchasing power by converting into international dollars; however, the problem with such a strategy is that costs reported in international dollars lack meaning for local policy makers since they co not reflect actual budgetary implications (nevertheless the conversions are provided in Additional file 1: Table S2 for reference). The inclusion of hospital length of stay as an explanatory variable and the likelihood of it being highly correlated with cost is a potential weakness in the modelling [23], as we may not be able to identify factors that affect the cost through the hospital length of stay. However, it is an important variable of interest and its inclusion is justified as it allows us to estimate the direct effect of other factors included in the model. Finally, without accounting for clustering in the analysis, variance and confidence intervals could be slightly underestimated. However, in international studies of this kind, it is conventional that such adjustments are not made.

Conclusion

The present analysis highlights the drivers of high-cost treatment for ACS in Asia. It represents an advance in this area by examining factors beyond the clinical drivers of costs. The study further identifies health-system factors including hospital type, and health insurance and socioeconomic status, providing evidence to policy makers of the financial implications of current and future reforms; notably programs in Asia to expand health insurance coverage to underserved populations. The value of prevention programs in avoiding hospitalizations for ACS is also considered to highlight population groups (e.g. men, high-income groups, and uninsured) in whom effective prevention may yield the greatest financial savings.

Abbreviations

ACS: Acute coronary syndromes; CABG: Coronary artery bypass graft; CAD: Coronary artery disease; CAG: Coronary angiogram; CCU: Critical care unit; CI: Confidence interval; ECG: Electrocardiogram; NA: Not available; NSTEMI: Non-ST-elevation myocardial infarction; OR: Odds ratio; PCI: Percutaneous coronary intervention; STEMI: ST-elevation myocardial infarction; TIA: Transient ischemic attack; UA: Unstable angina; UGH: University general hospital

Acknowledgements

The authors would like to thank the patients, their families and all investigators involved in this study. Medical writing and editorial support, including assisting authors with incorporation of comments, fact checking, referencing, figure preparation, formatting, proofreading, and submission was provided by Carl V Felton PhD, Prime Global (Knutsford, Cheshire, UK), supported by AstraZeneca according to Good Publication Practice guidelines (Link). The Sponsor was involved in the study design, collection, analysis and interpretation of data, as well as data checking of information provided in the manuscript. However, ultimate responsibility for opinions, conclusions, and data interpretation lies with the authors.

Funding

The EPICOR Asia study and editorial support were supported by AstraZeneca.

Authors' contributions

All authors, SJ, SW-LL, JPPS, TKO; CTC; H-SK, RK, VTN, SJP, AMV, NH, and YH made substantial contributions to the analysis and interpretation of the data, and to the preparation, review and final approval of this manuscript. SJ led the analysis of the data and was the major contributor in writing the manuscript: SW-LL, JPPS, TKO; CTC; H-SK, RK, VTN, SJP, AMV, and YH all provided critical review and intellectual comment; and NH undertook statistical analysis and provided critical review. All authors read and approved the final manuscript.

Competing interests

JPSS has been a consultant or advisory board member for AstraZeneca, Lupin, and Intas. TKO has acted as a consultant or advisory board member for Sanofi-Aventis, Abbott Vascular, Boston Scientific, Boehringer Ingelheim, Novartis, and AstraZeneca. CTC has received research support from Eli Lilly, honoraria from Medtronic, and has been a consultant or advisory board member for AstraZeneca. RK has been a consultant or advisory board member for AstraZeneca and Boehringer Ingelheim. VTN has received research grants from AstraZeneca, Servier, Sanofi, and Boston Scientific, and has been a consultant or advisory board member for AstraZeneca, Pfizer, Sanofi, Boehringer Ingelheim, Servier, MSD, Abbott, Bayer, Novartis, Merck Serono, Biosensor, Biotronic, Boston Scientific, Terumo, and Medtronic. SJP receives research funds from AstraZeneca. AMV and NH are employees of AstraZeneca. All other authors declare that they have no competing interests.

Author details

[1]The George Institute for Global Health, Sydney Medical School, University of Sydney, King George V Building, 83–117 Missenden Rd, Camperdown, NSW 2050, Australia. [2]Queen Mary Hospital, Hong Kong, SAR, China. [3]Sir Ganga Ram Hospital, New Delhi, India. [4]Sarawak General Hospital, Kuching, Malaysia. [5]National Heart Centre Singapore, Singapore, Singapore. [6]Seoul National University Hospital, Seoul, South Korea. [7]Siriraj Hospital, Bangkok, Thailand. [8]Cho Ray Hospital, Ho Chi Minh City, Vietnam. [9]London School of Hygiene and Tropical Medicine, London, UK. [10]Observational Research Centre, Global Medical Affairs, AstraZeneca, Madrid, Spain. [11]AstraZeneca, Osaka, Japan. [12]Peking University First Hospital, Beijing, China.

References

1. Vedanthan R, Seligman B, Fuster V. Global perspective on acute coronary syndrome: a burden on the young and poor. Circ Res. 2014;114:1959–75.
2. Roggeri DP, Roggeri A, Rossi E, Cinconze E, De Rosa M, Maggioni AP, et al. Direct healthcare costs and resource consumption after acute coronary syndrome: a real-life analysis of an Italian subpopulation. Eur J Prev Cardiol. 2014;21:1090–6.
3. Wieser S, Ruthemann I, De Boni S, Eichler K, Pletscher M, Radovanovic D, et al. Cost of acute coronary syndrome in Switzerland in 2008. Swiss Med Wkly. 2012;142:w13655.
4. Kim J, Lee E, Lee T, Sohn A. Economic burden of acute coronary syndrome in South Korea: a national survey. BMC Cardiovasc Disord. 2013;13:55.
5. Xi B, Liu F, Hao Y, Dong H, Mi J. The growing burden of cardiovascular diseases in China. Int J Cardiol. 2014;174:736–7.
6. Wang S, Petzold M, Cao J, Zhang Y, Wang W. Direct medical costs of hospitalizations for cardiovascular diseases in Shanghai, China: trends and projections. Medicine. 2015;94:e837.
7. Page RL II, Ghushchyan V, Van Den Bos J, Gray TJ, Hoetzer GL, Bhandary D, et al. The cost of inpatient death associated with acute coronary syndrome. Vasc Health Risk Manag. 2016;12:13–21.
8. Roggeri A, Gnavi R, Dalmasso M, Rusciani R, Giammaria M, Anselmino M, et al. Resource consumption and healthcare costs of acute coronary syndrome: a retrospective observational administrative database analysis. Crit Pathw Cardiol. 2013;12:204–9.
9. Fan GQ, Fu KL, Jin CW, Wang XZ, Han L, Wang H, et al. A medical costs study of older patients with acute myocardial infarction and metabolic syndrome in hospital. Clin Interv Aging. 2015;10:329–37.
10. Zhao Z, Zhu B, Anderson J, Fu H, LeNarz L. Resource utilization and healthcare costs for acute coronary syndrome patients with and without diabetes mellitus. J Med Econ. 2010;13:748–59.

11. Srivastava A, Mohanty SK. Age and sex pattern of cardiovascular mortality, hospitalisation and associated cost in India. PLoS One. 2013;8:e62134.
12. Huo Y, Lee SW, Sawhney JP, Kim HS, Krittayaphong R, Nhan VT, et al. Rationale, design, and baseline characteristics of the EPICOR Asia study (long-tErm follow-uP of antithrombotic management patterns in acute CORonary syndrome patients in Asia). Clin Cardiol. 2015;38:511–9.
13. Mani K, Lundkvist J, Holmberg L, Wanhainen A. Challenges in analysis and interpretation of cost data in vascular surgery. J Vasc Surg. 2010;51:148–54.
14. Thompson SG, Barber JA. How should cost data in pragmatic randomised trials be analysed? BMJ. 2000;320:1197–200.
15. Ramsey S, Willke R, Briggs A, Brown R, Buxton M, Chawla A, et al. Good research practices for cost-effectiveness analysis alongside clinical trials: the ISPOR RCT-CEA task force report. Value Health. 2005;8:521–33.
16. Hurley J. Chapter 2: An overview of normative economics of the health care sector. In: Culyer A, Newhouse J, editors. Handbook of health economics: volume 1A. 1st ed. Amsterdam: Elsevier Science BV; 2000.
17. Glick H, Doshi J, Sonnad S, Polsky D. Economic evaluation in clinical trials. Oxford: Oxford University Press; 2007.
18. Breslow NE, Day NE, Halvorsen KT, Prentice RL, Sabai C. Estimation of multiple relative risk functions in matched case-control studies. Am J Epidemiol. 1978;108:299–307.
19. Li H, Ge J. Cardiovascular diseases in China: current status and future perspectives. IJC Heart & Vasculature. 2015;6:25–31.
20. Elsaesser A, Hamm CW. Acute coronary syndrome: the risk of being female. Circulation. 2004;109:565–7.
21. Cutler DM, Zeckhauser RJ. The anatomy of health insurance. In: Handbook of health economics: volume 1A. First edn. Edited by Culyer AJ and Newhouse JP: Elsevier, Oxford; 2000: 563–643.
22. Berenson K, Ogbonnaya A, Casciano R, Makenbaeva D, Mozaffari E, Lamerato L, et al. Economic consequences of ACS-related rehospitalizations in the US. Curr Med Res Opin. 2010;26:329–36.
23. Polverejan E, Gardiner JC, Bradley CJ, Holmes-Rovner M, Rovner D. Estimating mean hospital cost as a function of length of stay and patient characteristics. Health Econ. 2003;12:935–47.

19

Choosing between Enoxaparin and Fondaparinux for the management of patients with acute coronary syndrome

Pravesh Kumar Bundhun[1], Musaben Shaik[2] and Jun Yuan[3*]

Abstract

Background: Enoxaparin and Fondaparinux are potential anticoagulants which are used peri-operatively in the management of patients with Acute Coronary Syndrome (ACS). We aimed to compare the adverse clinical outcomes which are associated with the use of these anticoagulants in patients who were treated for ACS.

Methods: Online databases (PubMed/Medline, EMBASE, Cochrane library) were searched for studies which compared differences in clinical outcomes observed with the use of enoxaparin and fondaparinux in patients who were treated peri-operatively for ACS. Statistical analysis was carried out by Revman 5.3 software with odds ratio (OR) and 95% confidence intervals (CI) as the analytical parameters.

Results: Seven studies with a total number of 9618 patients (mainly composed of non-ST elevated myocardial infarction/NSTEMI) were included. This analysis showed mortality to be similarly observed between enoxaparin and fondaparinux with OR: 1.05, 95% CI: 0.67–1.63; $P = 0.84$. Myocardial infarction (MI) and stroke were also not significantly different throughout different follow up periods. However, minor, major and total bleeding were significantly lower with fondaparinux (OR: 0.40, 95% CI: 0.27–0.58; $P = 0.00001$), (OR: 0.46, 95% CI: 0.32–0.66; $P = 0.0001$) and (OR: 0.47, 95% CI: 0.37–0.60; $P = 0.00001$) respectively during the 10-day follow up period. Even during a follow up period of 30 days or a midterm follow up, major and minor bleeding still significantly favored fondaparinux in comparison to enoxaparin.

Conclusion: In patients who were treated for ACS, fondaparinux might be a better choice when compared to enoxaparin in terms of short to midterm bleeding events. This result was mainly applicable to patients with NSTEMI. However, due to a limited number of patients analyzed, further larger randomized trials should be able to confirm this hypothesis.

Keywords: Enoxaparin, Fondaparinux, Acute coronary syndrome, Major bleeding, Minor bleeding, Heparin

Background

Enoxaparin and Fondaparinux are potential anticoagulants which are used peri-operatively in the management of patients with Acute Coronary Syndrome (ACS) [1]. The Fifth Organization to Assess Strategies in Ischemic Syndromes (OASIS 5) trial showed fondaparinux to reduce the rate of major bleeding and net clinical benefit including death, Myocardial Infarction (MI), stroke and major bleeding in comparison to enoxaparin [2]. However, results from the French Registry of ST segment elevation and non-ST segment elevation MI (FAST-MI) 2010 showed a similar rate of bleeding and mortality between fondaparinux and enoxaparin [3]. Even though, FAST-MI cannot be compared to the OASIS 5 trial which consisted of a very large number of patients, we would still like to confirm the results through a meta-analysis by comparing the adverse clinical outcomes which were observed with enoxaparin and fondaparinux in patients who were treated for ACS.

* Correspondence: nnyuanjun@163.com
[3]Department of Cardiology, The People's Hospital of Guangxi Zhuang Autonomous Region, Nanning, Guangxi 530021, China
Full list of author information is available at the end of the article

Methods

Data sources and search strategy

Online databases (PubMed/Medline, EMBASE, Cochrane library) were searched for studies (English publications) which compared differences in clinical outcomes observed with the use of enoxaparin and fondaparinux in patients who were treated peri-operatively for ACS by using the searched terms 'enoxaparin and fondaparinux and acute coronary syndrome'. Later in this search process, the terms 'percutaneous coronary intervention, heparin' and the abbreviations 'ACS and PCI' were also used. Reference lists of suitable articles were also reviewed for relevant publications.

Inclusion criteria

Studies were included if they satisfied certain major criteria which were:

(a) They were randomized controlled trials or observational studies comparing enoxaparin with fondaparinux in patients who were treated for ACS or in patients who were undergoing percutaneous coronary intervention (PCI).
(b) They reported adverse outcomes (cardiovascular and bleeding outcomes) as their clinical endpoints.
(c) They involved relevant data which could be used in this current analysis.

Exclusion criteria

Studies were excluded if they did not satisfy certain major criteria which were:

(a) They were systematic reviews, meta analyses, case studies or letter to editors.
(b) They did not include patients with ACS.
(c) They did not report the previously mentioned clinical outcomes.
(d) They were duplicates of the same study or they were associated with the same trial or cohort.

Types of participants

This analysis mainly included patients with non-ST segment elevated myocardial infarction (NSTEMI), patients with unstable angina (UA) and a small percentage of patients with ST segment elevated myocardial infarction (STEMI).

Definitions, outcomes and follow ups

Endpoints which were assessed included:

(a) Mortality;
(b) MI;
(c) Stroke;
(d) Minor bleeding: any type of minor bleeding;
(e) Major bleeding: any type of major bleeding;
(f) All bleeding (major and minor bleeding combined) including thrombolysis in myocardial infarction (TIMI) defined major and minor bleeding [4].

The follow up periods were classified as:

- Less than 10 days (including in-hospital follow up period);
- 30 days follow up period;
- Mid-term follow up (6 months to 1 year) period.

These outcomes and follow up periods have been summarized in Table 1.

Data extraction and review

Information and data including the name of authors, year of article publication, period of patients' enrollment, number of patients collected from each group (enoxaparin and fondaparinux), type of study (RCT or observational study), baseline characteristics of the patients, the outcomes reported, the follow up periods, the medications used by the patients, and the number of events reported with enoxaparin and fondaparinux respectively, were independently collected/extracted by two authors (PKB and MS). Disagreements were resolved by discussion with the third author (JY). Since this is a meta-

Table 1 Reported Outcomes and follow up periods

Studies	Reported outcomes	Follow up period	Types of participants
FAST MI [3]	Death, MI, stroke, TIMI major and minor bleeding	In-hospital	NSTEMI
OASIS 5 [2]	Death, MI, stroke, TIMI major bleeding, total bleeding, major bleeding	9 days, 30 days, 6 months	NSTEMI, UA
Schiele 2010 [14]	Death, bleeding	30 days	STEMI, NSTEMI, UA
Shah 2014 [15]	Death, bleeding	9 days, 30 days	UA, NSTEMI
Zhao 2015 [12]	Death, MI, major bleeding, minor bleeding, stroke	7 days, 30 days, 6 months	NSTEMI
Zhao 2016 [16]	Death, MI, stroke, major bleeding, all bleeding	30 days, 1 year	STEMI, NSTEMI, UA
Soeiro 2016 [10]	Death, MI, major bleeding, stroke	In-hospital	NSTEMI

Abbreviations: *MI* myocardial infarction, *TIMI* thrombolysis in myocardial infarction, *STEMI* ST elevated myocardial infarction, *NSTEMI* non-ST elevated myocardial infarction, *UA* unstable angina

analysis, the PRISMA guideline [5] was followed and the bias risk among the trials was assessed with reference to the features which have been stated in the Cochrane Collaboration [6]. All the trials were rated as having a 'low to moderate' risk of bias.

Statistical analysis

The statistical analysis was carried out by Revman 5.3 software with odds ratio (OR) and 95% confidence intervals (CI) as the analytical parameters. Two simple statistical methods were used to assess heterogeneity [7] across the studies namely the Q statistic test and the I^2 test.

A *P* value of less or equal to 0.05 was considered as statistically significant whereas a *P* value greater than 0.05 was insignificant in this analysis.

On the other hand, a fixed effects model or a random effects model was used during the analysis depending on the value of I^2. A fixed effects model was recommended if an I^2 value <50% was obtained, whereas if the I^2 value was >50%, a random effects model was recommended.

In addition, this I^2 value was also used to predict heterogeneity. The lower the I^2 value, the lesser would be the heterogeneity whereas heterogeneity would increase with an increasing I^2 value.

Sensitivity analyses were also carried out by excluding each study one by one and a new analysis was carried out each time.

Publication bias was visually observed by analyzing the funnel plots which were generated through the RevMan software. Since this analysis did not involve a large volume of studies (only 7 studies were available), asymmetry of the funnel plots was sufficient to represent publication bias. Normally, if the total number of studies which were included was more than 10, other methods would have been more appropriate.

Ethical approval was not required for this type of study.

Results

Search results

Seven hundred and eighty-seven (787) articles were obtained using the above mentioned searched terms from electronic databases. After a careful check of the abstracts and titles by the same two authors (PKB and MS), 764 articles were eliminated (not related to this current idea). Twenty-three (23) full-text articles were assessed for eligibility. Among these 23 articles, further studies were eliminated because they were:

- Systematic reviews, case studies or letter to editors (2);
- Articles with data which were irrelevant for this current meta-analysis (1);
- Articles which did not report adverse clinical outcomes as their endpoints (4);
- Duplicates or studies which were associated with the same trials or cohorts (9).

Finally, 7 studies were selected and included in this analysis (Fig. 1).

General features of the studies which were included

Five (5) observational studies and 2 randomized trials were included with a total number of 9618 patients (6587 patients were treated with enoxaparin and 3031 patients were treated with fondaparinux). Regions of patients' enrollment included France, China, Brazil, and Canada with an enrollment period ranging between years 2003 to 2015. The general features of the studies which were included have been listed in Tables 2 and 3.

Baseline features of the studies which were included

The baseline features (Table 4) were as follow: mean age 57.3–67.0 years, majority of the patients were male patients, other co-morbidities and smoking history were also reported in both groups. Overall, there were no significant differences in the baseline features between patients who were treated with enoxaparin and fondaparinux.

The OASIS 5 trial had a large number of patients when compared to the other studies. However, in order for the current results not to be influenced by the results obtained in the OASIS 5 trial, the proportion of patients obtained from the OASIS 5 trial was reduced in order to adjust to this current analysis. To be more clear, only the percentage of female patients (20–30%) from the trial were included when analyzing the 30-day outcomes and only 11 to 12% of patients were included when assessing bleeding events. It should be noted that the total number of patients which were extracted was not reduced. For example, '10 events of death out of 100 patients' was represented as '1 event of death out of 10 patients'. Therefore, it is basically the same thing.

Table 5 summarized other anti-platelet and anticoagulant medications which were used by the patients. It can clearly be seen that almost all the patients were also being treated by aspirin and clopidogrel. Glycoprotein IIb/IIIa, prasugrel and unfractionated heparin were also being used by certain patients.

Less than 10-days follow up period (enoxaparin versus fondaparinux)

Results of this analysis showed that mortality was similarly observed between enoxaparin and fondaparinux with OR: 1.05, 95% CI: 0.67–1.63; *P* = 0.84. MI and stroke were also not significantly different with OR: 0.77, 95% CI: 0.59–1.02; *P* = 0.07 and OR: 1.12, 95% CI: 0.51–2.46; *P* = 0.78 respectively during this 10-day period. However, minor, major and total

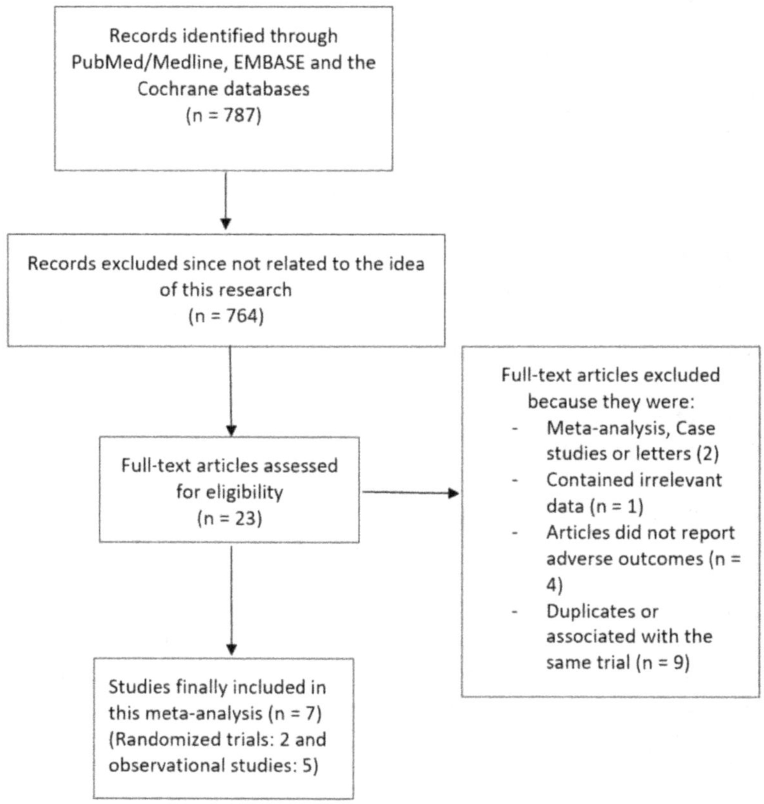

Fig. 1 Flow diagram representing the study selection

bleeding were significantly lower with fondaparinux (OR: 0.40, 95% CI: 0.27–0.58; P = 0.00001), (OR: 0.46, 95% CI: 0.32–0.66; P = 0.0001) and (OR: 0.47, 95% CI: 0.37–0.60; P = 0.00001) respectively. Results for this 10-day follow up period have been represented in Fig. 2.

When observational data were separately analyzed, MI and major bleeding significantly favored fondaparinux with OR: 0.61, 95% CI: 0.40–0.94; P = 0.02 and OR: 0.44, 95% CI: 0.23–0.86; P = 0.02 respectively (Fig. 3).

However, when randomized data were separately analyzed, mortality was not significantly different between these two drugs with OR: 1.00, 95% CI: 0.53–1.91; P = 0.99 whereas total bleeding still significantly favored fondaparinux with OR: 0.40, 95% CI: 0.30–0.55; P = 0.00001 (Fig. 4).

30-days follow up period (enoxaparin versus fondaparinux)

During this 30-days follow up period, mortality and MI were not significantly different with OR: 0.90, 95% CI: 0.57–1.42; P = 0.66 and OR: 1.00, 95% CI: 0.69–1.46; P = 1.00 respectively. However, major and minor bleeding significantly favored fondaparinux with OR:

Table 2 General features of the studies which were included

Studies	Type of study	Region	Patients' enrollment year	Total no of patients in Enoxaparin group (n)	Total no of patients in Fondaparinux group (n)
FAST MI	Observational	France	2010	1027	240
OASIS 5	RCT	Canada	2003–2005	1420	1414
Schiele2010	Observational	France	2006–2007	1418	301
Shah2014	RCT	-	2010	90	90
Zhao2015	Observational	China	2011–2012	232	229
Zhao2016	Observational	China	2010–2012	453	422
Soeiro2016	Observational	Brazil	2010–2015	1947	335
Total no of patients (n)				6587	3031

Abbreviations: *RCT* randomized controlled trials

Table 3 Procedures and duration of therapy

Studies	Procedures	PCI (%)	Type of CAD	Duration of therapy
	Eno/Fond	Eno/Fond	Eno/Fond	Eno/Fond
FAST MI	PCI	69.0/69.0	NSTEMI	2 days
OASIS 5	PCI	100/100	NSTEMI, UA	2–8 days
Schiele2010	PCI	84.0/72.0	STEMI, NSTEMI, UA	In hospital period
Shan2014	PCI	100/100	UA, NSTEMI	In hospital period
Zhao2015	PCI	100/100	NSTEMI	2–8 days
Zhao2016	PCI	100/100	STEMI, NSTEMI, UA	3–7 days
Speiro2016	PCI	100/100	NSTEMI	In hospital period

Abbreviations: *PCI* percutaneous coronary intervention, *Eno* enoxaparin, *Fond* fondaparinux, *CAD* coronary artery disease, *STEMI* ST segment elevated myocardial infarction, *NSTEMI* non-ST segment elevated myocardial infarction, *UA* unstable angina

0.49, 95% CI: 0.26–0.94; *P* = 0.03 and OR: 0.48, 95% CI: 0.27–0.85; *P* = 0.01 respectively. Results for the 30-days follow up period have been represented in Fig. 5.

When observational data were separately analyzed, mortality was not significantly different with OR: 0.84, 95% CI: 0.44–1.60; *P* = 0.60. However, even if major bleeding favored fondaparinux with OR: 0.41, 95% CI: 0.13–1.31; *P* = 0.13, the result was not statistically significant (Fig. 6).

Midterm follow up period (enoxaparin versus fondaparinux)

During this midterm follow up period, mortality, MI, and stroke were still not significantly different with OR: 0.79, 95% CI: 0.50–1.23; *P* = 0.30, OR: 1.05, 95% CI: 0.78–1.42; *P* = 0.73 and OR: 0.73, 95% CI: 0.38–1.41; *P* = 0.35 respectively. However, major, minor and total bleeding were significantly lower with fondaparinux with OR: 0.50, 95% CI: 0.28–0.89; *P* = 0.02, OR: 0.51, 95% CI: 0.31–0.84; *P* = 0.009 and OR: 0.48, 95% CI: 0.34–0.69; *P* = 0.0001 respectively (Fig. 7).

When observation studies were separately analyzed, mortality, MI and stroke were not significantly different with OR: 0.52, 95% CI: 0.19–1.39; *P* = 0.19, OR: 0.93, 95% CI: 0.52–1.65; *P* = 0.80 and OR: 0.85, 95% CI: 0.33–2.17; *P* = 0.74 respectively. However, even if major bleeding favored fondaparinux with OR: 0.43, 95% CI: 0.16–1.14; *P* = 0.09, the result was not statistically significant but total bleeding was significantly lower with fondaparinux with OR: 0.50, 95% CI: 0.33–0.78; *P* = 0.002 (Fig. 8).

Sensitivity analysis

Sensitivity analyses were carried out. During the 30-days follow up period, excluding study Zhang2016 resulted in a non-significant result associated with major bleeding with OR: 0.53, 95% CI: 0.27–1.04; *P* = 0.06. During the midterm follow up period, excluding trial OASIS 5 resulted in a non-significant major bleeding with OR: 0.43, 95% CI: 0.16–1.14; *P* = 0.09. For the other results, no significant change was observed.

In addition, when patients with STEMI were excluded, and an analysis was conducted based on patients with NSTEMI, major and minor bleeding were still significantly higher with enoxaparin, with OR: 0.46, 95% CI: 0.32–0.66; *P* = 0.0001 and OR: 0.40, 95% CI: 0.27–0.58; *P* = 0.00001 respectively during a 10-day follow up period. During a 30-day follow up period, only minor bleeding was significantly higher with enoxaparin, with OR: 0.48, 95% CI: 0.27–0.85; *P* = 0.01. In addition, during the mid-term follow up, major and minor bleeding were both significantly higher with enoxaparin, with OR: 0.55, 95% CI: 0.30–0.99; *P* = 0.05 and OR: 0.51, 95% CI:

Table 4 Baseline features of the studies which were included

Studies	Mean age	Males (%)	Ht (%)	Ds (%)	Cs (%)	DM (%)
	E/F	E/F	E/F	E/F	E/F	E/F
FAST MI	67.0/66.5	71.0/72.0	58.0/66.0	45.5/52.5	27.0/32.0	23.0/25.0
OASIS 5	64.5/64.6	69.1/71.7	-	-	-	23.1/23.5
Schiele2010	-	71.0/66.0	52.0/57.0	49.0/55.0	32.0/31.0	21.0/20.0
Shan2014	-	77.8/74.4	55.6/55.6	-	58.9/55.6	41.1/38.9
Zhao2015	59.8/60.1	73.3/76.9	65.5/66.8	-	68.5/68.1	39.6/37.1
Zhao2016	58.2/57.3	78.2/76.3	59.5/57.2	-	53.0/52.1	20.3/22.8
Speiro2016	61.8/61.0	62.6/65.7	73.6/67.8	51.2/48.9	30.5/24.2	46.9/55.8

Abbreviations: *E* enoxaparin, *F* fondaparinux, *Ht* hypertension, *Ds* dyslipidemia, *Cs* current smoker, *DM* diabetes mellitus

Table 5 Other anti-platelet and anticoagulant medications which were used by the participants

Studies	Aspirin	Clopidogrel	Glycoprotein IIb/IIIa	Prasugrel	U.heparin
	E/F	E/F	E/F	E/F	E/F
FAST MI	98.0/98.0	90.5/92.0	26.5/34.0	15.0/15.0	36.0/60.0
OASIS 5	98.9/98.6	92.3/91.1	38.8/40.4	-	-
Schiele2010	99.0/99.0	98.0/99.0	58.0/68.0	-	-
Zhao2015	96.5/96.1	100/100	-	-	100/100
Zhao2016	99.8/99.3	75.3/80.1	-	-	-
Soeiro2016	97.8/98.5	67.9/65.4	16.1/5.80	-	-

Abbreviations: *E* enoxaparin, *F* fondaparinux, data were represented in terms of %

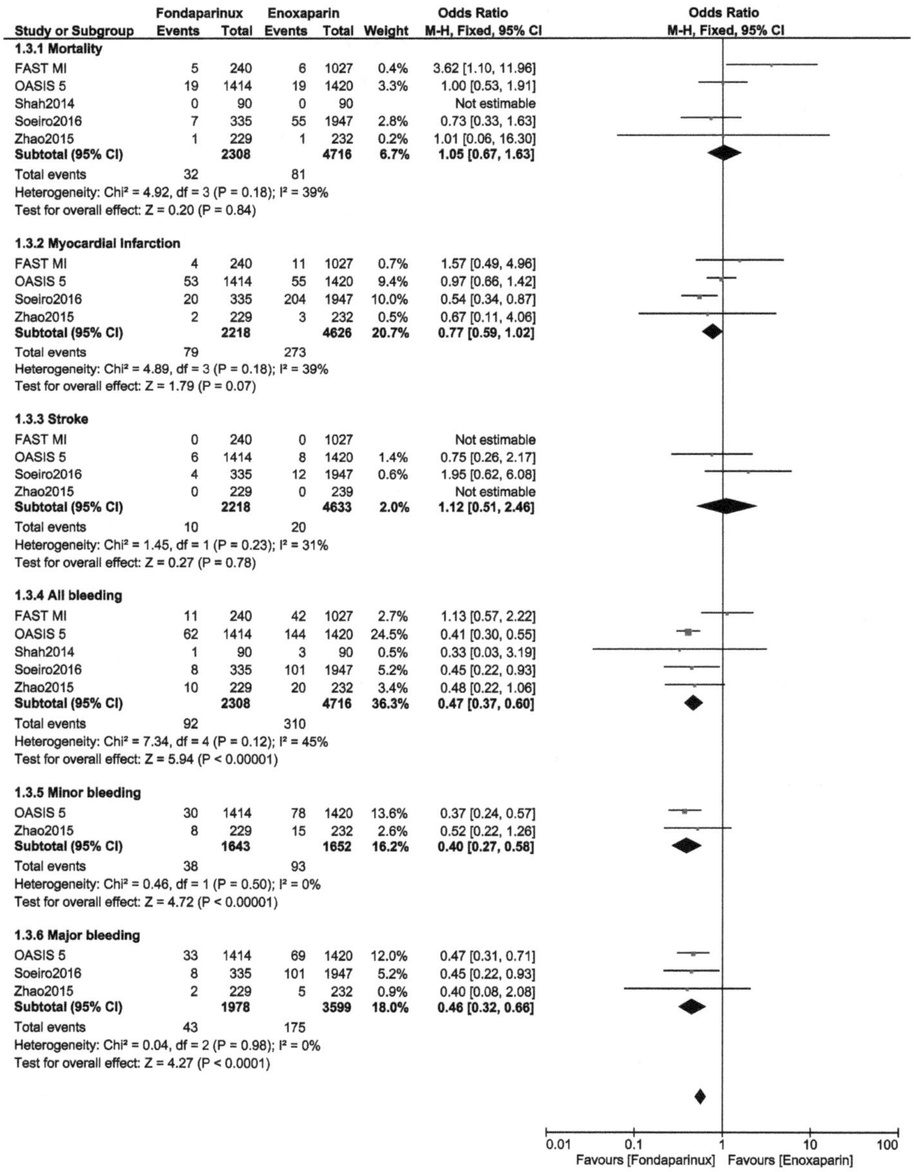

Fig. 2 Enoxaparin versus fondaparinux (10-day follow up)

Study or Subgroup	Fondaparinux Events	Fondaparinux Total	Enoxaparin Events	Enoxaparin Total	Weight	Odds Ratio M-H, Fixed, 95% CI
1.3.1 Myocardial Infarction						
FAST MI	4	240	11	1027	4.1%	1.57 [0.49, 4.96]
Soeiro2016	20	335	204	1947	55.9%	0.54 [0.34, 0.87]
Zhao2015	2	229	3	232	2.9%	0.67 [0.11, 4.06]
Subtotal (95% CI)		**804**		**3206**	**62.9%**	**0.61 [0.40, 0.94]**
Total events	26		218			
Heterogeneity: Chi² = 2.80, df = 2 (P = 0.25); I² = 29%						
Test for overall effect: Z = 2.25 (P = 0.02)						
1.3.2 Stroke						
FAST MI	0	240	0	1027		Not estimable
Soeiro2016	4	335	12	1947	3.5%	1.95 [0.62, 6.08]
Zhao2015	0	229	0	239		Not estimable
Subtotal (95% CI)		**804**		**3213**	**3.5%**	**1.95 [0.62, 6.08]**
Total events	4		12			
Heterogeneity: Not applicable						
Test for overall effect: Z = 1.15 (P = 0.25)						
1.3.3 Major bleeding						
Soeiro2016	8	335	101	1947	28.7%	0.45 [0.22, 0.93]
Zhao2015	2	229	5	232	4.9%	0.40 [0.08, 2.08]
Subtotal (95% CI)		**564**		**2179**	**33.6%**	**0.44 [0.23, 0.86]**
Total events	10		106			
Heterogeneity: Chi² = 0.01, df = 1 (P = 0.90); I² = 0%						
Test for overall effect: Z = 2.40 (P = 0.02)						

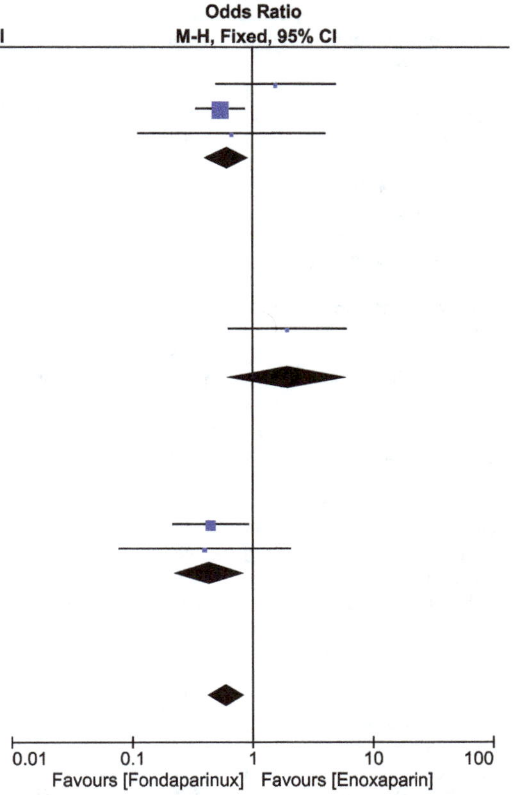

Fig. 3 Enoxaparin versus fondaparinux using data obtained only from observational studies (10-day follow up)

0.31–0.84; P = 0.009 respectively in these patients with NSTEMI.

Publication bias

This current analysis included of a total number of 7 studies (2 randomized and 5 observational studies) that assessed all the clinical endpoints with minimal evidence of publication bias which was visually observed through the funnel plots obtained (Figs. 9, 10, 11).

These funnel plots represented minimal publication bias. Possible reasons might be the presence of

Study or Subgroup	Fondaparinux Events	Fondaparinux Total	Enoxaparin Events	Enoxaparin Total	Weight	Odds Ratio M-H, Fixed, 95% CI
1.3.1 Mortality						
OASIS 5	19	1414	19	1420	11.8%	1.00 [0.53, 1.91]
Shah2014	0	90	0	90		Not estimable
Subtotal (95% CI)		**1504**		**1510**	**11.8%**	**1.00 [0.53, 1.91]**
Total events	19		19			
Heterogeneity: Not applicable						
Test for overall effect: Z = 0.01 (P = 0.99)						
1.3.4 All bleeding						
OASIS 5	62	1414	144	1420	86.4%	0.41 [0.30, 0.55]
Shah2014	1	90	3	90	1.9%	0.33 [0.03, 3.19]
Subtotal (95% CI)		**1504**		**1510**	**88.2%**	**0.40 [0.30, 0.55]**
Total events	63		147			
Heterogeneity: Chi² = 0.04, df = 1 (P = 0.85); I² = 0%						
Test for overall effect: Z = 5.82 (P < 0.00001)						

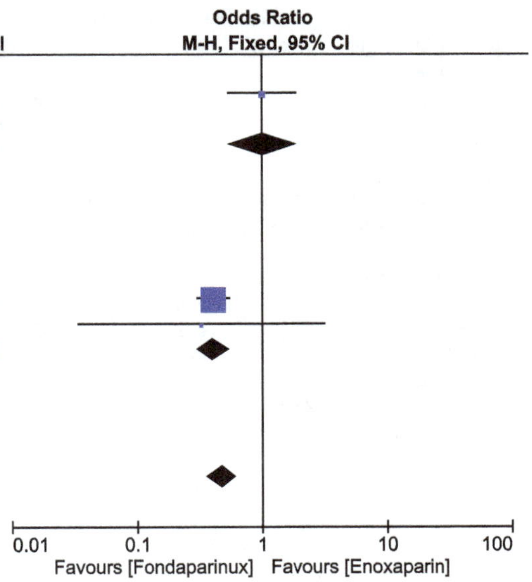

Fig. 4 Enoxaparin versus fondaparinux using only randomized patients (10-day follow up)

Study or Subgroup	Fondaparinux Events	Fondaparinux Total	Enoxaparin Events	Enoxaparin Total	Weight	Odds Ratio M-H, Fixed, 95% CI
1.1.1 Mortality						
OASIS 5	18	887	20	959	11.9%	0.97 [0.51, 1.85]
Schiele2010	10	301	51	1418	10.9%	0.92 [0.46, 1.84]
Shah2014	0	90	0	90		Not estimable
Zhao2015	2	229	4	232	2.5%	0.50 [0.09, 2.77]
Subtotal (95% CI)		**1507**		**2699**	**25.3%**	**0.90 [0.57, 1.42]**
Total events	30		75			
Heterogeneity: Chi² = 0.51, df = 2 (P = 0.78); I² = 0%						
Test for overall effect: Z = 0.44 (P = 0.66)						
1.1.2 Myocardial Infarction (MI)						
OASIS 5	51	887	53	957	30.4%	1.04 [0.70, 1.55]
Zhao2015	4	229	6	232	3.7%	0.67 [0.19, 2.40]
Subtotal (95% CI)		**1116**		**1189**	**34.1%**	**1.00 [0.69, 1.46]**
Total events	55		59			
Heterogeneity: Chi² = 0.42, df = 1 (P = 0.52); I² = 0%						
Test for overall effect: Z = 0.00 (P = 1.00)						
1.1.3 Major bleeding						
OASIS 5	11	376	18	341	11.6%	0.54 [0.25, 1.16]
Zhao2015	3	229	6	232	3.7%	0.50 [0.12, 2.02]
Zhao2016	1	422	4	453	2.4%	0.27 [0.03, 2.40]
Subtotal (95% CI)		**1027**		**1026**	**17.7%**	**0.49 [0.26, 0.94]**
Total events	15		28			
Heterogeneity: Chi² = 0.36, df = 2 (P = 0.84); I² = 0%						
Test for overall effect: Z = 2.16 (P = 0.03)						
1.1.4 Minor bleeding						
OASIS 5	6	376	15	341	9.8%	0.35 [0.14, 0.92]
Zhao2015	13	229	22	232	13.0%	0.57 [0.28, 1.17]
Subtotal (95% CI)		**605**		**573**	**22.8%**	**0.48 [0.27, 0.85]**
Total events	19		37			
Heterogeneity: Chi² = 0.64, df = 1 (P = 0.42); I² = 0%						
Test for overall effect: Z = 2.54 (P = 0.01)						

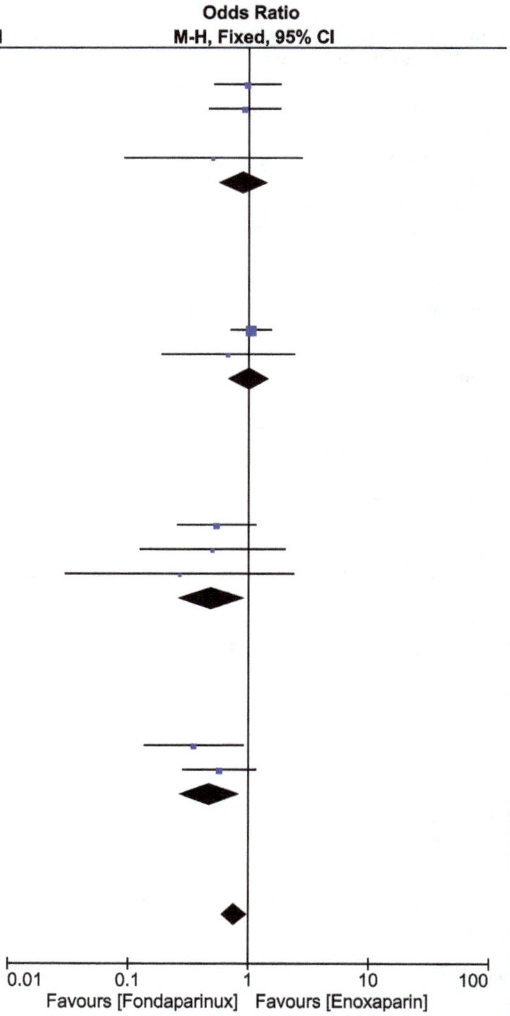

Fig. 5 Enoxaparin versus fondaparinux (30-day follow up)

Study or Subgroup	Fondaparinux Events	Fondaparinux Total	Enoxaparin Events	Enoxaparin Total	Weight	Odds Ratio M-H, Fixed, 95% CI
1.1.1 Mortality						
Schiele2010	10	301	51	1418	55.8%	0.92 [0.46, 1.84]
Zhao2015	2	229	4	232	12.7%	0.50 [0.09, 2.77]
Subtotal (95% CI)		**530**		**1650**	**68.5%**	**0.84 [0.44, 1.60]**
Total events	12		55			
Heterogeneity: Chi² = 0.42, df = 1 (P = 0.52); I² = 0%						
Test for overall effect: Z = 0.52 (P = 0.60)						
1.1.2 Major bleeding						
Zhao2015	3	229	6	232	19.0%	0.50 [0.12, 2.02]
Zhao2016	1	422	4	453	12.4%	0.27 [0.03, 2.40]
Subtotal (95% CI)		**651**		**685**	**31.5%**	**0.41 [0.13, 1.31]**
Total events	4		10			
Heterogeneity: Chi² = 0.23, df = 1 (P = 0.63); I² = 0%						
Test for overall effect: Z = 1.50 (P = 0.13)						

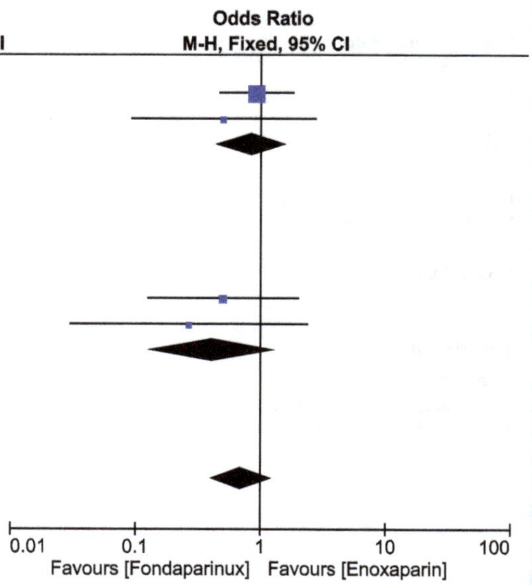

Fig. 6 Enoxaparin versus fondaparinux using data obtained only from observational studies (30-day follow up)

Study or Subgroup	Fondaparinux Events	Fondaparinux Total	Enoxaparin Events	Enoxaparin Total	Weight	Odds Ratio M-H, Fixed, 95% CI
1.2.1 Mortality						
OASIS 5	28	887	34	959	9.8%	0.89 [0.53, 1.47]
Zhao2015	4	229	5	232	1.5%	0.81 [0.21, 3.04]
Zhao2016	2	422	7	453	2.1%	0.30 [0.06, 1.47]
Subtotal (95% CI)		**1538**		**1644**	**13.4%**	**0.79 [0.50, 1.23]**
Total events	34		46			
Heterogeneity: Chi² = 1.62, df = 2 (P = 0.45); I² = 0%						
Test for overall effect: Z = 1.04 (P = 0.30)						
1.2.2 Myocardial Infarction						
OASIS 5	67	887	66	959	18.2%	1.11 [0.78, 1.57]
Zhao2015	7	229	9	232	2.7%	0.78 [0.29, 2.13]
Zhao2016	16	422	17	453	4.9%	1.01 [0.50, 2.03]
Subtotal (95% CI)		**1538**		**1644**	**25.8%**	**1.05 [0.78, 1.42]**
Total events	90		92			
Heterogeneity: Chi² = 0.43, df = 2 (P = 0.81); I² = 0%						
Test for overall effect: Z = 0.34 (P = 0.73)						
1.2.3 Stroke						
OASIS 5	7	887	12	959	3.6%	0.63 [0.25, 1.60]
Zhao2015	1	229	1	232	0.3%	1.01 [0.06, 16.30]
Zhao2016	7	422	9	453	2.7%	0.83 [0.31, 2.25]
Subtotal (95% CI)		**1538**		**1644**	**6.5%**	**0.73 [0.38, 1.41]**
Total events	15		22			
Heterogeneity: Chi² = 0.22, df = 2 (P = 0.90); I² = 0%						
Test for overall effect: Z = 0.94 (P = 0.35)						
1.2.4 Major bleeding						
OASIS 5	13	376	21	341	6.6%	0.55 [0.27, 1.11]
Zhao2015	5	229	9	232	2.7%	0.55 [0.18, 1.68]
Zhao2016	1	422	5	453	1.5%	0.21 [0.02, 1.83]
Subtotal (95% CI)		**1027**		**1026**	**10.8%**	**0.50 [0.28, 0.89]**
Total events	19		35			
Heterogeneity: Chi² = 0.69, df = 2 (P = 0.71); I² = 0%						
Test for overall effect: Z = 2.37 (P = 0.02)						
1.2.5 All bleeding						
OASIS 5	19	376	36	341	11.1%	0.45 [0.25, 0.80]
Zhao2015	24	229	40	232	11.1%	0.56 [0.33, 0.97]
Zhao2016	10	422	25	453	7.3%	0.42 [0.20, 0.88]
Subtotal (95% CI)		**1027**		**1026**	**29.5%**	**0.48 [0.34, 0.69]**
Total events	53		101			
Heterogeneity: Chi² = 0.51, df = 2 (P = 0.78); I² = 0%						
Test for overall effect: Z = 4.08 (P < 0.0001)						
1.2.6 Minor bleeding						
OASIS 5	7	376	16	341	5.1%	0.39 [0.16, 0.95]
Zhao2015	19	229	31	232	8.8%	0.59 [0.32, 1.07]
Subtotal (95% CI)		**605**		**573**	**13.9%**	**0.51 [0.31, 0.84]**
Total events	26		47			
Heterogeneity: Chi² = 0.58, df = 1 (P = 0.45); I² = 0%						
Test for overall effect: Z = 2.63 (P = 0.009)						

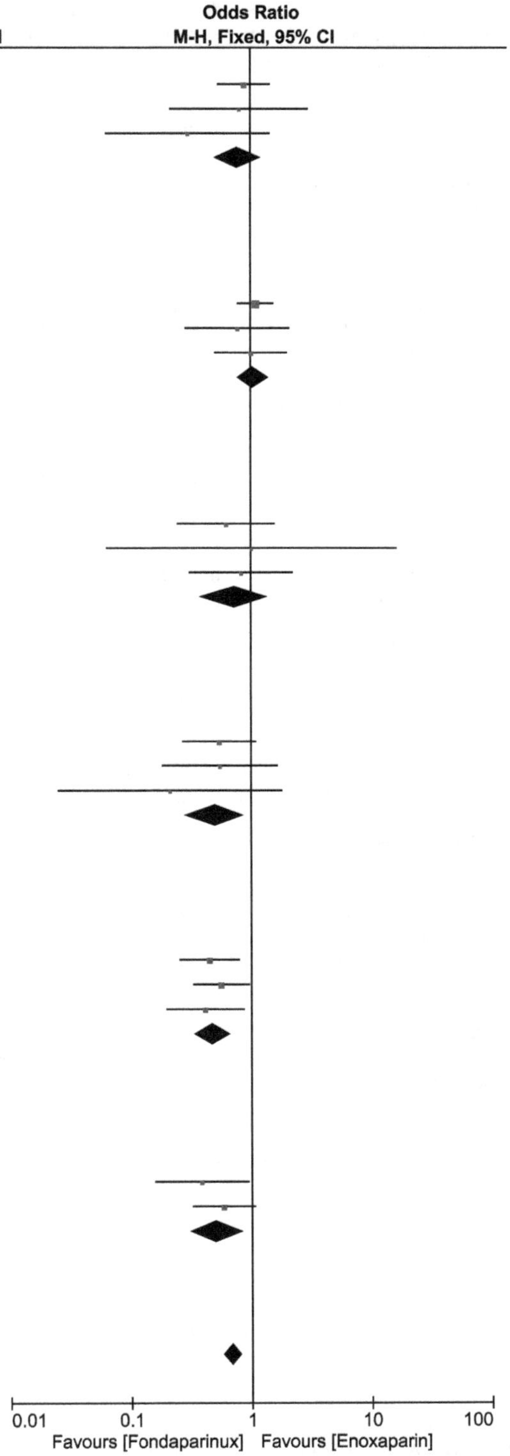

Fig. 7 Enoxaparin versus fondaparinux (mid-term follow up)

observational studies, and the selection of only English publications for this analysis.

Discussion

This analysis aimed to compare enoxaparin with fondaparinux. Current results showed both anticoagulants to have similar mortality and stroke rates. However, fondaparinux was associated with a significantly lower major and minor bleeding when compared to enoxaparin in majority of the bleeding subgroups which were analyzed.

Surprisingly, even if the use of glycoprotein IIb/IIIa was more in patients who used fondaparinux, a low

Study or Subgroup	Fondaparinux Events	Fondaparinux Total	Enoxaparin Events	Enoxaparin Total	Weight	Odds Ratio M-H, Fixed, 95% CI
1.2.1 Mortality						
Zhao2015	4	229	5	232	3.3%	0.81 [0.21, 3.04]
Zhao2016	2	422	7	453	4.6%	0.30 [0.06, 1.47]
Subtotal (95% CI)		**651**		**685**	**7.9%**	**0.52 [0.19, 1.39]**
Total events	6		12			
Heterogeneity: Chi² = 0.87, df = 1 (P = 0.35); I² = 0%						
Test for overall effect: Z = 1.31 (P = 0.19)						
1.2.2 Myocardial Infarction						
Zhao2015	7	229	9	232	5.9%	0.78 [0.29, 2.13]
Zhao2016	16	422	17	453	10.8%	1.01 [0.50, 2.03]
Subtotal (95% CI)		**651**		**685**	**16.7%**	**0.93 [0.52, 1.65]**
Total events	23		26			
Heterogeneity: Chi² = 0.17, df = 1 (P = 0.68); I² = 0%						
Test for overall effect: Z = 0.25 (P = 0.80)						
1.2.3 Stroke						
Zhao2015	1	229	1	232	0.7%	1.01 [0.06, 16.30]
Zhao2016	7	422	9	453	5.8%	0.83 [0.31, 2.25]
Subtotal (95% CI)		**651**		**685**	**6.5%**	**0.85 [0.33, 2.17]**
Total events	8		10			
Heterogeneity: Chi² = 0.02, df = 1 (P = 0.90); I² = 0%						
Test for overall effect: Z = 0.34 (P = 0.74)						
1.2.4 Major bleeding						
Zhao2015	5	229	9	232	6.0%	0.55 [0.18, 1.68]
Zhao2016	1	422	5	453	3.3%	0.21 [0.02, 1.83]
Subtotal (95% CI)		**651**		**685**	**9.3%**	**0.43 [0.16, 1.14]**
Total events	6		14			
Heterogeneity: Chi² = 0.61, df = 1 (P = 0.44); I² = 0%						
Test for overall effect: Z = 1.70 (P = 0.09)						
1.2.5 All bleeding						
Zhao2015	24	229	40	232	24.3%	0.56 [0.33, 0.97]
Zhao2016	10	422	25	453	16.1%	0.42 [0.20, 0.88]
Subtotal (95% CI)		**651**		**685**	**40.4%**	**0.50 [0.33, 0.78]**
Total events	34		65			
Heterogeneity: Chi² = 0.41, df = 1 (P = 0.52); I² = 0%						
Test for overall effect: Z = 3.07 (P = 0.002)						
1.2.6 Minor bleeding						
Zhao2015	19	229	31	232	19.3%	0.59 [0.32, 1.07]
Subtotal (95% CI)		**229**		**232**	**19.3%**	**0.59 [0.32, 1.07]**
Total events	19		31			
Heterogeneity: Not applicable						
Test for overall effect: Z = 1.73 (P = 0.08)						

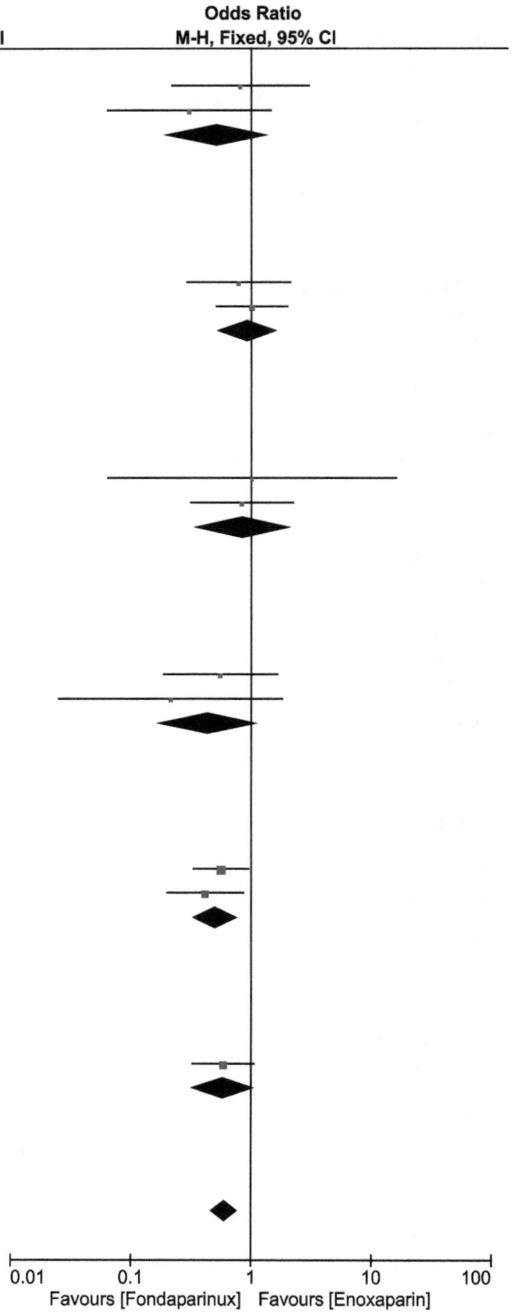

Fig. 8 Enoxaparin versus fondaparinux using data obtained only from observational studies (mid-term follow up)

bleeding was observed with this anticoagulant when compared to enoxaparin.

At this stage, it would be interesting to know the mechanisms of action of fondaparinux and enoxaparin. Fondaparinux is a factor Xa inhibitor and does not inhibit thrombin (IIa) [8]. Enoxaparin on the other hand, binds to antithrombin to form a complex molecule that can irreversibly inactivate clotting factor Xa and it has less activity against thrombin [9]. This is how these two anticoagulants work.

The Brazilian Registry Data which was a multicentered retrospective observational study including 2282 patients also supported the result of this current analysis which is similar to recently published data in international literature showing the superiority of fondaparinux to enoxaparin in the Brazilian population in terms of bleeding outcomes following PCI (40.1% of the patients in the fondaparinux group and 35.1% of patients in the enoxaparin group underwent PCI) [10].

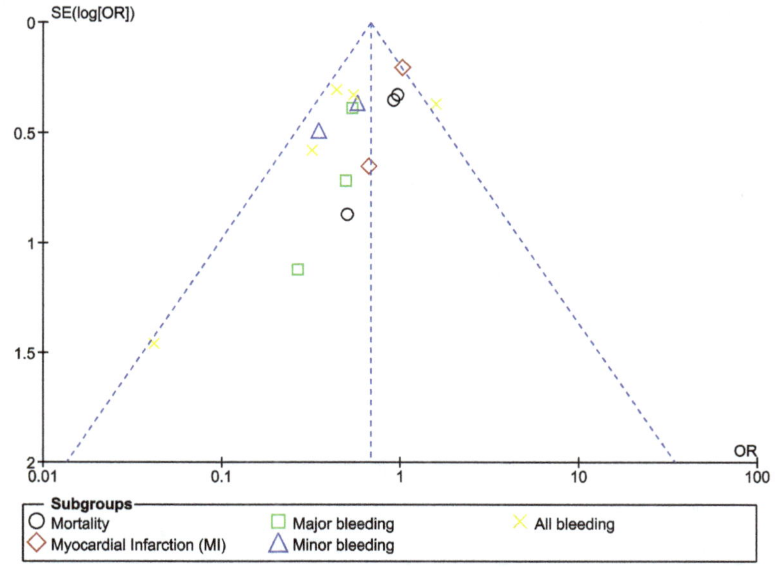

Fig. 9 Funnel plot representing publication bias

Similarly, the OASIS 5 trial which was a double blinded randomized trial comparing fondaparinux with enoxaparin in 6238 patients who underwent PCI showed reduced bleeding events to be associated with fondaparinux without any increase in mortality [2].

On the other hand, the OASIS 6 trial (12,092 patients obtained from 447 hospitals in 41 countries around the globe) which compared fondaparinux with placebo or unfractionated heparin in patients with STEMI showed that in patients who were not undergoing PCI, the former was associated with a lower mortality and re-infarction without increasing stroke or bleeding events [11]. However, our analysis showed no significant difference in mortality or stroke, but with significantly lower bleeding events following invasive procedures when fondaparinux was compared to enoxaparin. Could it be the invasive procedure which contributed to these different results obtained from OASIS 5 and 6?

To provide an answer to this question, a small Chinese study with NSTEMI patients who underwent PCI, showed no statistically significant difference in bleeding outcomes between fondaparinux and enoxaparin. However, it should not be ignored that both groups were also additionally treated with tirofiban [12] and the total

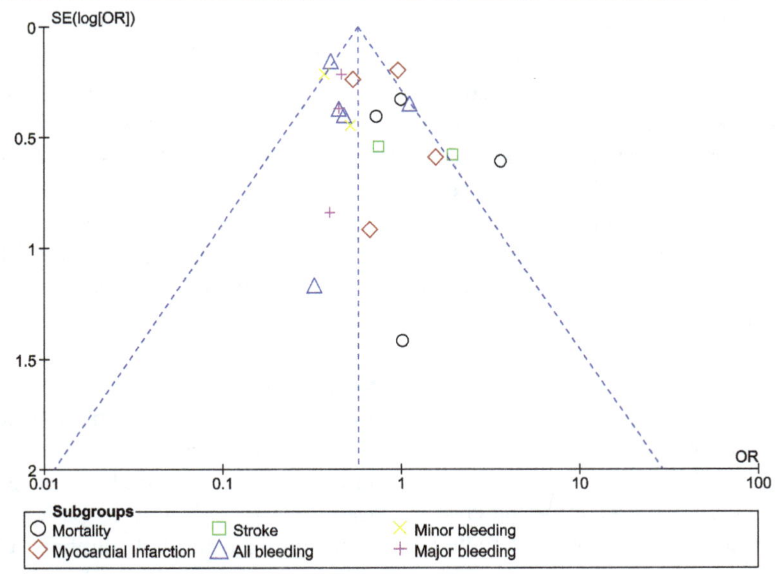

Fig. 10 Funnel plot representing publication bias

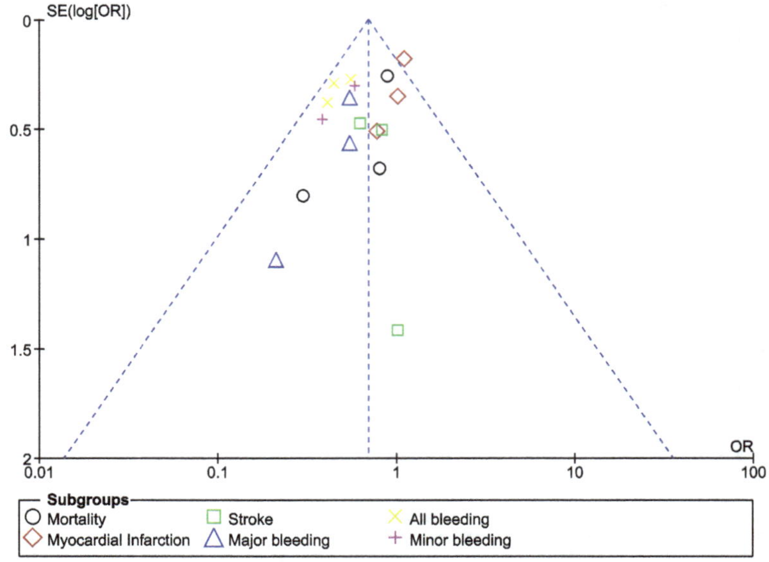

Fig. 11 Funnel plot representing publication bias

number of patients enrolled was less when compared to the OASIS 5 and 6.

Moreover, the French cohort of NSTEMI patients who were predominantly managed invasively did not show fondaparinux to be superior to enoxaparin in terms of bleeding outcomes [3]. However, similar to the results of this analysis, mortality was not significantly different between these two anticoagulants. Nevertheless, it was shown that during the propensity score matched cohorts, a lower number of patients used aspirin or clopidogrel before admission.

Finally, the fact that several factors such as comorbidities, age, use of anti-platelets and anticoagulants, as well as the dosage and whether these blood thinning agents were used before and after admission and the effect of plaque should all be taken into consideration when assessing bleeding risk and other adverse clinical outcomes in such patients. For example, a recent meta-analysis showed thin-cap fibro-atheroma to be highly associated with culprit plaque rupture [13]. This prevalence was higher in patients with STEMI compared to patients with NSTEMI or unstable angina. Therefore, clinical outcomes might vary from study to study due to the influence of such factors.

Novelty

This analysis is new in several ways:

- It is among the first meta-analyses comparing enoxaparin with fondaparinux in patients who were being treated for ACS.
- This interesting idea is very important clinically.
- A low to moderate level of heterogeneity was observed in several of the subgroups analyzing the outcomes, which might be a positive aspect of this analysis.
- Randomized patients and patients obtained from observational studies were combined as well as separately analyzed.

Limitations

Limitations were as follow:

- Due to the limited number of patients analyzed, the results might not be very accurate.
- This analysis concerned mainly patients suffering from NSTEMI.
- Classification of bleeding events was vast. Bleeding should be classified as TIMI defined bleeding, BARC defined bleeding and ACUITY defined bleeding and then analyzed.
- Use of other anti-platelets and anticoagulants and other factors might have influenced the results which were obtained.

Conclusion

In patients who were treated for ACS, fondaparinux might be a better choice when compared to enoxaparin in terms of short to midterm bleeding events. This result was mainly applicable to patients with NSTEMI. However, due to a limited number of patients analyzed, further larger randomized trials should be able to confirm this hypothesis.

Abbreviations
ACS: acute coronary syndrome; RCTs: randomized controlled trials; PCI: percutaneous coronary intervention

Acknowledgement
Not applicable.

Funding
There was no external source of funding for this research.

Authors' contributions
PKB, MS and JY were responsible for the conception and design, acquisition of data, analysis and interpretation of data, drafting the initial manuscript and revising it critically for important intellectual content. PKB wrote this manuscript. All authors read and approved the final manuscript.

Competing interests
The authors declare that they have no competing interests.

Author details
[1] Institute of Cardiovascular Diseases, the First Affiliated Hospital of Guangxi Medical University, Nanning, Guangxi 530027, People's Republic of China. [2] Department of Paediatrics, Pragati Children's Hospital, Ch Pet, Andhra Pradesh, India. [3] Department of Cardiology, The People's Hospital of Guangxi Zhuang Autonomous Region, Nanning, Guangxi 530021, China.

References
1. Weber K, Spirk D, Pieper M, Kucher N. Clinical efficacy and safety of enoxaparin in unselected Swiss patients undergoing primary or elective percutaneous coronary intervention: analysis of the RIVIERA study. Acta Cardiol. 2009;64(4):455–9.
2. Mehta SR, Granger CB, Eikelboom JW, Bassand JP, Wallentin L, Faxon DP, Peters RJ, Budaj A, Afzal R, Chrolavicius S, Fox KA, Yusuf S. Efficacy and safety of fondaparinux versus enoxaparin in patients with acute coronary syndromes undergoing percutaneous coronary intervention: results from the OASIS-5 trial. J Am Coll Cardiol. 2007;50(18):1742–51.
3. Puymirat E, Schiele F, Ennezat PV, Coste P, Collet JP, Bonnefoy-Cudraz E, Roul G, Richard P, Simon T, Danchin N. Impact of fondaparinux versus enoxaparin on in-hospital bleeding and 1-year death in non-ST-segmentelevation myocardial infarction. FAST-MI (French Registry of acute ST-elevation and non-ST-elevation myocardial infarction) 2010. Eur Heart J Acute Cardiovasc Care. 2015;4(3):211–9.
4. The Thrombolysis in Myocardial Infarction (TIMI) trial. Phase I findings. TIMI Study Group. N Engl J Med. 1985. 4;312(14):932–6.
5. Liberati A, Altman DG, Tetzlaff J, et al. The PRISMA statement for reporting systematic reviews and meta-analyses of studies that evaluate healthcareinterventions: explanation and elaboration. BMJ. 2009;339:b2700.
6. Higgins JP, Thompson SG, Deeks JJ, et al. Measuring inconsistency in meta-analyses. BMJ. 2003;327:557–60.
7. Higgins JPT, Thompson SG, Deeks JJ, Altman DG. Measuring inconsistency in meta-analyses. BMJ. 2003;327(7414):557–60.
8. Bauer KA. Fondaparinux sodium: a selective inhibitor of factor Xa. Am J Health Syst Pharm. 2001;58(Suppl 2):S14–7.
9. Yau JW, Stafford AR, Liao P, Fredenburgh JC, Roberts R, Weitz JI. Mechanism of catheter thrombosis: comparison of the antithrombotic activities of fondaparinux, enoxaparin, and heparin in vitro and in vivo. Blood. 2011; 118(25):6667–74.
10. Soeiro AM, Silva PG, Roque EA, Bossa AS, César MC, Simões SA, Okada MY, Leal TC, Pedroti FC, Oliveira MT Jr. Fondaparinux versus Enoxaparin - Which is the Best Anticoagulant for Acute Coronary Syndrome? - Brazilian Registry Data. Arq Bras Cardiol. 2016;107(3):239–244.
11. Yusuf S, Mehta SR, Chrolavicius S, Afzal R, Pogue J, Granger CB, Budaj A, Peters RJ, Bassand JP, Wallentin L, Joyner C, Fox KA, OASIS-6 Trial Group. Effects of fondaparinux on mortality and reinfarction in patients with acute ST-segment elevation myocardial infarction: the OASIS-6 randomized trial. JAMA. 2006;295(13):1519–30.
12. Zhao XM, Gao CY, Chu YJ, Yang L, Yang XZ, Xu WK, He WQ, Zhang PR, Liu XY, Tian LX. Fondaparinux vs. enoxaparin in patients with non-ST elevation acute coronary syndromes (NSTE-ACS) treated with percutaneous coronary intervention and tirofiban: an exploratory study in China. J Clin Pharm Ther. 2015.
13. Iannaccone M, Quadri G, Taha S, et al. Prevalence and predictors of culprit plaque rupture at OCT in patients with coronary artery disease: a meta-analysis. Eur Heart J Cardiovasc Imaging. 2016;17(10):1128–37.
14. Schiele F, Meneveau N, Seronde MF, Descotes-Genon V, Dutheil J, Chopard R, Ecarnot F, Bassand JP, Reseau de Cardiologie de Franche Comte. Routine use of fondaparinux in acute coronary syndromes: a 2-year multicenter experience. Am Heart J. 2010;159(2):190–8.
15. Shah S, Khajuria V, Tandon VR, Gillani ZH, Lal M. Comparative evaluation of efficacy, safety and haemostatic parameters of enoxaparin and fondaparinuxin unstable coronary artery disease. J Clin Diagn Res. 2014;8(1):31–4.
16. Zhao X, Yang XX, Ji SZ, Wang XZ, Wang L, Gu CH, Ren LL, Han YL. Efficacy and safety of fondaparinux versus enoxaparin in patients undergoing percutaneous coronaryintervention treated with the glycoprotein IIb/IIIa inhibitor tirofiban. Mil Med Res. 2016;3:13.

The cost-utility of point-of-care troponin testing to diagnose acute coronary syndrome in primary care

Michelle M. A. Kip[1*], Hendrik Koffijberg[1], Marco J. Moesker[1], Maarten J. IJzerman[1] and Ron Kusters[1,2]

Abstract

Background: The added value of using a point-of-care (POC) troponin test in primary care to rule out acute coronary syndrome (ACS) is debated because test sensitivity is inadequate early after symptom onset. This study investigates the potential cost-utility of diagnosing ACS by a general practitioner (GP) when a POC troponin test is available versus GP assessment only.

Methods: A patient-level simulation model was developed, representing a hypothetical cohort of the Dutch population (>35 years) consulting the GP with chest complaints. All health related consequences as well as cost consequences were included. Both symptom duration, selection of patients in whom the POC troponin test is performed, and test performance at different time points were incorporated. Health outcomes were expressed as Quality-Adjusted Life Years (QALYs). The main outcome parameters involve the effect of POC troponin testing on (in)correct hospital referrals, QALYs, and costs.

Results: The POC troponin strategy decreases the referral rate in non-ACS patients from 38.46% to 31.85%. Despite a small increase in non-referral among ACS patients from 0.22% to 0.27%, the overall health effect is negligible. Costs will decrease with €77.25/patient (95% CI €-126.81 to €-33.37).

Conclusions: The POC troponin strategy is likely cost-saving, by reducing hospital referrals. The small increase in missed ACS patients can be partly explained by conservative assumptions used in the analysis. Besides, current developments in POC troponin tests will likely further improve their diagnostic performance. Therefore, future prospective studies are warranted to investigate whether those developments make the POC troponin test to a safe and cost-effective diagnostic tool for diagnosing ACS in general practices.

Keywords: Cost-utility, Early health technology assessment, Point-of-care testing, Acute coronary syndrome

Background

Each year almost 200,000 patients in the Netherlands contact their general practitioner (GP) with chest pain [1]. Chest pain is a leading symptom of acute coronary syndrome (ACS), which encompasses both unstable angina pectoris (UAP) and acute myocardial infarction (AMI) [2]. Among AMI patients, two subgroups can be distinguished based on a deviation on the electrocardiogram (ECG), which are ST elevation myocardial infarction (STEMI) and non-ST elevation myocardial infarction (NSTEMI) [2]. However, only approximately 18% of all patients who present with chest pain to the hospital are eventually diagnosed with ACS [3]. Clinical management is a major challenge for GPs, because unnecessary referrals lead to unnecessary costs and patient distress. So, given the potentially life-threatening consequences, accurate and rapid diagnosis of ACS remains crucial.

Besides a patient's signs, symptoms, medical history, and the information obtained from the ECG, imaging modalities (for example coronary angiography), and laboratory biomarkers of myocardial necrosis (mainly involving high-sensitive troponin), provide additional diagnostic value [2]. As those diagnostic tools are often not readily available in primary care, current clinical guidelines recommend

* Correspondence: m.m.a.kip@utwente.nl
[1]Department of Health Technology and Services Research, MIRA institute for Biomedical Technology and Technical Medicine, University of Twente, Enschede, the Netherlands
Full list of author information is available at the end of the article

immediate hospital referral when ACS is suspected [4]. However, the introduction of point-of-care (POC) troponin tests, accompanied by a shorter turn-around-time, offers a low-cost diagnostic test for GPs. Although costs per tests are mostly higher for POC tests as compared to regular laboratory tests [5], the use of POC troponin as a diagnostic aid to rule out ACS might improve referral decisions and hence lead to overall cost savings [6]. This advantage needs however to be weighed against the lower sensitivity of this test especially in the early hours after symptom onset [2, 6–8]. Consequently, international guidelines do not give a recommendation on the use of POC troponin [2], while its use is discouraged in Dutch guidelines [9].

In addition to collecting clinical evidence, proper evaluation of the cost-utility of POC troponin testing in primary care is required. Although randomized controlled trials (RCTs) would provide the best source of evidence, these are commonly very expensive, time consuming, and often do not allow assessment of long-term outcomes or risks [10, 11]. Therefore, an early stage health economic model may provide a valid alternative to quantify the effect of POC troponin testing on costs, and on short and long term outcomes. In this paper, we present such model-based health economic analysis of the use of POC troponin testing to diagnose ACS in primary care, as compared to current practice.

Methods

Structure of the model

We developed a patient-level simulation model to reflect the diagnostic pathway of chest pain patients presenting to the GP (Fig. 1). This model was used to analyse the cost-utility of a POC troponin test to exclude ACS in addition to GP examination, as compared to GP examination without the test. As test and treatment decisions in this model are based (partially) on patient's characteristics and patient's history (including duration of symptoms, previous test outcomes, and previous management decisions) adequately reflecting the diagnostic pathway of patients requires simulating individual patients. Whereas such decisions are simulated for entire groups in a cohort (state-transition) model, they can be simulated on individual patient level when using a patient-level simulation model. The primary outcome measure was the incremental costs per quality-adjusted life year (QALY) gained for the POC strategy as compared to current practice. Secondary outcome measures were the percentage of chest pain patients that were either correctly or incorrectly referred to the hospital or sent home (expressed as true positives [TPs], true negatives [TNs], false positives [FPs], and false negatives [FNs]). Other secondary outcome measures included mortality and heart failure rates in both strategies. All costs and effects were evaluated from a societal point of view, over a lifelong time horizon.

Current evidence

The model was populated using data from literature. The following paragraphs present a summary of evidence used, for further details see Additional file 1. An overview of the assumptions used is provided in Additional file 2.

Patient pathways

In this patient-level model, each hypothetical patient was assigned an age, gender, and disease state (i.e. ACS or no ACS) based on the population distribution derived from a cross-sectional diagnostic study [12, 13]. For ACS patients in primary care, the probabilities of having either UAP, NSTEMI or STEMI were based on a prospective study [14].

Of all chest pain patients presenting to the GP, 14.7% was immediately referred to the hospital without diagnostic testing, because of a high perceived probability of ACS by the GP (Table 1) [15]. All patients that were referred to the hospital were assumed to be transported by ambulance. Among the patients that were not immediately referred, all GPs who had an ECG in their practice (45%) [16], were assumed to use it in those patients. In case the patient had a STEMI, there was a 50% probability that this was diagnosed in case an ECG was performed [17]. Those patients were also immediately referred to the hospital. In current practice, the GP decides on referral of the remaining patients without POC troponin. The sensitivity and specificity of this decision (i.e. 88.3% and 72.2%, respectively) were derived from Nilsson et al. [18]. For the POC strategy, the time from symptom onset to presentation was estimated for each patient separately [19], and then categorized according to time since symptom onset as a) <4.0 h, b) 4.0–5.5 h, c) 5.5–7.0 h, d) 7.0–10.0 h, and e) >10.0 h. As it is known that the performance of the POC troponin test is less in patients presenting shortly after symptom onset [7], it was assumed that this test was not performed in patients presenting with <4.0 h symptoms [7, 19]. In those patients, the referral decision was based on the judgment of the GP as in current practice [18]. In the remaining patients, it was assumed that the POC troponin test was performed, and the sensitivity and specificity for time categories b), c), d) and e) were derived from Diercks et al. [7]. In case the result of the POC troponin test did not correspond with what would have been the (initial) referral decision of the GP in current practice (i.e. without POC troponin), a probability of the GP revising the initial referral decision was incorporated in the model [15]. In both strategies, all patients who were not immediately referred to the hospital were assumed to be sent home without receiving medical care.

Mortality and heart failure rates were dependent on whether patients had ACS, and if present, whether ACS was correctly diagnosed. In addition, as the POC troponin test was assumed to delay time to treatment with 10 min, using this test would increase the mortality rate in AMI patients

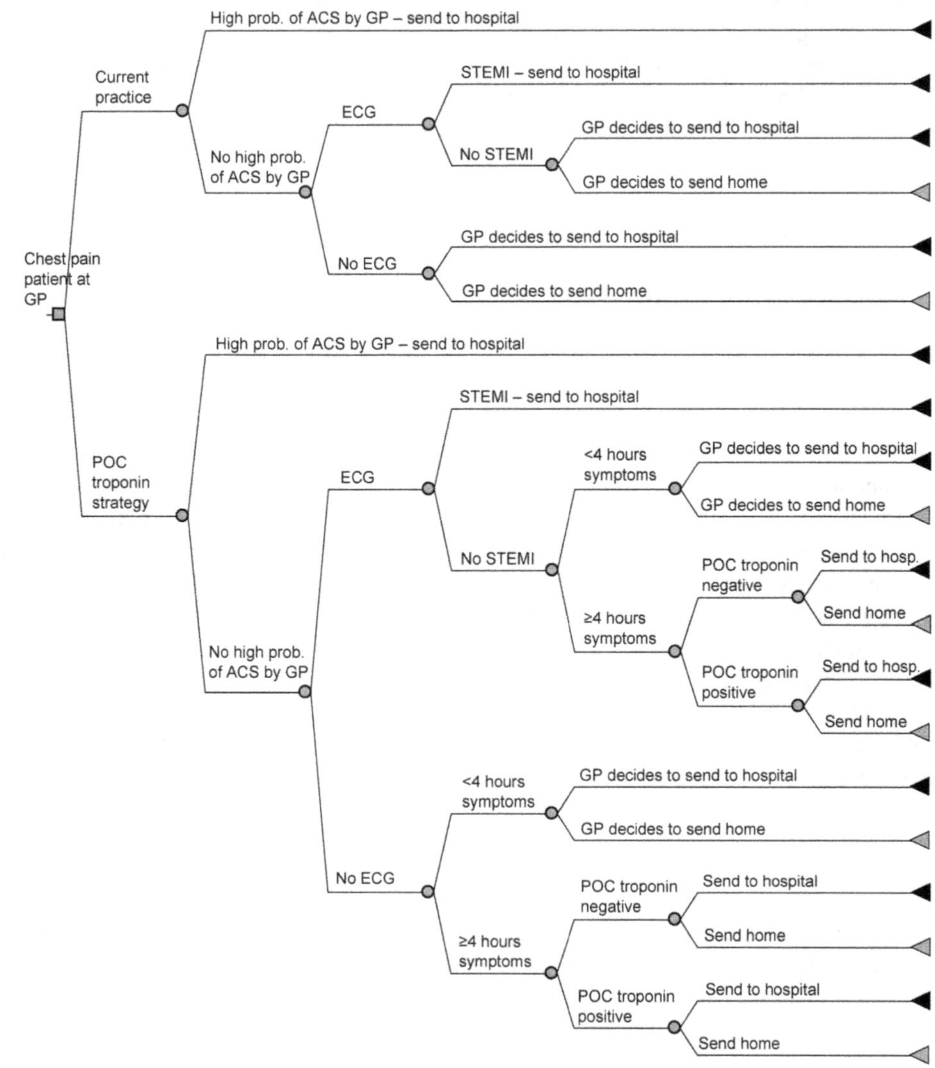

Fig. 1 structure of the decision tree. Black triangles represent braches in which patients are referred to the ED (because of suspected ACS), while grey triangles represent branches in which patients are send home. ACS = acute coronary syndrome, ECG = electrocardiogram, GP = general practitioner, hosp. = hospital, POC = point-of-care, prob. = probability, STEMI = ST elevation myocardial infarction

with 0.2% [20]. This 10 min duration of the POC troponin test was chosen as previous research has shown that GPs consider this the maximum acceptable duration of the POC troponin test [15]. Productivity losses incorporated lost working time due to GP visits, emergency department visits, and due to UAP, STEMI, NSTEMI, heart failure, and mortality [21–23].

Quality of life

The quality-adjusted life expectancy (QALE, based on combining expected quality of life with life expectancy) were obtained directly from a systematic review and economic model for STEMI, NSTEMI and UAP patients as well as for healthy patients [24–26]. Separate QALE estimates were used for categories of age and gender [24–26]. A missed diagnosis of ACS indirectly lowered quality of life by increasing the risk of heart failure and mortality. For heart failure patients, the QALEs were estimated by multiplying the reported utility of heart failure patients with their reported average life expectancy [27, 28].

Costs

Costs of both a GP consultation and ambulance transportation to the emergency department were derived from the Dutch cost manual [23], whereas costs of performing an ECG were derived from the Dutch Healthcare Authority [29]. As no tariff currently exists for the POC troponin test, and because a troponin test performed in a regular laboratory costs approximately €8 [29], the costs of a POC troponin test were conservatively estimated at €15. Average diagnosis and treatment costs per (suspected) ACS patient were derived from the Dutch Healthcare

Table 1 input parameters concerning patient pathways used in the model

Parameter	Category	Probability	95% CI	Distribution	Reference
Perceived probability of ACS by GP	High probability	14.7%	8.2% to 22.5%	Beta	[15]
ECG	Performed at GP's office	57.4%	56.0% to 58.7%	Beta	[16]
	Sensitivity for STEMI	50.0%	37.6% to 62.6%	Beta	[17]
Time from symptom onset to presentation (male)	< 4 h	47.5%	38.9% to 55.4%	Dirichlet	[19, 40]
	4–5.5 h	9.0%	5.2% to 14.5%	Dirichlet	[19, 40]
	5.5–7 h	7.3%	3.4% to 11.8%	Dirichlet	[19, 40]
	7–10 h	9.4%	5.2% to 14.9%	Dirichlet	[19, 40]
	> 10 h	26.8%	20.0% to 34.6%	Dirichlet	[19, 40]
Time from symptom onset to presentation (female)	< 4 h	54.8%	47.1% to 62.7%	Dirichlet	[19, 40]
	4–5.5 h	9.4%	5.1% to 13.9%	Dirichlet	[19, 40]
	5.5–7 h	6.5%	3.1% to 10.7%	Dirichlet	[19, 40]
	7–10 h	8.0%	4.6% to 13.1%	Dirichlet	[19, 40]
	> 10 h	21.2%	15.2% to 27.8%	Dirichlet	[19, 40]
Diagnostic performance of GP, without POC troponin	Sensitivity	88.3%	79.2% to 95.2%	Beta	[18]
	Specificity	72.2%	67.9% to 76.3%	Beta	[18]
Sensitivity of POC troponin at different duration of symptoms	4–5.5 h	66.7%	55.5% to 77.0%	Beta	[7]
	5.5–7 h	79.2%	69.3% to 87.5%	Beta	[7]
	7–10 h	84.7%	75.3% to 91.9%	Beta	[7]
	> 10 h	87.5%	78.8% to 94.2%	Beta	[7]
Specificity of POC troponin at different duration of symptoms	4–5.5 h	95.9%	94.2% to 97.3%	Beta	[7]
	5.5–7 h	94.4%	92.5% to 96.1%	Beta	[7]
	7–10 h	93.4%	91.3% to 95.3%	Beta	[7]
	> 10 h	92.6%	90.4% to 94.5%	Beta	[7]
Revise referral decision after discordant POC troponin	Negative troponin	80.6%	73.3% to 87.1%	Beta	[15]
	Positive troponin	83.3%	76.3% to 89.3%	Beta	[15]

This table shows the parameter, the value used in the model, the 95% confidence interval, the distribution used, and the data source. *ACS* acute coronary syndrome, *CI* confidence interval, *ECG* electrocardiogram, *GP* general practitioner, *POC* point-of-care, *STEMI* ST elevation myocardial infarction

Authority [3]. Healthcare costs for the remaining lifetime of STEMI, NSTEMI, and UAP patients were derived from Goodacre et al. [24–26]. Lifetime healthcare costs per patient with heart failure were based on Dutch data concerning the point prevalence of heart failure [30], the annual healthcare costs of those patients [31], and combined with the average remaining life expectancy [27]. All costs were converted to 2015 using the consumer price indices as reported by the Dutch Central Bureau of Statistics, and converted to Euros if necessary (exchange rate 1.271 GBP = €1.000, 31 March 2016) [32, 33]. All costs and effects were discounted at an annual rate of 4.0% and 1.5%, respectively, in accordance with Dutch costing guidelines [23]. An overview of all cost parameters, including costs of productivity losses, is shown in Additional file 1.

Probabilistic sensitivity analysis

A probabilistic sensitivity analysis was performed by means of Monte Carlo simulations, using 10,000 iterations of 20,000 hypothetical, unique patients. Distributions were assigned to all parameters under investigation [34]. An overview of the distributions and the 95% CI for each parameter is provided in Table 1, and Additional file 1.

Expected value of perfect information (EVPI) analysis

To determine the value of collecting additional information on this topic, and potentially enhance decision-making on the usefulness of POC troponin in primary care a value of information analysis was performed. The EVPI was calculated to estimate the expected costs of uncertainty in the current model, using a value of information tool developed by the University of Sheffield [35].

Cost-effectiveness acceptability curve (CEAC)

To evaluate the probability that the POC troponin strategy is cost-effective, a CEAC was constructed for a willingness-to-pay (WTP) threshold ranging from €0/QALY to €100,000/QALY. A separate CEAC was constructed under the assumption that use of the POC troponin test is only acceptable when it does not lead to health loss (i.e. does not increase the rate of missed ACS patients) and has acceptable cost-effectiveness.

Results

Probabilistic sensitivity analysis

The results indicate that the POC troponin strategy costs on average €1144 (95% CI €892 to €1451) per patient, as compared to €1221 (95% CI €955 to €1541) for current practice. The cost savings for the testing strategy are €77 [95% CI €-127 to €-33] per patient. The probability that patients were correctly not referred to the hospital (TNs) would increase from 57.90% to 64.51% (+6.61%). Consequently, unnecessary referrals (FPs) decreased with 6.61% (i.e. from 38.46% to 31.85%). However, the probability of patients being correctly referred to the hospital (TPs) showed a very small decrease from 3.42% to 3.37% (i.e. -0.05%), which in turn resulted in an increase of patients incorrectly not referred (FNs) from 0.22% to 0.27% (i.e. 54 vs. 45 per 20,000 simulated patients). In turn, this results in a very small increase in the probability of patients dying of ACS (i.e. 61 vs. 60 per 20,000 patients), as well as a small increase in the incidence of heart failure (i.e. 121 vs. 119 per 20,000 patients). The overall change in QALYs from POC troponin use is negligible (−0.0004 when rounded to 4 decimals, i.e. 3.5 h in full health).

Given the negligible impact on health outcomes, it is not useful to calculate an incremental cost utility ratio (ICUR), as this outcome is very unstable for tiny differences in health outcomes as estimated in this study. When combining differences in health outcomes with differences in costs, an incremental net monetary benefit of €69 was found. In the POC strategy, the POC troponin test was used in approximately 40% of all chest pain patients presenting to their GP. This strategy could result in annual cost savings in the Netherlands of approximately €14 million [1]. A detailed overview of all model outcomes, including the 95% CI, is shown in Table 2, and the incremental cost-effectiveness plane is shown in Fig. 2. In Table 2, the costs are divided in four categories: primary care costs involves the costs from presentation at the GP including potential hospital referral by ambulance. Hospital costs involves the costs from hospital admission until discharge. Lifetime costs involves the costs of follow-up after STEMI. Also, the effect on (correct) referral decisions, as well as the effect on the probability of heart failure and mortality is shown.

More specifically, the average cost savings of €77.25 per patient are mainly attributable to a decreased referral rate, resulting in a reduction in costs in primary care with €28.41 per patient (as caused by a decrease in hospital

Table 2 Outcomes of Monte Carlo simulations

Parameter	Without POC troponin (95% CI)	With POC troponin (95% CI)	Absolute effect (POC vs. non-POC) (95% CI)	Relative effect (POC vs. non-POC) (95% CI)
Primary care costs per patient	€290.52 (€188.99 to €421.09)	€262.10 (€173.63 to €375.33)	€-28.41 (€-50.38 to €-12.23)	−9.78% (−13.36% to −5.75%)
Hospital costs per patient	€446.00 (€307.80 to €620.41)	€398.38 (€277.19 to €551.81)	€-47.62 (€-77.28 to €-25.85)	−10.68% (−14.27% to −7.12%)
Lifetime costs per patient	€377.55 (€242.56 to €554.17)	€384.13 (€245.85 to €565.96)	€6.58 (€-17.25 to €33.47)	1.74% (−4.49% to 8.86%)
Costs of productivity loss per patient	€106.87 (€64.71 to €169.27)	€99.07 (€59.52 to €160.09)	€-7.80 (€-18.76 to €2.58)	−7.30% (−16.94% to 2.70%)
Total costs per patient	€1220.94 (€955.23 to €1540.85)	€1143.68 (€891.74 to €1451.12)	€ -77.25 (€-126.81 to €-33.37)	−6.33% (−9.80% to −2.85%)
Quality adjusted life expectancy	11.29 (9.41 to 13.33)	11.29 (9.41 to 13.33)	−0.00 (−0.00 to 0.00)	−0.00% (−0.02% to 0.01%)
Probability TP	3.42% (2.47% to 4.53%)	3.37% (2.44% to 4.47%)	−0.05% (−0.15% to 0.06%)	−1.37% (−4.08% to 1.64%)
Probability FP	38.46% (33.97% to 45.00%)	31.85% (28.29% to 38.70%)	−6.61% (−8.30% to −4.99%)	−17.19% (−20.86% to −12.66%)
Probability TN	57.90% (51.52% to 62.38%)	64.51% (57.82% to 68.14%)	6.61% (4.99% to 8.30%)	11.42% (8.34% to 15.06%)
Probability FN	0.22% (0.08% to 0.46%)	0.27% (0.14% to 0.46%)	0.05% (−0.06% to 0.15%)	20.91% (−15.72% to 135.02%)
Probability death	0.30% (0.19% to 0.45%)	0.30% (0.19% to 0.46%)	0.00% (−0.01% to 0.03%)	1.53% (−4.11% to 9.30%)
Probability HF	0.59% (0.40% to 0.83%)	0.60% (0.41% to 0.84%)	0.01% (−0.03% to 0.05%)	1.85% (−4.24% to 8.91%)

This table shows the results of 10,000 iterations of 20,000 patients, showing the costs and remaining quality-adjusted life expectancy per patient. Both the 95% CI and the absolute and relative effect are provided. *CI* confidence interval, *FN* false negative, *FP* false positive, *HF* heart failure, *POC* point-of-care, *TN* true negative, *TP* true positive

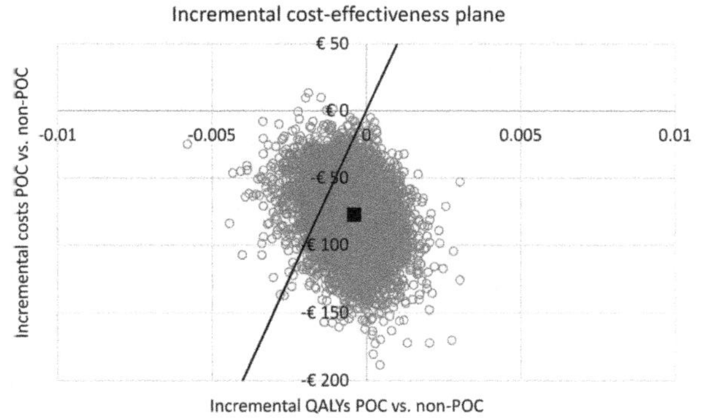

Fig. 2 Incremental cost-effectiveness plane, showing the result of 10,000 model iterations of 20,000 patients, the mean value, and the ICUR threshold of €20,000/QALY. ICUR = incremental cost-utility ratio, POC = point-of-care, QALY = quality-adjusted life year

referrals by ambulance), accompanied by a decrease in costs of hospital treatment of €47.62 per patient. Although the lifetime costs per patient are slightly higher (i.e. +€6.58), which is mainly attributable to a small increase in heart failure rates, those higher costs are compensated by a decrease in productivity loss per patient (−€7.80), caused by a decrease in hospital referral rates.

EVPI results

Results indicate that the overall EVPI per person presenting with chest pain in primary care is estimated to be €0.22. Based on a decision relevance of ten years, and an estimated 182,897 individuals presenting with chest pain in this period, this results in an overall EVPI per year of €403,364 in the Netherlands [1]. Thus, giving this low EVPI, it is unlikely that performing more research, to decrease uncertainty, would be considered an efficient use of resources. An overview of the expected value of partial perfect information for groups of model input parameters is shown in Additional file 3.

CEAC results

The CEAC indicates that the probability of the POC troponin strategy to be cost-effective ranges from 100.0% to 52.7%, for a WTP threshold of €0 to €200,000/QALY. For a WTP of €20,000/QALY, this probability was 98.4% (Fig. 3). Thus, when society is unwilling to pay any money for an increase in health outcomes (i.e. a WTP of €0/QALY), the POC troponin strategy has to be cheaper compared to current practice to be considered cost-effective, regardless of the effect on health outcomes. On the other hand, a very high WTP indicates that society is unwilling to accept any loss in QALYs. Therefore, an increase in WTP decreases the probability that the POC troponin strategy is cost-effective. However, when the POC test was also required to provide equal or better health outcomes compared with usual care (non-inferiority), the probability of the POC troponin strategy to be cost-effective remained stable at 28.2% for a WTP ranging from €0 to €200,000/QALY (Fig. 3). Although this suggests that the POC troponin strategy has a large chance of resulting in health loss, it should be noted that the actual absolute health loss is likely to be vanishingly small. For example, previous research has indicated that a change in health utility of 0.03 is the minimum clinically important difference, and that smaller differences can be considered to be not clinically important [36]. In our analysis the difference in utility is much smaller than 0.03, as even over the lifetime horizon the accumulated corresponding health loss equals only −0.0004. Indeed, when a very small decrease of 0.002 QALYs is chosen as cut-off for the maximum acceptable health loss, the probability that the POC troponin strategy is cost-effective already remains very high, decreasing only from 100.0% to 97.3% for a WTP ranging from €0 to €200,000/QALY (Fig. 3).

Discussion

Using a POC troponin test in primary care is expected to increase the probability at which the GP is able to correctly exclude ACS (TNs), accompanied by a decrease in unnecessary hospital referrals (FPs). However, the rate of correct referrals (TPs) decreases slightly, while the rate at which ACS patients are incorrectly not referred (FNs) shows a small increase. Despite this, the average per patient effect on QALYs is very small (i.e. -0.0004). Costs per chest pain patient are expected to decrease with approximately €77, indicating that the POC troponin strategy is likely cost-saving as compared to current practice.

Strengths

The main strength of the current study is that it was designed to accurately represent the current work-up of GPs, in chest pain patients. To achieve this, three real decisions were built into the model, in which the POC troponin test is unlikely to be used: 1) when the GPs considers a patient at high risk of ACS, 2) when the GP diagnoses STEMI using an ECG, or 3) when a patient presents <4 h after symptom onset. Consequently, the POC troponin test is only used in approximately 40% of all chest pain patients presenting to the GP. Furthermore, as it is unlikely that GPs base their referral decision solely on a POC troponin test result, the probability of GPs adhering to this result was also incorporated. Although those assumptions inevitably limit the potential impact of the POC troponin test, they are crucial to obtain a realistic estimate of the test's potential cost-utility.

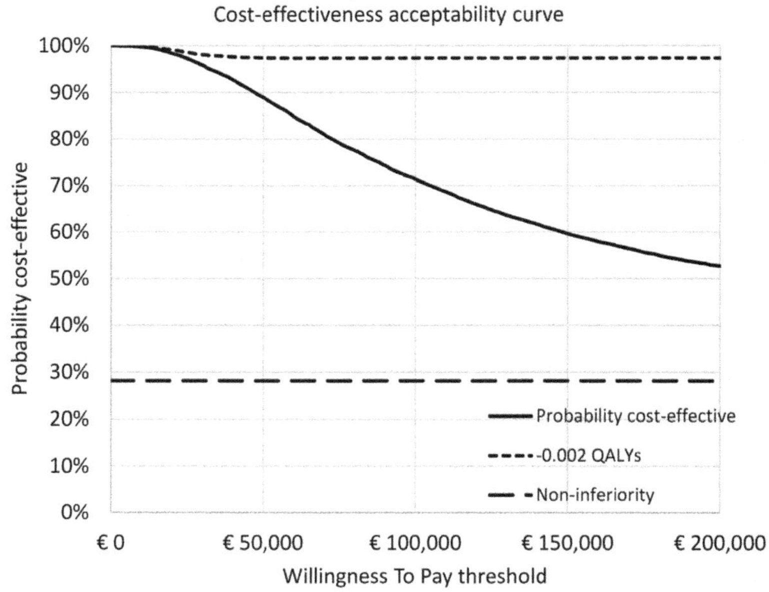

Fig. 3 Cost-effectiveness acceptability curve of the POC troponin strategy versus current practice, for a WTP ranging from €0/QALY to €200,000/QALY. The black line represents the base case cost-effectiveness acceptability curve. The 'non-inferiority' and '-0.002 QALYs' line represent scenarios in which POC troponin has acceptable cost-utility, and is either at least equally effective, or does not involve a decrease of ≥0.002 QALYs. QALYs = quality-adjusted life years

Secondly, the use of a patient-level model has several advantages. First of all, probabilities of ACS are both age and gender specific, allowing to estimate costs, QALYs and productivity losses at the individual patient level. In addition, a duration of symptoms was assigned to each patient, allowing to incorporate time-dependent sensitivities and specificities, which is an important characteristic of the POC troponin test [7].

Furthermore, all assumptions used in the analysis were conservative regarding the potential impact of POC troponin, which may have led to underestimating both cost savings and health benefits. First, the delay by POC troponin testing was set at 10 min, thereby assuming that the test is performed after the consultation by the GP, whereas it is likely that the test can already be performed during the patient's anamnesis and physical examination. Besides cost savings, this work-up would also prevent the potential negative health impact caused by a delay in treatment. Second, it was assumed that GPs would perform the test in all remaining chest pain patients, and therefore also in patients that are not actually suspected of having ACS. However, GPs can probably exclude ACS with certainty in some patients without using the POC troponin test, thereby saving costs. Third, it was assumed that the 14.7% of patients that are perceived to be at high risk of ACS by their GP (and who are immediately referred), corresponded to the patients with the highest actual probability of ACS. This assumption most likely overestimates the ability of the GP to identify high-risk patients.

Limitations

There are two limitations to be mentioned. First, evidence on the correlation between several input parameters were lacking. For example, no evidence was available on the relationship between a) the pre-test probability of ACS, b) diagnostic accuracy of the GP in current practice, and c) the diagnostic accuracy of the POC troponin test. Similarly, no evidence was available on the potential influence of patient's characteristics, such as age and gender, on the probability that the GP revises his or her initial referral decision following a discordant POC troponin result. Therefore, changes in referral decisions made in practice may concern different patients than those with a change in referral decision in our model. However, results of a systematic review and meta-analysis indicate that it was not possible to define an important role for signs and symptoms in diagnosing AMI or ACS [37]. Accordingly, it is unlikely that this limitation strongly affects model outcomes.

Second, as this study is based on a hypothetical cohort of patients, the impact of POC troponin testing on health outcomes is dependent on the literature used in the model. However, evidence regarding the diagnostic performance of GPs (without the use of POC) is limited. The drawback of the study used in the current analysis, is that the sensitivity of the GP was based on their 'action in daily practice' in chest pain patients. This definition however, included besides referral to the hospital, also exercise testing, prescribing medication, and requesting a second opinion [18]. In addition, the diagnostic performance may also be dependent on the type of POC analyzer used, but the number of studies that report the diagnostic performance of POC troponin for (a) specific time(s) since symptom onset is limited. Furthermore, more sensitive POC troponin tests have already become available [38]. All in all, the current model may thus have overestimated the rate of missed ACS patients due to POC troponin use. In absence of real-life patient data, this model-based analysis gives a first insight in to the potential cost-effectiveness of the POC troponin test. Our results indicate that future prospective studies into the safety and efficacy of using POC troponin in primary care are warranted.

Implications for practice

Results from a previous study indicate that GPs' main requirements regarding POC troponin tests are a) test result within 10 min, b) a test performed with a finger prick, and c) reimbursement of the POC analyzer [15]. Recently developed POC troponin tests may already comply with the desired turn-around-time and the finger prick blood sample [39]. In addition, literature indicates that the diagnostic performance of recently developed POC troponin tests is comparable to the results obtained in a routine laboratory. Consequently, the accompanying increase in negative predictive value likely prevents that ACS patients are missed, thereby making use of the POC troponin test a cost-effective strategy. In turn, further research is necessary to investigate whether this lower limit of detection may allow use of this test to rule out ACS in patients presenting within four hours after symptom onset. In addition, including the expected improvement on patient's well-being (and consequently on QALYs) as achieved by decreasing unnecessary hospital referrals would further increase the potential benefit of this test.

Conclusion

Owing to the expected reduction in hospital referrals, the POC troponin strategy is likely cost-saving. The potential (accompanying) small increase in missed ACS patients can partly be explained by conservative assumptions used in the analysis. In addition, ongoing developments in POC troponin tests will likely further improve their diagnostic performance. Therefore, the use of a POC troponin testing strategy is likely to become cost-effective in the nearby future. When data from new prospective (randomized) studies into the safety and diagnostic accuracy of the use of POC troponin tests become available, the health economic model presented here allows rapid reassessment into the benefits of such a diagnostic tool for diagnosing ACS in general practices.

Additional files

Additional file 1: Model input parameters. This file contains an overview of all model input parameters, including the value used in the model, the 95% confidence interval, the distribution used, and the data source (DOCX 73 kb)

Additional file 2: Overview of model assumptions. This file contains an overview of all assumptions that have been used in the health economic analysis (DOCX 18 kb)

Additional file 3: Results of partial perfect value of information analysis. This file contains an overview of the results of the partial perfect value of information analysis (DOCX 13 kb)

Abbreviations

ACS: acute coronary syndrome; CEAC: cost-effectiveness acceptability curve; CI: confidence interval; ECG: electrocardiogram; EVPI: expected value of perfect information; FN: false negative; FP: false positive; GP: general practitioner; NSTEMI: non-ST elevation myocardial infarction; POC: point-of-care; QALY: quality-adjusted life year; RCT: randomized controlled trial; STEMI: ST elevation myocardial infarction; TN: true negative; TP: true positive; UAP: unstable angina pectoris; WTP: willingness-to-pay

Acknowledgements

Not applicable.

Funding

This study was not funded.

Authors' contributions

MK, HK, MM and RK were involved the conception and design of the study. MK, HK, and MM designed the health economic model. All authors were involved in analyzing the health economic model and interpretation of the model outcomes. MK drafted the manuscript, and HK, MM, MIJ and RK were major contributors in critically reviewing the manuscript. All authors read and approved the final manuscript.

Competing interests

The authors declare that they have no competing interests.

Author details

[1]Department of Health Technology and Services Research, MIRA institute for Biomedical Technology and Technical Medicine, University of Twente, Enschede, the Netherlands. [2]Laboratory for Clinical Chemistry and Haematology, Jeroen Bosch Ziekenhuis, Den Bosch, the Netherlands.

References

1. Okkes IM, Oskam SK, van Boven K, Lamberts H: Continue morbiditeitsregistratie Nijmegen. Episodes of care in family practice. Epimiological data based on the routine use of the International Classification of Primary Care (ICPC) in the Transition project of the Academic Medical Center/University of Amsterdam (1985–2003), Amsterdam; 2005.
2. Authors/Task Force Members, Roffi M, Patrono C, Collet JP, Mueller C, Valgimigli M, Andreotti F, Bax JJ, Borger MA, Brotons C, et al. 2015 ESC guidelines for the management of acute coronary syndromes in patients

presenting without persistent ST-segment elevation: task force for the Management of Acute Coronary Syndromes in patients presenting without persistent ST-segment elevation of the European Society of Cardiology (ESC). Eur Heart J. 2016;37:267–315.

3. Nederlandse Zorgautoriteit (2016, March 1, 2016). Open data van de Nederlandse Zorgautoriteit. Retrieved March 29, 2016. http://www.opendisdata.nl/.
4. Bruins Slot MH, Rutten FH, van der Heijden GJ, Geersing GJ, Glatz JF, Hoes AW. Diagnosing acute coronary syndrome in primary care: comparison of the physicians' risk estimation and a clinical decision rule. Fam Pract. 2011; 28:323–8.
5. St John A, Price CP. Economic evidence and point-of-care testing. Clinical Biochemist Rev/Aust Assoc Clin Biochemists. 2013;34:61–74.
6. Nilsson S, Andersson A, Janzon M, Karlsson JE, Levin LA. Cost consequences of point-of-care troponin T testing in a Swedish primary health care setting. Scand J Prim Health Care. 2014;32:241–7.
7. Diercks DB, Peacock WF, Hollander JE, Singer AJ, Birkhahn R, Shapiro N, Glynn T, Nowack R, Safdar B, Miller CD, et al. Diagnostic accuracy of a point-of-care troponin I assay for acute myocardial infarction within 3 hours after presentation in early presenters to the emergency department with chest pain. Am Heart J. 2012;163:74–80. e74
8. Bruins Slot MH, van der Heijden GJ, Stelpstra SD, Hoes AW, Rutten FH. Point-of-care tests in suspected acute myocardial infarction: a systematic review. Int J Cardiol. 2013;168:5355–62.
9. Rutten FH, Bakx JC, Bruins Slot MHE, Van Casteren BCAM, Derks CJT, Rambharose VR, Burgers JS, Wiersma Tj, Mensink PAJS, Bouma M: NHG-Standaard Acuut coronair syndroom (eerste herziening). Huisarts en Wetenschap. 2012;55:564–570.
10. Bossuyt PM, Lijmer JG, Mol BW. Randomised comparisons of medical tests: sometimes invalid, not always efficient. Lancet. 2000;356:1844–7.
11. Moons KG. Criteria for scientific evaluation of novel markers: a perspective. Clin Chem. 2010;56:537–41.
12. Bosner S, Haasenritter J, Hani MA, Keller H, Sonnichsen AC, Karatolios K, Schaefer JR, Baum E, Donner-Banzhoff N. Gender differences in presentation and diagnosis of chest pain in primary care. BMC Fam Pract. 2009;10:79.
13. Bosner S, Becker A, Haasenritter J, Abu Hani M, Keller H, Sonnichsen AC, Karatolios K, Schaefer JR, Seitz G, Baum E, Donner-Banzhoff N. Chest pain in primary care: epidemiology and pre-work-up probabilities. Eur J Gen Pract. 2009;15:141–6.
14. Bruins Slot MH, Rutten FH, van der Heijden GJ, Doevendans PA, Mast EG, Bredero AC, van der Spoel OP, Glatz JF, Hoes AW. Diagnostic value of a heart-type fatty acid-binding protein (H-FABP) bedside test in suspected acute coronary syndrome in primary care. Int J Cardiol. 2013;168:1485–9.
15. Kip MMA, Noltes AM, Koffijberg H, IJzerman MJ, Kusters R. Improving early exclusion of acute coronary syndrome in primary care: the added value of point-of-care troponin as stated by general practitioners. Prim Health Care Res Dev. 2017;18:386–97.
16. van Hassel D, Korevaar J, Batenburg R, Schellevis F. De Toekomstvisie Huisartsenzorg 2011, waar staat de huisartsenzorg anno 2014? NIVEL. 2015;1–85.
17. Martin TN, Groenning BA, Murray HM, Steedman T, Foster JE, Elliot AT, Dargie HJ, Selvester RH, Pahlm O, Wagner GS. ST-segment deviation analysis of the admission 12-lead electrocardiogram as an aid to early diagnosis of acute myocardial infarction with a cardiac magnetic resonance imaging gold standard. J Am Coll Cardiol. 2007;50:1021–8.
18. Nilsson S, Ortoft K, Molstad S. The accuracy of general practitioners' clinical assessment of chest pain patients. Eur J Gen Pract. 2008;14:50–5.
19. Bruins Slot MH, Rutten FH, van der Heijden GJ, Doevendans PA, Mast EG, Bredero AC, Glatz JF, Hoes AW. Gender differences in pre-hospital time delay and symptom presentation in patients suspected of acute coronary syndrome in primary care. Fam Pract. 2012;29:332–7.
20. Nallamothu B, Fox KA, Kennelly BM, Van de Werf F, Gore JM, Steg PG, Granger CB, Dabbous OH, Kline-Rogers E, Eagle KA, Investigators G. Relationship of treatment delays and mortality in patients undergoing fibrinolysis and primary percutaneous coronary intervention. The global registry of acute coronary events. Heart. 2007;93:1552–5.
21. Mourad G, Alwin J, Stromberg A, Jaarsma T. Societal costs of non-cardiac chest pain compared with ischemic heart disease–a longitudinal study. BMC Health Serv Res. 2013;13:403.
22. Ghushchyan V, Nair KV, Page RL 2nd. Indirect and direct costs of acute coronary syndromes with comorbid atrial fibrillation, heart failure, or both. Vasc Health Risk Manag. 2015;11:25–34.
23. Hakkaart-van Roijen L, van der Linden N, Bouwmans C, Kanters T, Tan SS Bijlage 1. Kostenhandleiding: methodologie van kostenonderzoek en referentieprijzen voor economische evaluaties in de gezondheidszorg: Institute for Medical Technology Assessment, Erasmus Universiteit Rotterdam; Rotterdam. 2015:1–120.
24. Goodacre S, Thokala P, Carroll C, Stevens JW, Leaviss J, Al Khalaf M, Collinson P, Morris F, Evans P, Wang J. Systematic review, meta-analysis and economic modelling of diagnostic strategies for suspected acute coronary syndrome. Health Technol Assess. 2013;17(v-vi):1–188.
25. Polanczyk CA, Kuntz KM, Sacks DB, Johnson PA, Lee TH. Emergency department triage strategies for acute chest pain using creatine kinase-MB and troponin I assays: a cost-effectiveness analysis. Ann Intern Med. 1999;131:909–18.
26. Ward S, Lloyd Jones M, Pandor A, Holmes M, Ara R, Ryan A, Yeo W, Payne N. A systematic review and economic evaluation of statins for the prevention of coronary events. Health Technol Assess. 2007;11:1–160. iii-iv
27. Alter DA, Ko DT, Tu JV, Stukel TA, Lee DS, Laupacis A, Chong A, Austin PC. The average lifespan of patients discharged from hospital with heart failure. J Gen Intern Med. 2012;27:1171–9.
28. Sullivan PW, Ghushchyan V. Preference-based EQ-5D index scores for chronic conditions in the United States. Med Decis Making. 2006;26:410–20.
29. Nederlandse Zorgautoriteit: Tarieventabel DBC zorgproducten en overige producten per 1 januari 2016 (bijlage bij TB-CU-2066-01). 2016. Retrieved March 31, 2016.[https://www.nza.nl/regelgeving/bijlagen/Tarieventabel_DBC_zorgproducten_en_overige_producten_per_1_januari_2016_bijlage_bij_TB_CU_2066_01].
30. Poos MJJC, Van Dis I, Engelfriet PM, Deckers JW: Hoe vaak komen coronaire hartziekten voor en hoeveel mensen sterven eraan? In: Volksgezondheid Toekomst Verkenning, Nationaal Kompas Volksgezondheid. RIVM, Bilthoven: 2014. Retrieved November 20, 2015. [http://www.nationaalkompas.nl/gezondheid-en-ziekte/ziekten-en-aandoeningen/hartvaatstelsel/coronaire-hartziekten/omvang/].
31. Volksgezondheidenzorg.info: Cijfertool Kosten van Ziekten. 2015. Retrieved November 20, 2015.[https://kostenvanziektentool.volksgezondheidenzorg.info/tool/nederlands/?ref=kvz_v2l1b1p4r3c0i0t1j0o3y6a-1g0d207s54f0z0w2].
32. Centraal Bureau voor de Statistiek: Consumentenprijzen; prijsindex 2006 = 100. 2016. Retrieved March 31, 2016.[http://statline.cbs.nl/Statweb/publication/?DM=SLNL&PA=71311NED&D1=0&D2=0&D3=64,77,90,103,116,129,142,155,168,181,194,219,232,245,258,l&HDR=G1,T&STB=G2&VW=T].
33. Belastingdient: Wisselkoersen. 2016. Retrieved March 31, 2016. [http://www.belastingdienst.nl/rekenhulpen/wisselkoersen/].
34. Briggs A, Claxton K. Sculpher M. Decision Modelling for health economic evaluation. Oxford University Press; New York; 2006.
35. Strong M, Oakley JE, Brennan A. Estimating multiparameter partial expected value of perfect information from a probabilistic sensitivity analysis sample: a nonparametric regression approach. Med Decis Making. 2014;34:311–26.
36. Drummond M. Introducing economic and quality of life measurements into clinical studies. Ann Med. 2001;33:344–9.
37. Bruyninckx R, Aertgeerts B, Bruyninckx P, Buntinx F. Signs and symptoms in diagnosing acute myocardial infarction and acute coronary syndrome: a diagnostic meta-analysis. Br J Gen Pract. 2008;58:105–11.
38. Aldous S, Mark Richards A, George PM, Cullen L, Parsonage WA, Flaws D, Florkowski CM, Troughton RW, O'Sullivan JW, Reid CM, et al. Comparison of new point-of-care troponin assay with high sensitivity troponin in diagnosing myocardial infarction. Int J Cardiol. 2014;177:182–6.
39. Philips In-vitro Diagnostics: Minicare I-20, Enabling near patient blood testing in the acute care setting.2016. Retrieved April 21, 2016. [http://www.philips.nl/healthcare/product/HCNOCTN496/minicare-i20-enabling-near-patient-blood-testing-in-the-acute-care-setting].
40. R Core Team: R: A languange and environment for statistical computing. R Foundation for Statistical Computing; Vienna; 2015.

Acute coronary syndrome secondary to allergic coronary vasospasm (Kounis Syndrome)

Jing Li*, Jingang Zheng, Yifeng Zhou, Xiaofei Liu and Wenhua Peng

Abstract

Background: Kounis syndrome (KS) is the concurrence of acute coronary syndrome associated with mast-cell and platelet activation in the setting of hypersensitivity and allergic or anaphylactic insults. Many drugs and environmental exposures had been reported as inducers, but various inducers and the mechanism of KS remained unknown till now. The widely used traditional Chinese medicine (TCM) as a potential sensitizer were scarcely reported to induce allergic vasospasm due to the ignorance of the linkage between traditional medicine allergy and vasospasm.

Case presentation: We described 5 rare cases of KS including unreported triggers of TCM and abortion, reported the treatment strategy and 1~4 years' follow-up results, and tried to probe into the etiology of KS. Case 1 and case 2 for the first time reported acute ST-segment elevation myocardial infarction (STEMI) caused by Chinese herbs related allergic coronary vasospasm. Case 3 reported recurrent angina following allergen contact and wheezing, indicating the internal linkage of coronary vasospasm and allergic asthma. Case 4 described a childbearing-age woman suffered refractory ischemic chest pain due to coronary vasospasm in a special period of post-abortion, the attacks suddenly disappeared when her menopause recovered. Case 5 described an isolated episode of allergic coronary vasospasm under exposure of smoking and stress, which was successfully prevented by avoiding the exposures.

Conclusion: Kounis syndrome is not rare but rarely recognized and under-diagnosed. It is necessary to recognize KS and various inducers, especially for the patients suffering refractory vasospastic cardiac attacks concentrating in special periods. Blood test of eosinophil might contribute to diagnose KS and anti-allergic agents might be helpful for controlling KS attacks.

Keywords: Kounis Syndrome, Anaphylaxis, Coronary vasospasm, Cardiac attack

Background

KS was initially defined as the acute coronary syndrome (angina and myocardial infarction) associated with allergic reaction in 1991 [1]. After that, over 300 cases of KS had been described, researchers emphasizing the existence and association of this syndrome with coronary inflammation and vasospasm. In 2016, Dr. Kounis revised the definition of KS as the concurrence of acute coronary syndrome associated with mast-cell and platelet activation in the setting of hypersensitivity and allergic or anaphylactic insults [2]. Till now, diagnosis of KS is based on clinical manifestations. Many cases may be missed or underdiagnosed due to the unawareness of physicians, determining the prevalence or true incidence of KS is difficult with ore current state of knowledge. Helbling et al. reported an incidence of 7.9-9.6 per 100,000 inhabitants of anaphylaxis with circulatory symptoms per year, and the case-fatality rate was 0.0001% [3], the incidence of KS in the emergency

* Correspondence: nami2003@163.com
Department of Cardiology, China-Japan Friendship Hospital, No. 2, Yinghua Road, Beijing 100029, China

department among all admissions and allergy patients was 19.4 per 100,000 and 3.4%, respectively [1]. Recent reports have shown that KS has been observed in every race, age group (from 9 to 90-year-old) and geographic location, the most common affected age is 40-70 years old (68%). Risk factors of KS include history of previous allergy, hypertension, smoking, diabetes and hyperlipidemia. The number of causes that have been implicated to induce KS is increasing rapidly; of the various identified triggers, the most common triggers were antibiotics (27.4%) and insects' bites (23.4%) [4], yet more triggers are still beyond detection.

KS is recognized to be "not rare but underdiagnosed", new triggers are continuously being reported, while unrecognized triggers or circumstances that might induce KS are believed to be identified. We recognized 5 cases of KS induced by different allergens or circumstance, especially TCM. TCM is believed to have few side effects by a large amount of people in China. However, Chinese materia medica (CMM) derived from serious plants, animal components and other sources might contain bioactivators and cause anaphylaxis. Here we report three common CMM: Ma-Huang (plant of ephedra), Di-Long (dried earthworm) and injection cervus and cucumis polypeptide (CCP, the combined extracts from deer horn and sweet melon seeds), which could induce KS.

Methods

From March, 2011 to January, 2018, we recognized 8 cases of highly suspected KS in the admitted patients of cardiology department of China-Japan Friendship Hospital and collected the data during hospitalization. After discharge, for the first year, the patients were followed up by one cardiologist (the first author of this report) in the cardiology clinic every month, their symptoms, physical examination and ECG were collected. After the first year, the patients were followed every 3 months till January, 2018. Besides these follow-up time, patients could inform the cardiologist of the onset of ischemic chest pain by cell phone. 3 of the 8 patients were lost of follow-up after one year while 5 patients were intact followed up.

Case presentation

Case 1

A 56 year-old male without known cardiac risk factors presented to the emergency room complaining of retrosternal chest pain radiating to his back with excessive sweating, vertigo and mild dyspnea for about 30 minutes. Physical examination revealed scattered wheezing and a little shortness of breath. The first electrocardiogram (ECG) (18:18) demonstrated ST segment elevation of 2 mm in leads I, aVL, and ST depression in leads II, III and aVF (Fig. 1). The second ECG at 18:22 indicated that all ST segments recovered to baseline. 2 hours later, the chest pain relapsed, ECG showed ST segment elevation of 3-4mm in leads II, III, aVF, V3R~V5R (Fig. 2). Emergency coronary angiography revealed 50% stenosis in the middle segment of left anterior descending(LAD), 50% stenosis in the proximal segment of LCX, 90% stenosis in the middle and subocclusion in the distal segment of right coronary artery (RCA) all the stenosis disappeared after 200μg intracoronary nitroglycerin (Fig. 3). He was diagnosed as coronary vasospasm and given oral isosorbidemononitrate and diltiazem as well as atrovastatin and double anti-platelet therapy (DAPT), chest pain seemed to be controlled. 11 days later, severe substernal chest pain attacked again at 2:40 during sleep, ECG showed ST segment elevation of 4mm in leads V1~V4 and ST depression of 3mm in leads V5 and V6 (Fig. 4). The frequent onset of chest pain was not controlled by doubled anti-vasospasm drugs during hospitalization.

The frequent onset of ischemic chest pain pushed us to probe into the inducer of coronary vasospasm, and detailed medical history enquiry provided new information pointing to anaphylaxis: the patient had experienced bronchial asthma for 6 months. Seven days before the first attack of cardiac event, he was given Chinese traditional decoction called "Ma-Xing shi gan tang", which was boiled with Ephedra (Ma-Huang), earthworm (Di-Long) and other herbs. He suffered skin allergy with flushing, itching, erythematous rashes and urticaria on the exact day taking the decoction and experienced several episodes of mild chest pain. Therefore, discontinuation of the traditional herbs

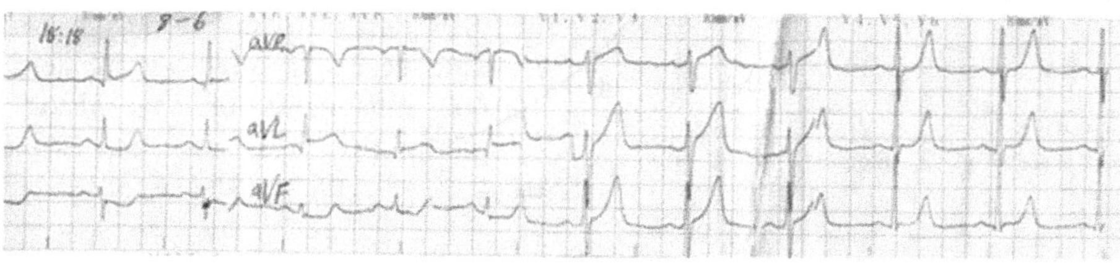

Fig. 1 The first ECG demonstrated ST segment elevation of 2 mm in leads I, aVL, and ST depression in leads II, III and aVF

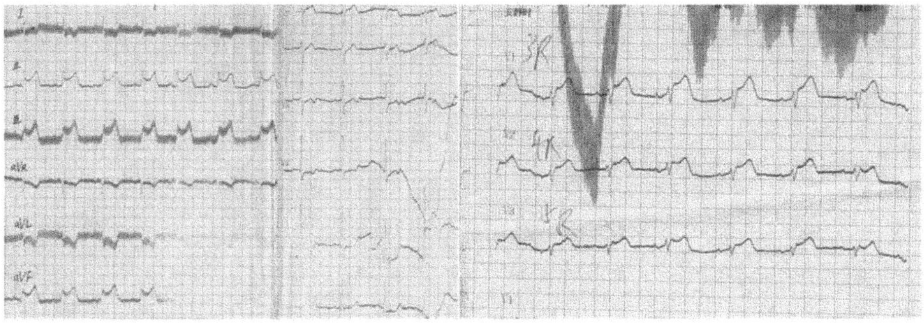

Fig. 2 ECG at 20:30 revealed ST elevation of 3-4 mm in leads II, III, aVF, V3R~V5R with a specular changes in leads I, aVL, V4~V6

therapy (which was the suspicious sensitizer of coronary vasospasm) accompanied by oral loratadine were performed to cure anaphylaxis, this treatment strategy seemed to be effective because the onset of chest pain turned rare and mild in the following 1 month, and the patient kept symptomless for the next 2 months. However, he then attempted to resume the herbs and suffered the 3rd cardiac event, presenting extremely strong chest pain, tall and peaked T waves in leads V3~V6 in ECG (Fig. 5) and obvious elevation of blood eosinophil of 23.4%. This time he completely discarded the herbs and complied to anti-vasospasm therapy for 6 months, he felt no more attacks and discontinued the anti-vasospasm drugs. During the 3 years' follow-up, he kept free of ischemic chest pain without any anti-vasospasm drugs, although wheezing still relapsed intermittently.

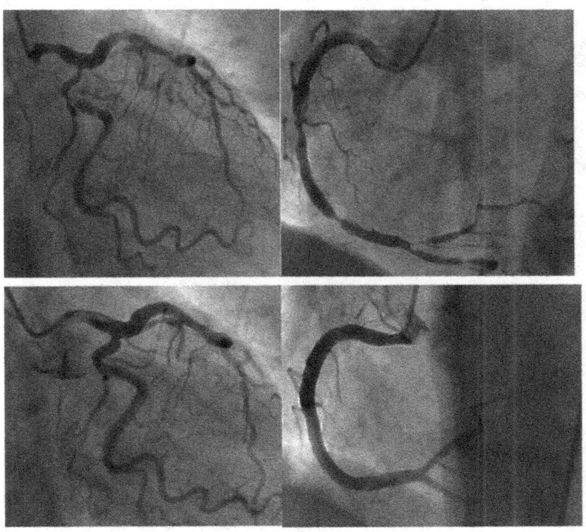

Fig. 3 Coronary angiography of: Upper left: left coronary artery spasm; Lower left: left coronary artery relaxed after intracoronary nitroglycerin; Upper right: right coronary artery spasm; Lower right: right coronary artery relaxed after intracoronary nitroglycerin

Case 2

A 57 year-old male suffered anaphylactic shock and loss of consciousness when Given Intravenous administration of cervus and cucumis polypeptide for treatment of low back pain in a local hospital. His vital signs recovered in 30 minutes after successful salvage, but then he developed tightening central chest pain and dyspnea, the ECG showed ST segment elevation of 0.5 mm in leads II, III and avF (Fig. 6). He was suspected acute myocardial infarction and sent to our hospital. He had no cardiac risk factors and history of cardiovascular disease (CVD). On admission, his symptom had partly relieved, ECG showed ST segment recovered and Q wave in leads III (Fig. 7). Emergency coronary angiography (5 hours after the event) showed 50% stenosis in the proximal and middle segments of LAD, 25–50% stenosis in the middle segment of LCX and 25–50% stenosis in the middle segment of Without evidence of thrombosis or trace of dissolved thrombosis in the coronary arteries. Chest pain did not relapse during hospitalization, T waves inversion persisted in leads II, III and Q wave in leads III in subsequent ECGs (Fig. 8). His troponin I was 2.27ng/mL on the 5th hour of onset and reached to the peak of 3.0 ng/mL on the 18th hour, and blood eosinophil was 15.5% on arrival. Echocardiography showed regional wall motion abnormality in the inferior left ventricular wall. The patient was diagnosed as acute ST-segment elevation myocardial infarction due to allergic coronary vasospasm, the allergen was recognized as injection cervus and cucumis polypeptide. He had neither injected cervus and cucumis polypeptide nor suffer any attack of chest pain during the 1-year follow-up.

Case 3

A 68 year-old male without known cardiac risk factors had suffered bronchial asthma for 2 years, aggregating for 3 months with the suspected allergen of detergent and pesticide sprays since he moved from south China to Beijing, accompanied by recurrent precordial squeezing pain, dyspnea and excessive sweating several hours

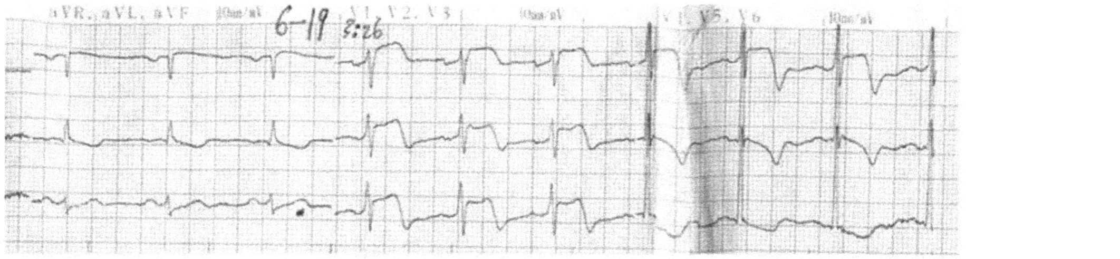

Fig. 4 ECG at 3:26on the ambulance revealed ST segment elevation of 4mm in leads V1~V4 and ST depression of 3 mm in leads V5 and V6

after the episodes of wheezing and spontaneously resolved in 10~15 minutes. After admitted to the cardiology unit, he complained allergy to the smell of pesticide sprays and suffered chest pain for several times at 1:00~3:00 in the morning which was relieved by intravenous administration of nitroglycerin. ECG showed ST segments depression of 0.2-0.3 mv in leads V1-V6 on attack and resolution of ST segments when symptom was resolved, Holter showed non-sustained ventricular tachycardia at the time he felt dyspnea, while repeated tests of troponin I were negative. Coronary angiography was performed on the third day after admission, revealing a 90% stenosis in the proximal segment of LAD, a 75% stenosis in the middle segment of LAD and a 50% stenosis in the proximal segment of LCX respectively, and all stenosis disappeared after 200ug intracoronary administration of nitroglycerin. The patient was diagnosed as coronary vasospasm and was given oral isosorbidemononitrate and diltiazem for long-term therapy. The attacks of chest pain developed less frequently but still relapsed after wheezing, he could predict the midnight chest pain by the preceding contact of allergen and wheezing, and experimentally taking loratadine (which is a non-sedating anti-histamine drug that inhibit the release of histamine from mast cells) could effectively prevent or alleviate the episodes of chest pain.

Case 4

A 42 year-old female without history of atopy and cardiovascular risks received surgical abortion under intravenous anesthesia of Propofol in February, 2013. At 7:30 on the 7th morning of the surgery, she suffered a sudden severe pressure-like pain of 10 minutes in the left subclavian and retrosternal area when she was lying in bed. After that, such pain recurrently occurred in the midnight and early morning. She was diagnosed as angina pectoris in the local hospital and given aspirin, clopidogrel, atorvastatin and nitrates, but chest pain still relapsed. After a serious attack of 15 minutes with heavy sweating at 2:00, she was sent to our hospital. On admission, her blood pressure was 150/100 mmHg, heart rate was 76 beat per minute, physical examination revealed no abnormalities. ECG on admission was normal (Fig. 9), troponin I was negative and the rate of eosinophil was 2.5%, coronary angiography revealed a plaque in the proximal segment of LAD without stenosis and other coronary arteries were normal. She was suspected as coronary vasospasm and was given mononitrate, nifedipine, aspirin, clopidogrel and atrovastatin. However, ischemic chest pain continued attacking in the morning during hospitalization. On the 3rd morning after angiography, she suffer a 5-minute episode, ECG showed downsloping ST segments depression of 1~3mm in leads

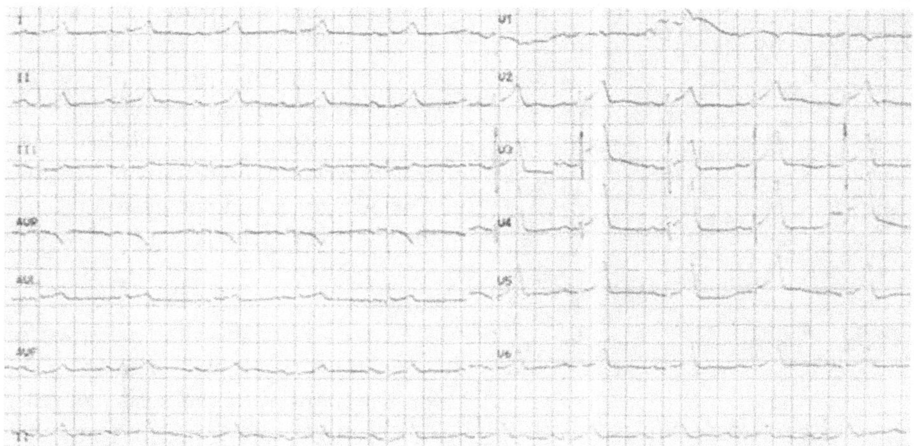

Fig. 5 Tall and peaked T waves in leads V3~V6

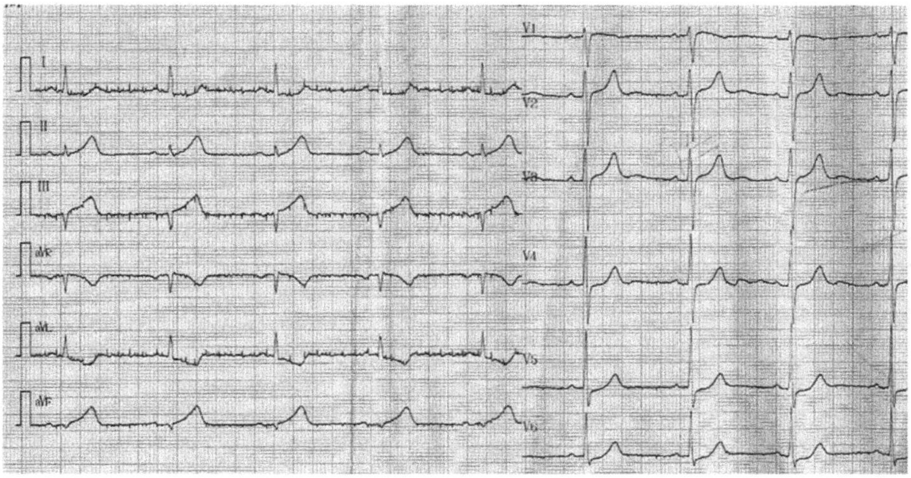

Fig. 6 ECG in the local hospital revealed ST segment elevation of 0.5 mm and peaked T wave in leads II, III and avF

I, aVL, II, III, aVF and V2-V6 (Fig. 10), the symptom was relieved by one dose (0.5 mg) of sublingual nitroglycerin and ST segments recovered, whereas another two attacks occurred 2 hours and 4 hours later, respectively, with the same ECG presentation. After continuous 48-hour intravenous administration of nitroglycerin, as well as added dose of mononitrate and nifedipine before night sleep, chest pain seemed to calm down, she kept symptomless for 5 days and discharged. She occasionally suffered early morning chest pain for 5-10 minutes in the first 4 months though adhering to drugs. Interestingly, the episodes suddenly stopped when her menopause recovered in August, 2013, and her chest pain never relapsed during the 4 years follow-up.

Case 5

A 45 year-old male developed flushing and urticaria 15 minutes after eating pineapple, then he felt precordial squeezing pain radiating to the left shoulder, lasting for several minutes, accompanied by palpitation and excessive sweating. He is a smoker with no other cardiac risk factors and no history of CVD, he was allergic to pineapple before but only manifested as slight itching and skin rashes which spontaneously disappeared in hours. Before this onset, he had been working day and night for 1 month with doubled tabacco smoking, though he did not smoke after eating pineapple. The patient was sent to the emergency room, on arriving, his symptoms had been relieved by sublingual nitroglycerin, his blood pressure was 120/70mmHg, pulse rate was 80 beat per minute, and ECG revealed no abnormalities while the symptom had relieved. 24h Holter (Figs. 11, 12 and 13) revealed ST segment elevation for 2~3 mm in leads II, III, aVF, V5, V6 at 13:40-13:42 (when he felt malaise, chest pain and palpitation at rest) and 20:20-20:22 (when he was driving, he felt chest pain and left arm numb), as well as ventricular bigeminy and nonsustained ventricular tachycardia at 13:20 and 13:42. He was admitted to cardiology department, blood test showed normal troponin I level and elevated eosinophil of 7.6% on the first day of admission. Coronary angiography showed subocclusion in the proximal segment of LCX with TIMI grade 3 flow, which was relieved by 3 times of 200μg intracoronary nitroglycerin. He was diagnosed as coronary vasospasm on the basis of anaphylaxis to pineapple, and received anti-vasospasm therapy of mononitrate and

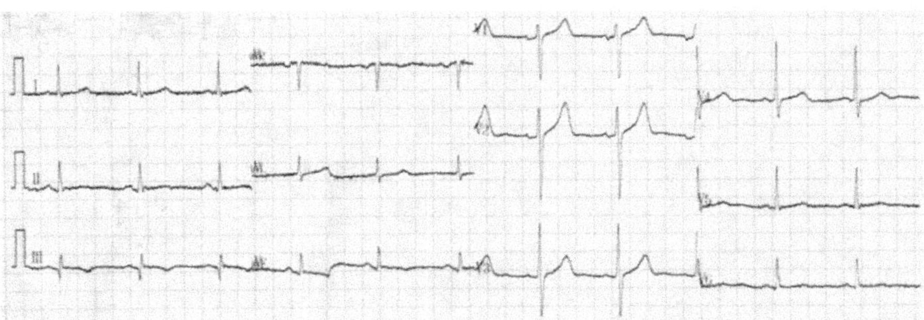

Fig. 7 ECG on arrival in our hospital revealed ST segment recovered to baseline in leads II, III and avF and Q wave in lead III

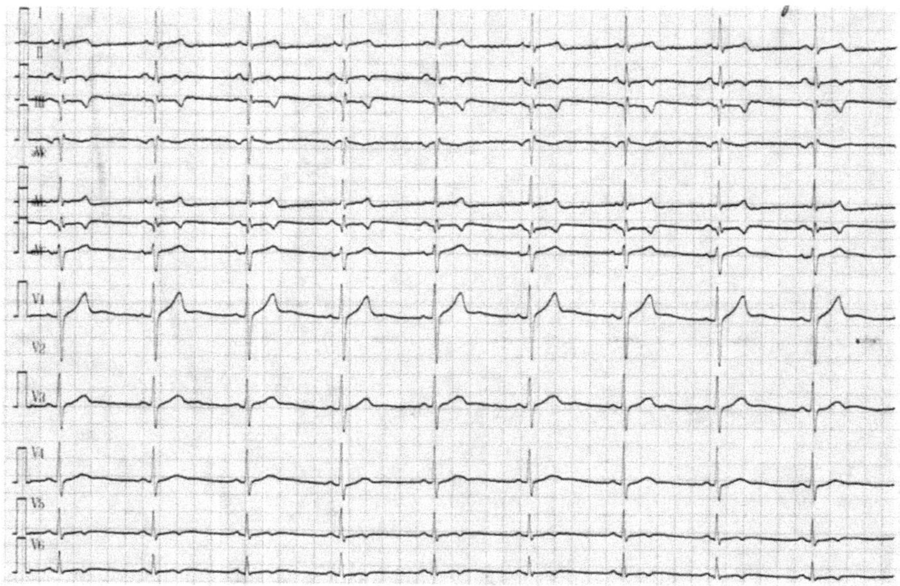

Fig. 8 ECG showed ST segment and T wave evolution in leads II, III and avF

nifedipine as well as antiallergic agent, the eosinophil rate declined to 6.1% on the 7th day, chest pain didn't relapse during hospitalization. After 12 months of mononitrate and nifedipine medication, anti-vasospasm therapy was discontinued. During 3 years follow-up, he kept free of cardiac events.

Discussion

We report 5 rare cases of KS induced by unreported exposures or circumstances. To our knowledge, this is the first time reporting Chinese traditional herbs as the sensitizer of allergic coronary vasospasm.

The two patients had no cardiovascular risk factors and pre-existing atherosclerotic diseases, they experienced recurrent coronary vasospasm and acute myocardial infarction, accompanied by definite manifestations of anaphylaxis obviously elevated level of blood eosinophil, supporting the diagnosis of allergic coronary vasospasm based myocardial infarction. Angiography revealed no stenosis after the vasospasm relieved, indicating the diagnosis of type I KS [5].

In case 1, both asthma and the decoction were the possible culprit responsible for coronary vasospasm. Wheezing may be associated with an increased risk of

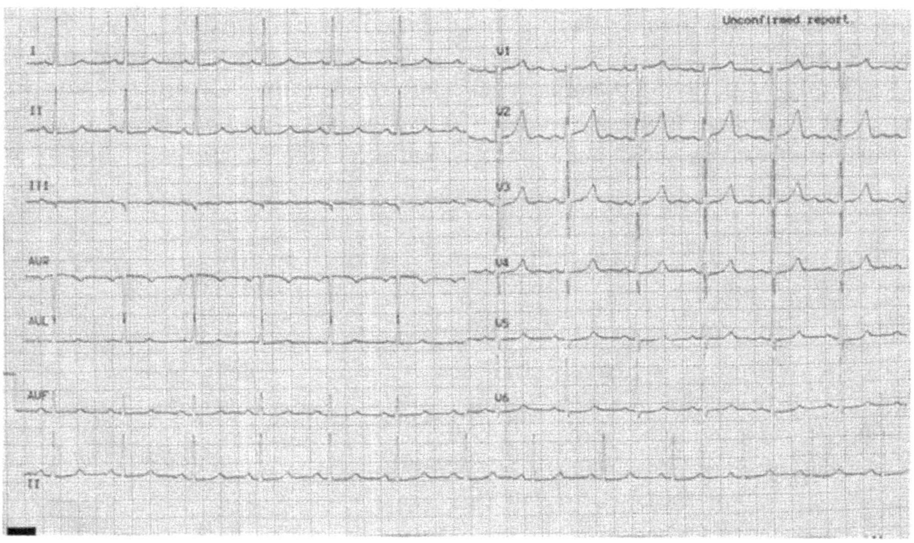

Fig. 9 ECG on admission was normal

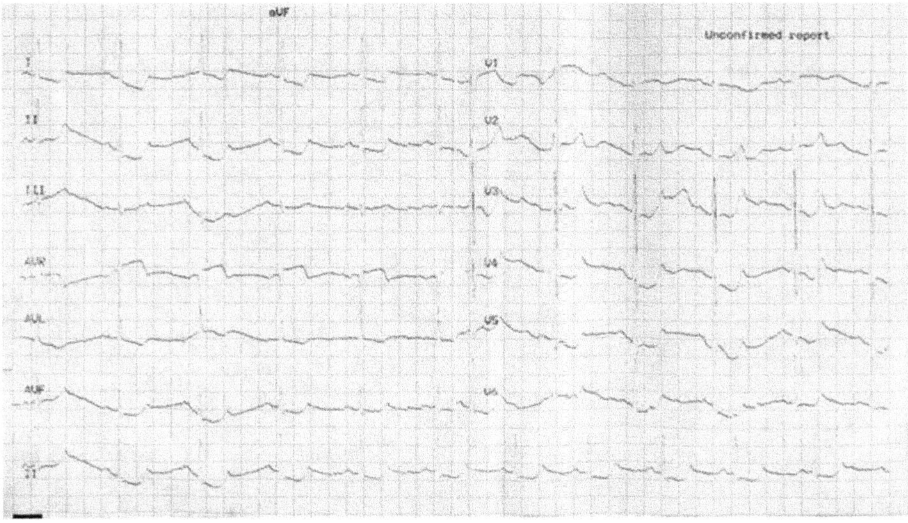

Fig. 10 Downsloping ST segments depression of 1-3 mm in leads I, aVL, II, III, aVF, V2-V6

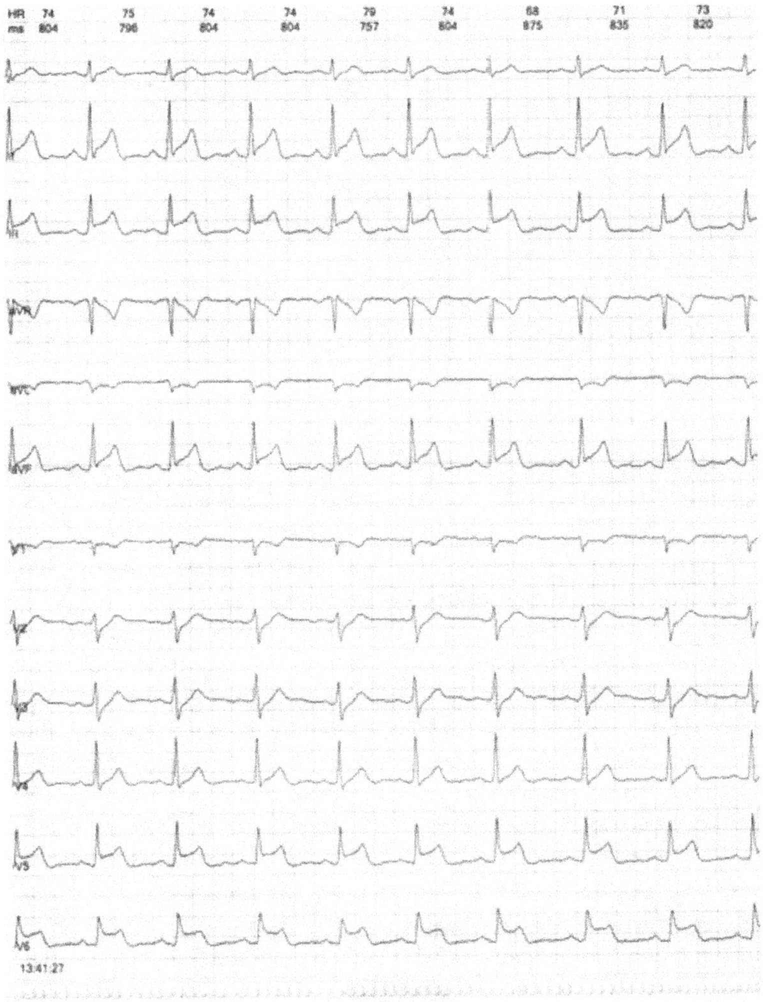

Fig. 11 ST segment elevation for 2-3 mm in leads II, III, aVF, V5, V6 at13:40-13:42 in Holter

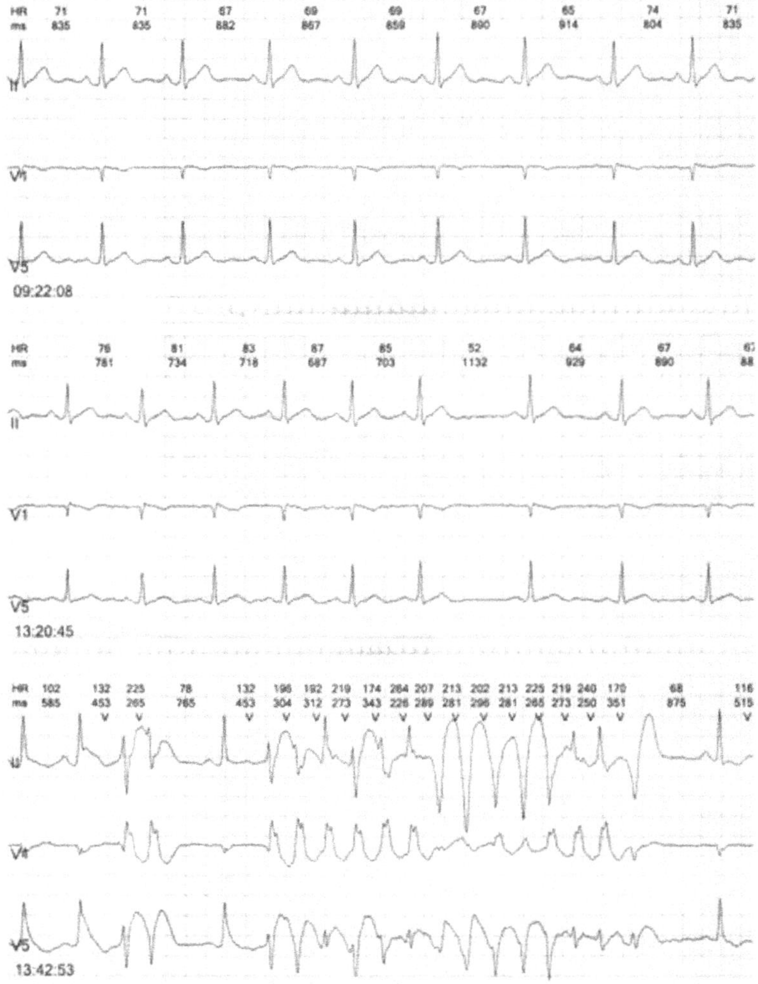

Fig. 12 Nonsustained ventricular tachycardia at 13:42 in Holter

coronary vasospasm, both the status of asthma and the allergic factors may cause the onset of vasospasm [6]. However, the onset of asthma was 6 months earlier than coronary vasospasm, during the recurrent episodes of wheezing in this 6 months, there were no attacks of ischemic chest pain; during the 4 years follow-up, wheezing still occurred although the chest pain had disappeared, indicating that the time window of coronary vasospasm was not consistent with the status of wheezing. On the contrary, the patient suffered skin allergy (which provided the evidence of anaphylaxis induced by herbs) as well as recurrent ischemic chest pain on the first day taking the decoction, chest pain was relieved by the discontinuation of the decoction and relapsed when the patient resume the decoction again, strongly indicating the close relationship between TCM-induced anaphylaxis and coronary vasospasm, supporting the point that the anaphylaxis induced by Chinese decoction rather than the status of asthma should responsible for the frequent episodes of coronary vasospasm. Furthermore, the status of asthma might put the patient into an exposure of hypersensitivity, and the decoction induced anaphylaxis on the basis of this hypersensitivity.

"Ma-Xing Shi Gan Tang" is a classical decoction for asthma which is boiled in water with 16 plants and animal composition. We considered the whole decoction as the inducer of KS, but it's difficult to precisely tell which one of the 16 components or their compound (formed during boiling) should be the culprit. Ephedra (Ma-Huang) and earthworm (Di-Long) are the two main effective components in the decoction, so we analyzed these two components in detail.

Ma-Huang is a classical bronchodilator in TCM with a history of medical use for over 5000 years, ephedra is the effective constituent. In the western countries, ephedra as a mainstream treatment for asthma reached its zenith in the late 1950s, and then moved into the

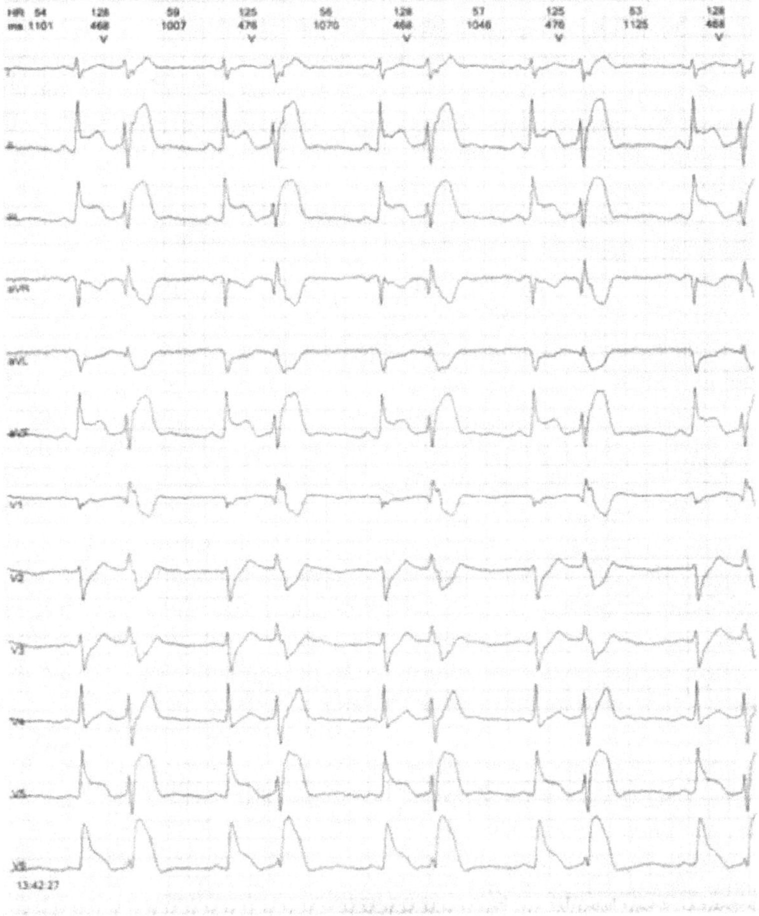

Fig. 13 Ventricular bigeminy at 13:40 in Holter

twilight zone with the emergence of other drug groups. Ephedra contains 1~2% of ephedrine, which is its primary active ingredient. Ephedrine is a predominantly indirectα-and β-adrenoceptor agonist for heart and blood vessels, could cause peripheral vasoconstriction and coronary vasospasm [7, 8]. In the US, there are more than 16,000 reports about the adverse events associated with ephedra-containing dietary supplements, especially acute myocardial infarction and stroke [9]. However, the procedure we manage ephedra in Chinese decoction is different from the procedure of chemical isolation and purification in western countries, the plant of ephedra (Ma-Huang) is mixed with other plants and boiled in water, so the concentration of effective constituent should be much lower, this might explain the rare reports about Ma-Huang related coronary vasospasm in Chinese medicine. In case 1, we suppose the coronary artery was hypersensitive to ephedrine and experienced anaphylaxis that lead to skin allergy and coronary vasospasm.

Di-Long, also known as common earthworm (*lumbricusterrestris),* is one of the most common component of Chinese decoction for asthma therapy. The earthworm peptides were demonstrated to regulate immune-responsiveness and relieve bronchial spasm [10], but it's also a source of foreign protein reasonable to be a suspicious allergen. Several case reports had described patients suffering allergic angioedema, conjunctivitis, rhinitis and urticarial caused by common earthworm *L.terrestris* (used as fish baits), type I hypersensitivity mechanism was demonstrated to be responsible [11–13]. Carreñoet et al [14] recognized 1 allergen of around 15.5kDa in 13cases allergic to *L terrestris,* which provided a molecular proof for earthworm allergy. We consider earthworm as a probable culprit allergen for the coronary vasospasm in this case.

In case 2, Allergy is evidenced by anaphylactic shock and raised blood eosinophil count; the patient had no cardiac risk factors, no history of coronary heart disease and no such episodes during follow-up, while the isolated coronary event happened exactly 30 minutes after the allergic shock, which logically highly pointed to the link of allergy and coronary event. There are two reasonable explanation for this coronary event: (1) allergic vasospasm (type 1 KS) or vasospasm triggered plaque rupture (type 2 KS) might be a logically reasonable explanation. (2) However, the coronary angiography was performed 5 hours after the event, we have no direct evidence of vasospasm. Thrombus formed over a ruptured yet subcritical plaque might be another reasonable explanation, which could have dissolved after 5 hours when coronary angiography was performed, and the eosinophil raise could be linked to a reaction to the traditional medication. The anaphylactic shock and coronary vasospasm based STEMI had a definitely close relation with injection CCP. CCP is the combined extracts from deer horn and sweet melon seeds, which has gained popularity in orthopedic clinics in China, with the aim to promote fracture healing and treat osteoarthritis and rheumatoid arthritis. Till now, we have not found any reports about CCP induced anaphylaxis.

Decoction is a kind of liquid mixture made of various Chinese materia medica (CMM) including medical plants, insects and animal components under the procedure of soak, boil and steam. There are thousands of CMM in China, a decoction usually contains twenty kinds of CMM, the prescriptions are fairly different according to different patients, diagnosis or symptoms. CMM are proved to effectively modulate constriction-dilation of blood vessels, modulate oxygen reply-demand and influence the stability of plaques [15]. The functional components are proved to be the various bioactivators (proteins, alkaloids) rooted from herbs [16], which also might act as allergens and toxicants, although reports about CMM induced allergy are very rare. We suppose that allergic coronary artery spasm is not a rare condition but a rarely suspected and under-diagnosed condition, our reports may remind physicians of the linkage between ischemia chest pain and the anaphylaxis induced by TCM.

Kounis syndrome, also known as allergic angina syndrome, was described in 1991 by Kounis and Zavras [17] as "the concurrence of chest pain and allergic reactions, accompanied by clinical and laboratory findings of classical angina pectoris caused by inflammatory mediators released during the allergic insult". Allergic angina could progress to acute myocardial infarction which was named allergic myocardial infarction [18]. The main pathophysiological mechanism is vasospasm of epicardial coronary arteries due to increased inflammatory mediators that are released during a hypersensitivity reaction.

KS should be kept in mind especially when diagnosing patients without CV risk factors and pre-existing CVD who experience acute coronary syndrome and report ingestion of a drug accompanied by symptoms of anaphylaxis. Ruptured plaques, a traditional known reason for acute coronary syndrome, may not be the explanation for this case. It seems that atopic individuals are at higher risk of acute coronary syndromes than normal people [19]. A population based study revealed a causal role of IgE in the development of cardiovascular disease [20], mast cell degranulation inhibitors might prevent acute thrombotic events [21], this may explain why administration of clopidogrel helped to cease the episodes of ischemic chest pain in our cases.

Several pathophysiological mechanisms have been described to explain the involvement of the heart in anaphylactic reactions. The existence of mastocytes in heart tissue and their participation in the anaphylactic reaction that triggers coronary vasoconstriction, dysfunctional ventricular contractility and blockade of atrioventricular conduction is well known. These abnormalities are attributed to the release of inflammatory mediators such as histamine, thrombin, prostaglandins, leukotrienes and platelet activation factors, as well as the release of rennin during episodes of anaphylaxis and its involvement [22]. The factors released from mastocytes and other interacting inflammatory cells during the anaphylactic activation and manifests as vasospastic angina, acute myocardial infarction and stent thrombosis. A subset of platelets bearing, in their surface, FCγRI, FCγTII, FCεRII receptors are also involved in this activation cascade [23].

In Case 3, KS is a reasonable explanation, but not the only. We consider two explanations: (1). The patient showed bronchial hypersensitivity to the exposure of pesticide sprays, followed by episodes of coronary vasospasm, it's reasonable to consider that there might be systemic hypersensitivity involved in both bronchus and coronary artery. Bronchial and myocardial involvement with early severe bronchoconstriction and vasospasm-induced coronary blood flow reduction manifesting as KS respectively should be always considered. Combined bronchoconstriction with interstitial edema and tissue suppression from arterial involvement and peripheral vasodilatation, perhaps, occur simultaneously [24]. (2). The coronary artery is not a direct target organ of hypersensitivity, the coronary spasm might be secondary to smooth muscle contraction reflex caused by the irritation of the bronchial epithelium by molecules, the bronchial smooth muscle contraction reflex induced the epithelium derived inflammatory molecules accumulation, and cause coronary vasospasm through this pathway.

In Case 4, after surgical abortion under anesthesia of propofol, a childbearing woman experienced refractory angina, which was highly suspected as coronary vasospasm evidenced by classical clinical manifestations of angina and nearly normal coronary artery in angiography. Several case reports described transient coronary vasospasm based cardiac events under the administration of

Propofol [25], but in our case, the first onset of angina occurred 7 days after the administration of propofol, and the following refractory relapse had no relation with propofol, indicating the little causality between propofol administration and angina. Another explanation might be as below: the surgery had injured her endometrium and disturbed the ovarian function, evidenced by the significant delay of menstruation recovery. Because endogenous estrogens are involved in the regulation of vascular tone and protect premenopausal women from development of coronary disease [26, 27], the post-abortion disorder of estrogen/progestin might lead to the imbalance between coronary vasoconstriction and vasodilation, therefore cause refractory vasospastic angina. The refractory vasospasm occurred synchronously with the loss of menstruation and spontaneously disappeared when the ovarian function returned, supporting our assumption that the exposure to disturbance of ovarian function induced by surgical abortion might be the inducer of KS.

Case 5 displayed a patient suffering ST-elevated ACS and malignant ischemic ventricular arrhythmia due to allergic coronary vasospasm, the allergen seemed to be pineapple, to which he only had slight skin allergy history, it's interesting why severe coronary vasospasm was involved this time. One reasonable explanation may be that the anaphylaxis exploded on the basis of "preconditioning" of the exposure to tabacco smoking and stress, causing explosive release of inflammatory mediators and trigger anaphylactic reaction in the heart. In fact, stress could precipitate allergies and trigger coronary mast cells leading to cardiac events [28]. Though smoking exposure is a recognized risk factor for coronary vasospasm in susceptible individual [29], this patient did not suffer vasospastic angina when he doubled smoking, whereas he did not smoke when the pineapple-induced angina broke out, implying that smoking was not the direct inducer of vasospasm. Thus neither pineapple-induced anaphylaxis nor smoking independently triggered vasospasm events. Our explanation is: the exposure of smoking and stress provided "preconditioning" status for the realization of anaphylactic coronary vasospasm induced by pineapple.

Conclusion

Allergic coronary vasospasm is not rare but rarely recognized and under-diagnosed. It is necessary to recognize KS and various inducers, especially for the patients suffering refractory vasospatic cardiac attacks concentrating in special periods. Blood test of eosinophil might contribute to diagnose KS and anti-allergic agents might be helpful for controlling KS attacks.

Abbreviations

ECG: Electrocardiogram; KS: Kounis syndrome; STEMI: ST-segment elevation myocardial infarction; TCM: Traditional Chinese medicine

Acknowledgements

These case reports was supported by doctors working in the cardiology department, China-Japan Friendship Hospital in acquisition, analysis and interpretation of data.

Funding

No source of funding.

Authors' contributions

LJ observed the manifestations of KS in the patients, collected and analyzed the cases, and followed up all the patients. ZJG performed coronary angiography for all the patients, and analyzed the angiography data. ZYF helped to follow up the patients and collected data. LXF helped to revise the manuscript. PWH helped with the literature review. All authors read and approved the final manuscript.

Competing interests

The authors declare that they have no competing interests.

References

1. Kounis NG, Zavras GM. Histamine-induced coronary artery spasm: the concept of allergic angina. Br J Clin Pract. 1991;45(2):121–8.
2. Kounis NG. Kounis syndrome: an update on epidemiology, pathogenesis, diagnosis and therapeutic management. Clin Chem Lab Med. 2016;54(10):1545–59.
3. Helbling A, Hurni T, Mueller UR, Pchler WJ. Incidence of anaphylaxis with circulatory symptoms: a study over a 3-year period comprising 940000 inhabitants of the Swiss Canton Bern. Clin Exp Allergy. 2004;34:285–90.
4. Abdelghany M, Subedi R, Shah S, Kozman H. Kounis syndrome: a review article on epidemiology, diagnostic findings, management and complications of allergic acute coronary syndrome. Int J Cardiol. 2017;232:1–4.
5. Kounis NG, Mazarakis A, Tsigkas G, et al. Kounis syndrome: a new twist on an old disease. Future Cardiol. 2011;7(6):805–24.
6. Kim J, Purushottam B, Chae YK, et al. Relation between common allergic symptoms and coronary heart disease among NHANES III participants. Am J Cardiol. 2010;106:984–7.
7. Kranjec I, Cerne A, Noc M. Ephedrine-induced acute myocardial infarction in a young athlete: a case of thrombus management. Angiology. 2009;60(2):254–8.
8. Khavandi A, Gatward JJ, Whitaker J, Walker P. Myocardial infarction associated with the admisistration of intravenous ephedrine and metaraminol for spinal-induced hypotension. Anaesthesia. 2009;64:563–6.
9. Haller CA, Benowitz NL. Adverse cardiovascular and central nervous system events associated with dietary supplements containing ephedra alkaloids. N Engl J Med. 2000;343(25):1833–8.
10. Huang CQ, Li W, Wu B, Chen WM, Chen LH, Mo GW, Zhang QF, Gong L, Li J, Zhang HC, Zhu HM, Zeng QZ. Pheretima aspergillum decoction suppresses inflammation and relieves asthma in a mouse model of bronchial asthma by NF-kB inhibition. J Ethnopharmacol. 2016;189:22–30.
11. McMorrow NY, Goodman GM, Moeller KR, et al. Fisherman's rhinitis: IgE mediated sensitivity to earthworms (Lumbricusterrestris). J Allergy Clin Immunol. 1993;93:301.
12. Tripodi S, Falangiani P, Perinelli T, et al. Allergy to fishing bait. Allergy. 2002;57:653.
13. Porcel S, Cámara C, Rodríguez A, et al. IgE-mediated hypersensitivity to common earthworm. Characterization of allergens evolved. Allergy Clin Immunol Int. 2005;17:246–8.
14. Porcel Carreño SL, Pineda de la Losa F, Fronteracarrion EM, Sánchez González AB, et al. Allergen profile of Protophormiaterraenovae, other species of Calliphoridae, and Lumbricusterrestris in anglers allergic to maggots in Cáceres. Spain. J Investig Allergol Clin Immunol. 2013;23(3):176–82.
15. Dou Y, Chen Y, Zhang X, Xu X, Chen Y, Guo J, Zhang D, Wang R, Li X,

Zhang J. Non-proinflammatory and responsive nanoplatforms for targeted treatment of atherosclerosis. Biomaterials. 2017;143:93–108.
16. Tan F, Chen Y, Tan X, Ma Y, Peng Y. Chinese material medica used in medicinal diets. J Ethnopharmacol. 2017;206:40–54.
17. Kounis NG, Zavras GM. Histamine-induced coronary artery spasm: the concept of allergic angina. Br J Clin Pract. 1991;45:121–8.
18. Kounis NG, Zavras GM. Allergic angina and allergic myocardial infarction. Circulation. 1996;94:1789.
19. AV-Tejedor, Espinosa MA, Cuesta J, et al. Kounis syndrome secondary to amoxicillin use in an asthmatic patient. Inter J Cardiol. 2011;150:e113–5.
20. Criqui MH, Lee ER, Mamburger RN, et al. IgE and cardiovascular disease. Results from a population-based study. Am J Med. 1987;82:964–8.
21. Nemmar A, Hoet PHM, Vermylen J, et al. Pharmacological stabilization of mast cells abrogates late thrombotic events induced by diesel exhaust particles in hamsters. Circulation. 2004;110:1670–7.
22. Reid A, Silver R, Levi R. Renin: at the heart of the mast cell. Immunol Rev. 2007;217:123–40.
23. Kounis NG. Kounis syndrome: a monster for the atopic patient. CardiovascDiagn and Ther. 2013;3(1):1–4.
24. Kounis NG, Soufras GD, Hahalis G. Anaphylactic shock: Kounis hypersensitivity-associated syndrome seems to be the primary cause. N Am J Med Sci. 2013;5(11):631–6.
25. Arakawa K, Himeno H, Gondo T, Kirigaya J, Otomo F, Matsushita K, et al. Refractory vasospasms of the coronary arteries due to multiple factors: an autopsy case. Intern Med. 2014;35(9):963–7.
26. Meyer MR, Haas E, Barton M. Gender differences of cardiovascular disease: new perspectives for estrogen receptor signaling. Hypertension. 2006;47:1019–26.
27. White RE. Estrogen and vascular function. Vascul Pharmacol. 2002;38:73–80.
28. Alevizos M, Karagkouni A, Panagiotidou S, Vasiadi M, Theoharides TC. Stress triggers coronary mast cells leading to cardiac events. Ann Allergy Asthma Immunol. 2014;112(4):309–16.
29. Maouad J, Fernandez F, Hebert JL, Zamani K, Barrillon A, Gay J. Cigarette smoking during coronary angiography: diffuse or focal narrowing (spasm) of the coronary arteries in 13 patients with angina at rest and normal coronary angiograms. Cathet CardiovascDiagn. 1986;**12**:366–75.

22

Electrocardiographic changes mimicking acute coronary syndrome in a large intracranial tumour: A diagnostic dilemma

Nilukshana Yogendranathan*, H.M.M.T.B. Herath, S.P. Pahalagamage and Aruna Kulatunga

Abstract

Background: ST elevation Myocardial infarction is a medical emergency. A variety of noncardiac conditions had been known to mimic the ECG changes that are seen in acute coronary syndrome. Although the common ECG changes that are documented with raised intracranial pressure are T inversions, prolongation of QT interval and sinus bradycardia, ST elevation or depression, arrhythmias and prominent U waves have also been recognized. However, ST elevations in association with primary intracranial tumours are rarely reported.

Case presentation: A 68-year-old female patient with a large left sided frontoparietal sphenoidal ridge meningioma with mass effect developed sudden onset shortness of breath while awaiting surgery. Her ECG showed ST segment elevations in the inferior leads along with reciprocal T inversions in anterior leads. The patient was treated with dual antiplatelet therapy and unfractionated heparin. The ST elevations in the ECG remained static and the cardiac Troponin assay was repeatedly negative. 2D ECHO, coronary angiogram and CT pulmonary angiography were normal. The repeat noncontract CT scan of the brain revealed two small areas of haemorrhage in the tumour.

Conclusion: The two mechanisms for ECG changes described in subarachnoid haemorrhage are the neurogenic stunned myocardium due to the catecholamine surge on the myocytes and stress cardiomyopathy. The same mechanisms could be the reasons for the ECG changes seen in intracranial tumours. These ECG changes could be easily misdiagnosed as acute coronary syndrome. This case emphasizes the importance of the cardiac biomarkers, 2D ECHO and coronary angiogram when confronted with such a diagnostic dilemma. Thus a more holistic analysis should be practiced in diagnosing acute coronary events in patients with intracranial pathologies to obviate a myriad of unnecessary investigations, interventions, costly treatment strategies which may well be detrimental to the patient.

Keywords: Inferior ST segment elevated myocardial infarction, Intracranial tumour, ECG changes

Background

Myocardial infarction (MI) is defined as a clinical or pathological event due to myocardial ischaemia causing myocardial injury or necrosis. The electrocardiogram (ECG) is the mainstay in the initial diagnosis of patients with suspected acute coronary syndrome (ACS). ST elevation myocardial infarction (STEMI) is a medical emergency, as the beneficial effects of therapy with reperfusion are greatest when performed early. But a variety of noncardiac conditions have been known to mimic the ECG changes seen in ACS. It is well recognized that certain neurological diseases present with such alterations in the ECG. The common ECG changes that are documented with raised intracranial pressure are T inversions, prolongation of QT interval and sinus bradycardia. Yet ST elevation or depression, arrhythmias, neurogenic T waves, J waves and prominent U waves have all been recognized [1–4].

However the occurrence of ST elevations in association with primary intracranial tumours is not a frequent finding in the literature. We intend to report a patient with a large meningioma presenting with ST elevations in the inferior leads on ECG with no echocardiographic

* Correspondence: ynilu6@gmail.com
National Hospital, Colombo, Sri Lanka

(ECHO) or coronary angiographic evidence of myocardial infarction.

Case presentation

A 68-year-old female patient with the background of hypertension, hypothyroidism and dyslipidaemia was diagnosed with a large left sided frontoparietal sphenoidal ridge meningioma with mass effect (Fig. 1). She developed sudden onset shortness of breath while she was awaiting surgery in the neurosurgical ward. There was no clear history of chest pain. She was febrile and hypoxic in the room air maintaining an oxygen saturation of 90% and had bilateral diffuse crepitations in the lungs. The CXR revealed bilateral haziness of the lung fields. White cell count, C reactive protein and Erythrocyte Sedimentation Rate (ESR) were elevated (14.85 × 10^9/L; 30 mg/L; 85 mm at 1st hour respectively). She was commenced on intravenous broad spectrum antibiotics due to the suspicion of aspiration pneumonia. However an urgent ECG was done to exclude an acute coronary event and showed ST segment elevations in the inferior leads along with reciprocal T inversions in anterior leads (Fig. 2). Her baseline ECG on admission had been normal (Fig. 3).

Then she was taken over to our acute medical unit, in liaison with the cardiology team was given loading doses of anti platelet therapy (Aspirin 300 mg and Clopidogrel 300 mg) with Atorvastatin 40 mg and then commenced on unfractionated heparin (UFH) after three hours duration from the onset of symptoms pending the results of Troponin assay. Fibrinolytic agents were not given as they are contraindicated in the presence of intracranial tumours. UFH was given as a bolus of 5000 units followed by 700 units/ h. Surprisingly the ST elevations on the ECG were static; cardiac Troponin assay done immediately and repeated three times at 4 h, 12 h and 36 h from the onset of symptoms remained negative. The Glasgow coma scale of the patient slightly deteriorated while on UFH and she was then subjected to an urgent noncontrast CT scan of the brain which revealed two small areas of haemorrhage in the tumour (Fig. 4). The UFH was discontinued by the end of 12 h and a thromboelastographic (TEG) analysis was performed with the intension to revert the coagulation abnormalities. However there was no derangement in the analysis as it was done around 12 h after the cessation of UFH. An ECHO done at 36 h from the onset of initial symptoms revealed normal sized chambers with an ejection fraction of 55%, normal aortic and mitral valves. It did not show any wall motion abnormality to suggest MI. Coronary angiography done on day 5 of the event revealed only a minor coronary artery disease with mild plaques on left circumflex artery. The D dimers too became positive with a value of 10.34 mg/L. An urgent CT pulmonary angiogram performed failed to reveal evidence of pulmonary embolism.

Discussion

ACS is due to ischaemia of the cardiac muscles and is a medical emergency. The first step in the management is prompt recognition with proper history taking along with an ECG and cardiac biomarkers. Despite of the variety of diagnostic tests available, the ECG remains the mainstay in the initial diagnosis, categorization and the localization of the vascular territory in patients with suspected ACS. Furthermore a recent meta-analysis had suggested that presence of ST segment elevation in lead aVR as a powerful predictor of left main coronary

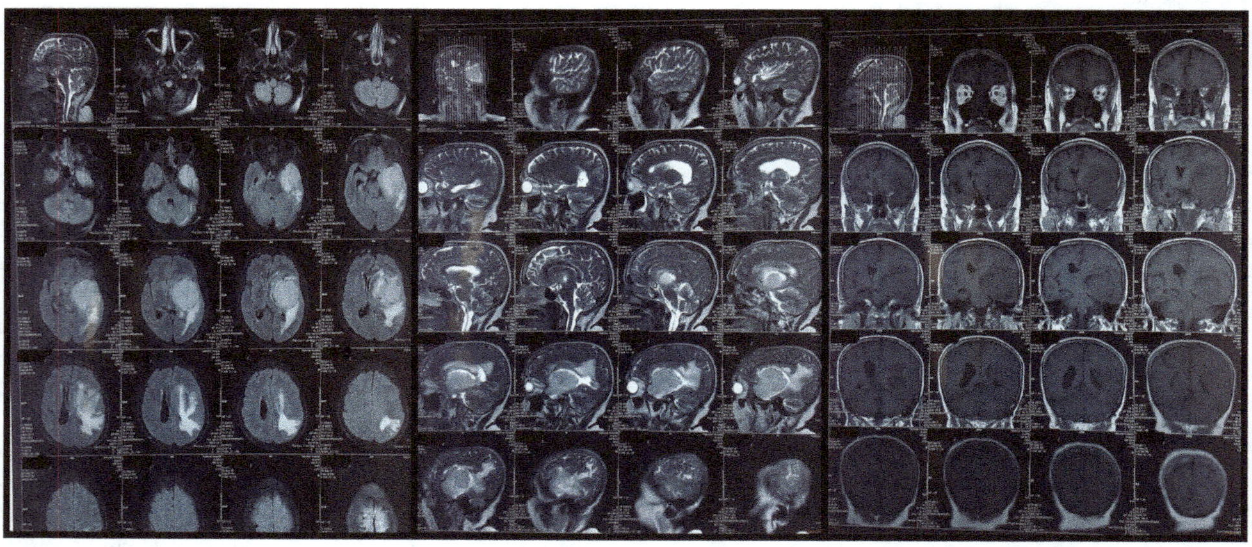

Fig. 1 MRI images of the large left sided frontoparietal sphenoidal ridge meningioma with mass effect (Axial, sagittal and coronal view)

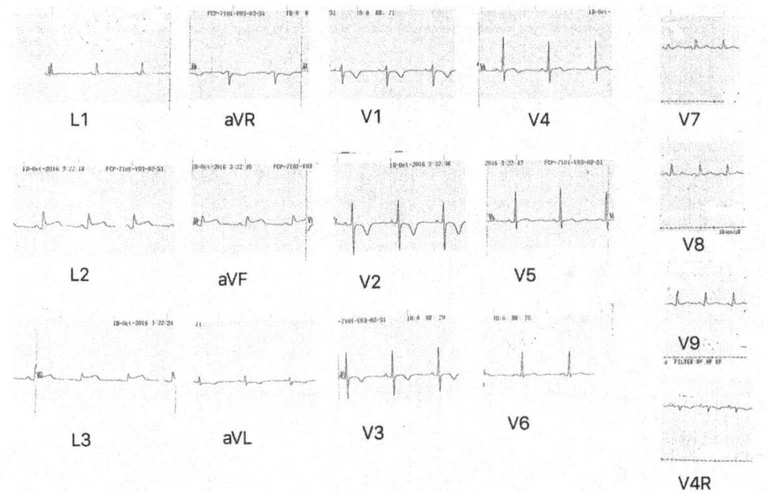

Fig. 2 Electrocardiogram showing ST segment elevations in the inferior leads along with reciprocal T inversions in anterior leads

disease and triple vessel disease [5]. Our patient had ST segment elevations confined to the inferior leads on ECG. However there had been numerous studies that concluded that there could be a myriad of ECG changes in association with raised intra cranial pressure.

A study conducted among a group of patients with elevated intracranial pressure (ICP) but without cardiac comorbidities revealed ECG changes such as ST segment elevation, T wave inversion, shortening or prolongation of QT interval, prominent U waves and notched T waves. The ICP was monitored using Konigsburg extradural transducer and the ECG changes reverted with the reduction in ICP [6].

Although the repolarisation abnormalities in ECG are more frequent after subarachnoid hemorrhages (SAH) they are also reported in brain tumours. It is believed that such changes are generally reversible and the prognostic value is limited [7]. The two mechanisms described for the ECG changes in SAH are the neurogenic stunned myocardium due to the catecholamine surge on the myocytes [8] and stress cardiomyopathy [9]. However the exact mechanisms for ST segment elevations in intracranial tumours is unclear.

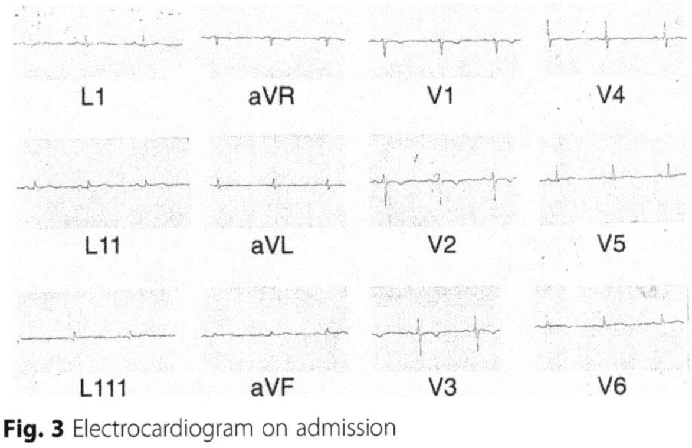

Fig. 3 Electrocardiogram on admission

There had been very few cases of intracranial tumours reported presenting with ST segment elevation. Povoa and Cavichio had concluded in a study done in Brazil that 2 out of 66 patients with intracranial tumours (3%) had ST segment elevations on ECG [10]. Hersch concluded in another study done in South Africa that 3 out of 20 (15%) patients with intracranial space occupying lesions including tumours, cerebral abscesses, subdural haematoma and tuberculoma had significant ST segment elevation in precordial leads [11].

Furthermore there had been ECG changes associated with perioperative periods of intracranial tumours [12]. Nevertheless a study conducted in Sweden had suggested that such ECG changes are more associated with SAH (15%) than intracranial tumours (13%) [13]. However, there had been recent studies concluding that the ECG changes in neurological diseases are not as frequent as reported in the literature and such changes are "non-specific" [10].

The presence of an intracranial tumour is an absolute contraindication for administration of fibrinolytic agents such as Streptokinase. Thus misdiagnosis of such ST elevations as STEMI would invariably lead to the decision to anticoagulate with short acting heparin which inturn may culminate intracranial bleeding and resulting deterioration of the neurological condition as in our patient.

Conclusion

We present a female patient with a large intracranial tumour who presented with an ECG mimicking inferior ST elevation MI. The same mechanisms which cause ECG changes in SAH and increased ICP might be responsible for the ECG changes seen in intracranial

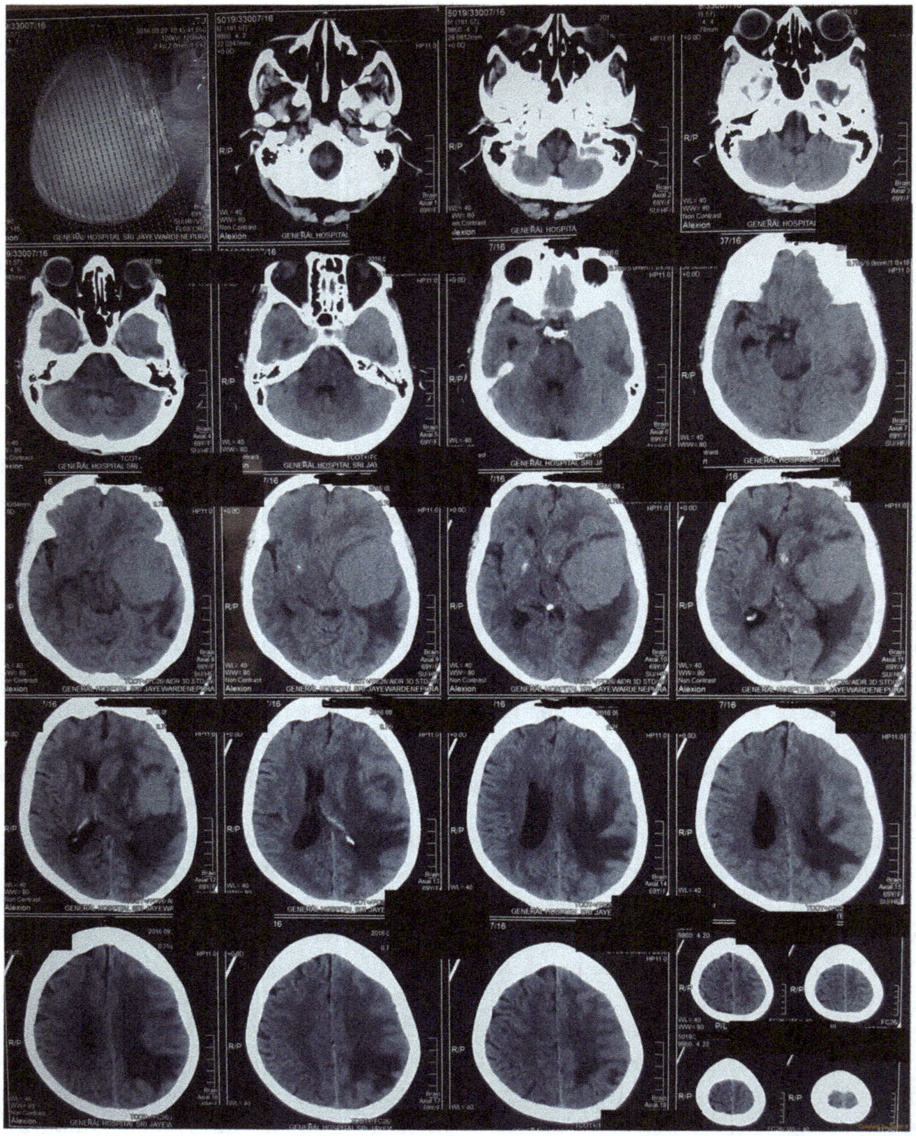

Fig. 4 Noncontrast CT scan of the brain revealing two small areas of haemorrhage in the tumour

tumours. This case also emphasises the importance of cardiac biomarkers, 2D ECHO and coronary angiogram in the diagnosis of ACS when faced with diagnostic dilemma. The ECG changes could be misleading in patients with intracranial pathologies. Thus, a more holistic analysis should be practised in diagnosing acute coronary events in such patients to obviate a myriad of unnecessary investigations, interventions, costly treatment strategies.

Abbreviations

MI: Myocardial infarction; ECG: Electrocardiogram; ACS: Acute coronary syndrome; STEMI: ST elevation myocardial infarction;
ECHO: Echocardiography; ESR: Erythrocyte sedimentation rate;
UFH: Unfractionated heparin; GCS: Glasgow Coma Scale; CT: Computer tomography; TEG: Thromboelastographic analysis; ICP: Intracranial pressure; SAH: Subarachnoid hemorrhages; SDH: Subdural haemorrhages

Acknowledgement

This case report was supported by ward doctors in acquisition, analysing and interpretation of data. We are thankful to the patient's relatives for the support given in providing data.

Funding

No source of funding.

Authors' contributions

Dr. N.Y. and Dr.H.M.M.T.B.H. collected data, followed up the patient and did the literature review and drafted the manuscript. Dr.S.P. and Dr.A.K. corrected the manuscript. All authors read and approved the final manuscript.

Competing interests

The authors declare that they have no competing interests.

References

1. Library E, Library T, 100 T, Burns E. Raised Intracranial Pressure - Life in the Fast Lane ECG Library. LITFL: Life in the Fast Lane Medical Blog. 2016 [cited 23 October 2016]. Available from: http://lifeinthefastlane.com/ecg-library/raised-intracranial-pressure/
2. Lindberg D, Jauch E. Neurogenic T Waves preceding acute ischemic stroke. Circulation. 2006;114(9):e369–70.
3. Pinto W, Barros L, Souza P, Pedroso J, Barsottini O. Neurogenic T waves as clues for diagnosing hemorrhagic stroke. Arq Neuropsiquiatr. 2014;72(6):472.
4. Milewska A, Guzik P, Rudzka M, Baranowski R, Jankowski R, Nowak S, et al. J-wave formation in patients with acute intracranial hypertension. J Electrocardiol. 2009;42(5):420–3.
5. D'Ascenzo F, et al. Prevalence and non-invasive predictors of left main or three-vessel coronary disease: evidence from a collaborative international meta-analysis including 22 740 patients. Heart. 2012;98(12):914–9.
6. Jachuck S, Ramani P, Clark F, Kalbag R. Electrocardiographic abnormalities associated with raised intracranial pressure. BMJ. 1975;1(5952):242–4.
7. Clinical Disorders - ECGpedia. en.ecgpedia.org. 2016 [cited 23 Oct 2016]. Available from: http://en.ecgpedia.org/index.php?title=Clinical_Disorders
8. Coppola G, Carità P, Corrado E, Borrelli A, Rotolo A, Guglielmo M, et al. ST segment elevations: always a marker of acute myocardial infarction? Indian Heart J. 2013;65(4):412–23.
9. Manikandan S. Heart in the brain injured. J Neuroanaesthesiol Crit Care. 2016;3(4):12.
10. Póvoa R, Cavichio L, Almeida A, Viotti D, Ferreira C, Galvão L et al. Electrocardiographic abnormalities in neurological diseases. Arq Bras Cardiol. 2003;80(4):355-6 .
11. Hersch C. Electrocardiographic changes in subarachnoid Haemorrhage, meningitis, and intracranial space-occupying lesions. Heart. 1964;26(6):785–93.
12. López-Lluva M, Arizón-Muñoz J, Gonzalez-Ruiz de la Herran F, Marina-Breysse M. Electrocardiographic changes underlying central nervous system damage. Rev Esp Cardiol (English). 2012;65(10):958–60.
13. Rudehill A, Olsson G, Sundqvist K, Gordon E. ECG abnormalities in patients with subarachnoid haemorrhage and intracranial tumours. J Neurol Neurosurg Psychiatry. 1987;50(10):1375–81.

Compared efficacy of clopidogrel and ticagrelor in treating acute coronary syndrome

Dong Wang, Xiao-Hong Yang*, Ji-Dong Zhang, Rui-Bin Li, Min Jia and Xiao-Ran Cui

Abstract

Background & Aims: Ticagrelor has been acknowledged as a new oral antagonist of P2Y12-adenosine diphosphate receptor, as a strategy with more rapid onset as well as more significant platelet inhibition function in acute coronary syndrome (ACS) patients. The clinical benefit of ticagrelor compared with clopidogrel remains controversial. The current meta-analysis was conducted to better evaluate the role of ticagrelor in comparison of clopidogrel in treating ACS patients.

Methods: The publications involving the safety as well as the efficacy of clopidogrel versus ticagrelor were screened and identified updated to June 2018. After rigorous review, eligible randomized controlled trials (RCTs) were extracted and propensity score matching (PSM) analysis was conducted. To analyze the summary odds ratios (ORs) of the endpoints of interest, we applied Meta-analysis Revman 5.3 software.

Results: There were a total of 10 studies that met our inclusion criteria, of which the risk of bleeding rate ($P = 0.43$), MI ($P = 0.14$), and stroke ($P = 0.70$) had no association with significant differences between patients receiving ticagrelor or clopidogrel. Nonetheless, higher rate of dyspnea was observed in ticagrelor group (OR = 1.87, 95% CI: 1.70–2.05, $P<0.00001$ = .

Conclusions: Our present findings suggest similar efficacy and safety profiles for clopidogrel and ticagrelor Ticagrelor should be considered as a valuable option to reduce the risk of bleeding, MI and stroke, whereas potentially increases the incidence of dyspnea. Given the metabolic process, ticagrelor may be a valid and even more potent antiplatelet drug than clopidogrel, as an alternative strategy in treating patients with clopidogrel intolerance or resistance.

Keywords: Ticagrelor, Clopidogrel, Acute coronary syndrome, Meta-analysis

Introduction

Acute coronary syndrome (ACS) is a series of urgent clinical syndromes in the coronary arteries because of decreased blood flow. It has been acknowledged that occurrence as well as the development of ACS has a strong link to platelet aggregation. Therefore, standard treatment has been established with the use of dual antiplatelet therapy (DAPT) with P2Y12 receptor inhibitor and aspirin for ACS patients regardless previous treatments, such as medical management or percutaneous coronary intervention (PCI) [1, 2].

Clopidogrel, a P2Y12 receptor antagonist as a valid antiplatelet drug for patients ACS patients, has been extensively used worldwide for over a decade. As a prodrug, it often requires hepatic conversion and leads to onset delay of metabolites with a wide variability of platelet inhibition between individuals, and more than one-third of them display minimal platelet inhibition or "clopidogrel non responders" [3–5]. Moreover, the high bleeding risk, stent thrombosis, myocardial infarction (MI) and poor response of patients with the use of clopidogrel show the limitation of its efficacy [6–8]. Hence, slow onset and low potency of

* Correspondence: 13933058601@163.com
Department of Sixth Cardiovascular Medicine, Second Hospital of Hebei Medical University, No. 309 North Zhonghua Street, Shijiazhuang 05400, Hebei, China

platelet inhibition of clopidogrel has been found based on previous publications [9].

Ticagrelor is a direct-acting oral antagonist of P2Y12-adenosine diphosphate (ADP) receptor blocker with reversibility and without catabolite activation, which can have a substantial impact on faster and greater platelet inhibition than clopidogrel [10, 11]. Ticagrelor has more remarkable beneficial outcomes in reversible long-term P2Y12 inhibition than clopidogrel in the total death, cardiovascular prevention, stent thrombosis as well as myocardial infarction without increasing the major bleeding rates in a wide ACS patient population with timely intervention, according to the Phase III PLATO (Platelet Inhibition and Patient Outcomes) trial [12]. Thus, several clinical management guidelines suggested that ticagrelor could be a valid strategy and associated with superior effects over clopidogrel for P2Y12 inhibition in ACS patients [13, 14].

Earlier studies have been published for the assessment of safety and efficacy of ticagrelor versus clopidogrel in ACS patients Nevertheless, given the differences of genetic backgrounds, comorbidities, disease patterns, and demographics, patients tend to show various prognostic results with uncertain bleeding risk [15, 16].

Therefore, attempts have been made in the present study in order to offer conclusive clinical evidence on the controversial results through this meta-analysis that evaluates the safety and efficacy profile of ticagrelor versus clopidogrel in ACS patients.

Methods and materials

Search strategy

An electronic search of literature using Embase, PubMed, and the Cochrane Library was conducted by two reviewers separately up to June 2018. All publications with the following keywords were included: "Ticagrelor"; "Clopidogrel" and "Acute coronary syndrome". We also applied the associated Medical Subject Heading (MeSH) terms. References from relevant studies and review literatures were further searched to confirm retrieval of all possible pertinent trials.

Eligibility criteria

Qualified Studies were assessed based on the following criteria [1]: the studies are designed as random control trials (RCTs) and propensity score matching (PSM) control trials comparing clopidogrel versus ticagrelor [2]; inclusion of patients with ACS [3]; the incidence of vascular effects as well as major adverse cardiovascular were considered as the primary efficacy end point, which was also defined as the composite events of stroke, myocardial infarction(MI), bleeding and dyspnea.

Quality assessment

The quality of retrieved studies was rated and collected separately by two studiers (Dong Wang and Xiao-Hong Yang). And the quality of observational studies was under assessment with the use of Newcastle- Ottawa Quality Assessment Scale [17]. RCTs were graded using the Jadad scale [18].

Data extraction

Data from each included study were checked and collected for consistency by two investigators. Any arising disagreements were settled through discussion to reach general consensus. The main categories from each of the eligible studies were included on the basis of the following parameters: family name of first author, year of publication, study design, dose and method of drugs, number of patients, follow-up time, and clinical outcome.

Statistical analysis

The statistical analyses were carefully conducted through the use of Review Manager version 5.3 software (Revman; The Cochrane collaboration Oxford, United Kingdom). We used the inverse variance method for the calculation of endpoints of interest based on ORs with their 95% confidence intervals (CIs); the individual estimate of the OR was weighted through endpoint outcomes across each study.

The heterogeneity across studies was examined through the I^2 statistic to evaluate the sensitivity [19], describing as follows respectively: low, $I^2<50\%$; moderate or high, $I^2 \geq 50\%$ [20]. We applied the fixed-effect models when low heterogeneity showed in studies. In other cases, we used the random effects model. Studies with a P value less than 0.05 was thought to have statistical significance.

Results

Searched outcomes and general features of the trials

Electronic search of literatures resulted in a total number of 369 publications originally. On the basis of the abovementioned criteria, assessment of detail was carried out and 14 publications were included, whereas some articles were excluded due to the lack of outcomes of two approaches. Hence, there were a total number of 10 studies with eligibility [12, 21–29]. Figure 1 revealed the detailed search process.

The abovementioned studies were based on evidence with moderate to high quality. Table 1 described the major characteristics of the qualified studies in more detail.

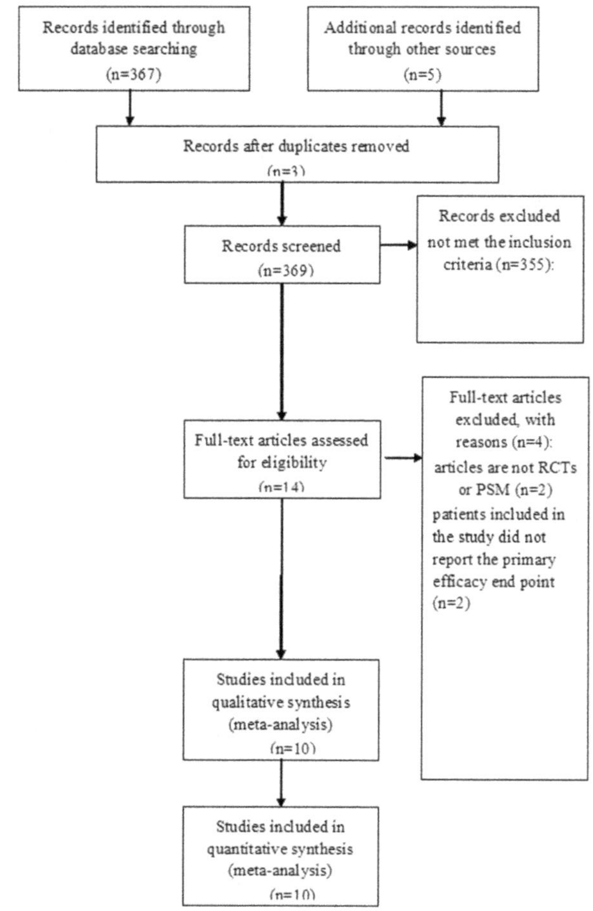

Fig. 1 PRISMA flow chart of selection process to identify eligible studies

Clinical and methodological heterogeneity

Pooled analysis of the risk of bleeding

Pooled data from 8 studies showed no differences in the risk of bleeding (OR = 1.07, 95%CI: 0.91–1.26, *P* = 0.43) when comparing ticagrelor and clopidogrel group (Fig. 2).

Pooled analysis of stroke Stroke rate was available for 7 trials. No significant differences were observed when comparing ticagrelor and clopidogrel (OR = 0.93, 95% CI: 0.64–1.34, *P* = 0.70) (Fig. 3).

Pooled analysis of MI

In the analysis of MI in patients who were treated with ticagrelor or clopidogrel, eight studies were included. Pooled data revealed that ticagrelor was not associated with higher trend of rate than clopidogrel, with the pooled OR being 0.87 (95% CI 0.72–1.05, *P* = 0.14) (Fig. 4).

Pooled analysis of dyspnea events The incidences of dyspnea events in patients with ACS were available for four studies (Fig. 5). The pooling analysis revealed that ticagrelor was linked to a higher rate of dyspnea (OR = 1.87, 95% CI: 1.70–2.05, *P*<0.00001).

Discussion

Dual antiplatelet therapy, usually accompanied with a P2Y12 receptor antagonist and aspirin, is generally acknowledged as a vital approach in treating ACS patients, partly because of the increased occurrence of thrombogenesis. Dual antiplatelet therapy has been also regarded as a standard therapy especially after PCI according to several clinical guidelines [14, 30].

Clopidogrel, a P2Y12 receptor antagonist, has been generally utilized with aspirin as prescribed antiplatelet agents in an attempt to decrease the MI risk and stent thrombosis

Table 1 Major characteristics of the included studies

Study	Publication year	Study design	No. Patients		Drug Dose		Follow-up, mo	Clinical Outcome
			Ticagrelor	Clopidogrel	Ticagrelor, mg.q.d	Clopidogrel, mg.q.d		
Cannon	2007	RCT	6732	6676	90 mg.bid	LD: 300 MD: 75	3	1、2、3、4
Lars Wallentin	2009	RCT	9333	9291	LD: 180 mg.bid MD: 90 mg.bid	LD: 300–600 MD: 75	12	1、2、3、4
Cannon	2010	RCT	663	327	LD: 180 mg.bid MD: 90 mg.bid	LD: 300 MD: 75	12	1、2、3
Laurent Bonello	2014	RCT	30	30	LD: 180 mg.bid MD: 90 mg.bid	LD: 600 MD: 75	N	4
Y. Hiasa	2014	RCT	93	46	90/45 mg.bid	75	3	3
Shinya Goto	2015	RCT	401	400	LD: 180 mg.bid MD: 90 mg.bid	LD: 300 MD: 75	12	1、2、3
Huidong Wang	2016	RCT	100	100	LD: 180 mg.bid MD: 90 mg.bid	LD: 300 MD: 75	12	1、2、3
Ran Xiong	2015	RCT	112	112	LD: 180 mg.bid MD: 90 mg.bid	LD: 600 MD: 150	12	1
I-Chih Chen	2016	PSM	224	224	/	/	12	1、2、3、4
Cheng-Han Lee	2018	PSM	2389	19,112	LD: 180 mg.bid MD: 90 mg.bid	LD: 300–600 MD: 75	18	1、2、3

RCT random control trial, *PSM* propensity score matching, *LD* loading dose, *MD* maintenance dose
Outcome [1]: MI [2]; stroke [3]; TIMI-defined bleeding [4]; Dyspnea

Study or Subgroup	Experimental Events	Experimental Total	Control Events	Control Total	Weight	Odds Ratio M-H, Random, 95% CI
Cannon 2007	67	663	30	327	8.8%	1.11 [0.71, 1.75]
Cannon 2010	675	6651	678	6585	23.9%	0.98 [0.88, 1.10]
Cheng-Han Lee 2018	70	2389	712	19112	16.6%	0.78 [0.61, 1.00]
Huidong Wang 2016	14	100	21	100	4.1%	0.61 [0.29, 1.29]
I-Chih Chen 2016	44	224	32	224	7.7%	1.47 [0.89, 2.41]
Lars Wallentin 2009	657	9235	638	9186	23.9%	1.03 [0.92, 1.15]
Shinya Goto 2015	92	387	56	381	11.4%	1.81 [1.25, 2.61]
Y. Hiasa 2014	30	93	10	46	3.5%	1.71 [0.75, 3.91]
Total (95% CI)		**19742**		**35961**	**100.0%**	**1.07 [0.91, 1.26]**
Total events	1649		2177			

Heterogeneity: $Tau^2 = 0.03$; $Chi^2 = 19.70$, df = 7 (P = 0.006); $I^2 = 64\%$

Test for overall effect: Z = 0.79 (P = 0.43)

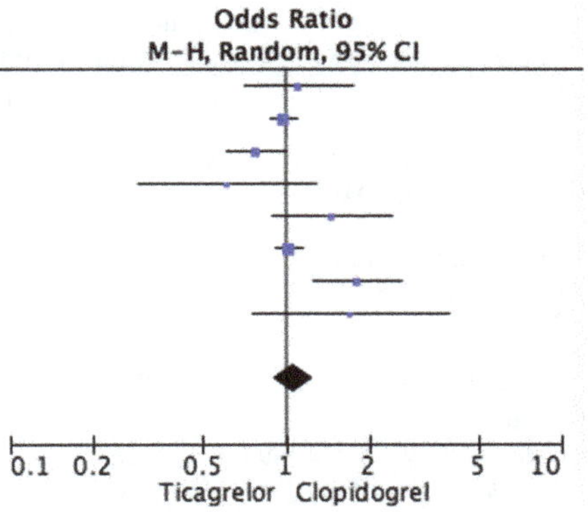

Fig. 2 Pooled analysis of the risk of bleeding between ticagrelor and clopidogrel

in patients with acute coronary syndromes with or without ST elevation [22]. However, clopidogrel requires 2-step hepatic metabolism as an inactive pro-drug that has a strong link to delayed onset and various responses [31, 32].

Ticagrelor is a direct-acting oral antagonist of P2Y12-receptor antagonist with reversibility and without catabolite activation, which can have a substantial impact on faster with consistent greater platelet inhibition than clopidogrel [10, 12].

However, previous trial supported by some studiers demonstrated no remarkable difference in terms of the bleeding rate with the use of ticagrelor in comparison of clopidogrel. Additionally, results of ventricular pauses on Holter monitoring as well as the dose-related episodes of dyspnea were found with high occurrence when using ticagrelor [12]. We conducted the study to evaluate the function of ticagrelor in terms of its superior effect to clopidogrel for ACS patients.

The present analysis showed no statistical reduction of bleeding incidence, MI as well as stroke in ticagrelor in comparison of clopidogrel. Nonetheless, dyspnea was more common in the ticagrelor group.

Although susceptibility of higher bleeding risk was affected by platelet inhibition, controversy existed regarding to the link of bleeding risk and platelet inhibition level, of which the risk of major bleeding based on platelet inhibition level has not been estimated [33, 34]. As shown in human race, there is variation in the drug response with different populations. Comparing with non-Asian patients, Asian patients tend to be more susceptive with high bleeding risk in terms of the lower body weight, different genetic background, disease patterns as well as comorbidities [35]. Higher bleeding risk in Asian population has gained interests with standard doses of new P2Y12 inhibitors, especially in East Asian patients [36]. Furthermore, on basis of clinical experience and evidence, there may be a dissimilarity between the Chinese and Japanese patients [37, 38]. It is always important to take different genetic predisposition into consideration in order to perform proper antiplatelet therapy if clopidogrel is applied

Study or Subgroup	Experimental Events	Experimental Total	Control Events	Control Total	Weight	Odds Ratio M-H, Random, 95% CI
Cannon 2007	2	657	1	327	2.2%	1.00 [0.09, 11.02]
Cannon 2010	75	6732	69	6676	26.5%	1.08 [0.78, 1.50]
Cheng-Han Lee 2018	42	2389	564	19112	26.9%	0.59 [0.43, 0.81]
Huidong Wang 2016	3	100	2	100	3.7%	1.52 [0.25, 9.27]
I-Chih Chen 2016	1	224	6	224	2.8%	0.16 [0.02, 1.36]
Lars Wallentin 2009	125	9333	106	9291	28.8%	1.18 [0.91, 1.53]
Shinya Goto 2015	9	401	6	400	9.1%	1.51 [0.53, 4.28]
Total (95% CI)		**19836**		**36130**	**100.0%**	**0.93 [0.64, 1.34]**
Total events	257		754			

Heterogeneity: $Tau^2 = 0.10$; $Chi^2 = 15.77$, df = 6 (P = 0.02); $I^2 = 62\%$

Test for overall effect: Z = 0.39 (P = 0.70)

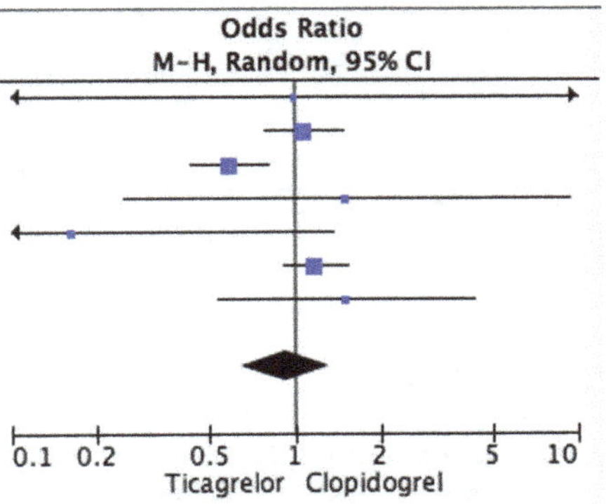

Fig. 3 Pooled analysis of stroke between ticagrelor and clopidogrel

Study or Subgroup	Experimental Events	Experimental Total	Control Events	Control Total	Weight	Odds Ratio M-H, Random, 95% CI
Cannon 2007	20	663	15	327	5.9%	0.65 [0.33, 1.28]
Cannon 2010	328	6732	406	6676	25.8%	0.79 [0.68, 0.92]
Cheng-Han Lee 2018	180	2389	1726	19112	25.2%	0.82 [0.70, 0.96]
Huidong Wang 2016	15	100	6	100	3.1%	2.76 [1.03, 7.45]
I-Chih Chen 2016	7	224	6	224	2.6%	1.17 [0.39, 3.54]
Lars Wallentin 2009	504	9333	539	9291	27.2%	0.93 [0.82, 1.05]
Ran Xiong 2015	8	112	23	112	4.1%	0.30 [0.13, 0.70]
Shinya Goto 2015	24	400	15	395	6.2%	1.62 [0.84, 3.13]
Total (95% CI)		**19953**		**36237**	**100.0%**	**0.87 [0.72, 1.05]**
Total events	1086		2736			

Heterogeneity: Tau² = 0.03; Chi² = 18.66, df = 7 (P = 0.009); I² = 62%
Test for overall effect: Z = 1.49 (P = 0.14)

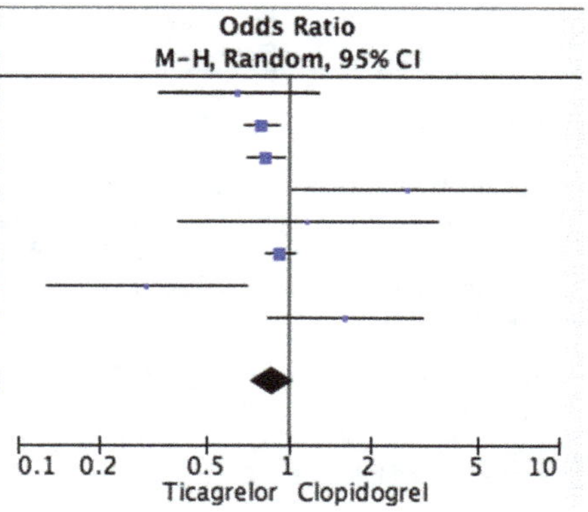

Fig. 4 Pooled analysis of MI between ticagrelor and clopidogrel

as a control. Compared with clopidogrel, ticagrelor is less likely to be influenced by CYP2C19 polymorphism [39]. The role of platelet inhibition in ticagrelor may gain popularity among Asian patients who are prone to have higher prevalence of loss of CYP2C19 function polymorphism, which may be associated with the remarkable decrease of ischemic events [40].

Increased risk of cardiovascular events usually leads to bleeding [41]. However, the risk factors of subsequent cardiovascular events were associated with major bleeding with differences in degree between Asian and non-Asian patient individuals. Debates exists concerning the reason for the susceptibility of Asian patients to subsequent cardiovascular events. Asian patients who suffer numerically higher subsequent ischemic events are those who are associated with major bleeding than without bleeding [40]. In addition, another strong predictor of adverse prognosis after ACS is the age of patients [42, 43]; ACS patients with older age tend to be accompanied with drug-related bleeding complications and increased risk of CV death. Previous clinical prognosis of older age with ACS is often further complicated by more common comorbidity [44, 45]. The abovementioned findings need further evaluation to offer strong evidence.

Dyspnea is another pivotal parameter as adverse effect in addition to bleeding. In our study, ticagrelor exerted increased dyspnea incidence in comparison of clopidogrel, which mainly due to its function in increasing the inhibition of P2Y12 on sensory neurons and the endogenous adenosine concentration [46–48].

The main strength of our study is the use of a well-maintained and updated database including studies that were designed as random control trials (RCTs) and propensity score matching (PSM) control trials. Nevertheless, potential bias exists by the intrinsic retrospective study and the imbalance in baseline demographics and clinical characteristics which may impact the comparison of relevant outcomes. More large-scale studies with greater statistical significance are warranted for the confirmation of the safety as well as efficacy profile of ticagrelor and clopidogrel.

Conclusion

In summary, we present a meta-analysis with evidence-based data comparing ticagrelor and clopidogrel in treating ACS patients. Aggregated results showed no increase in major bleeding rate, MI and stroke with the use of ticagrelor except for dyspnea rate. However, considering ticagrelor is less likely to be influenced by metabolic

Study or Subgroup	Experimental Events	Experimental Total	Control Events	Control Total	Weight	Odds Ratio M-H, Fixed, 95% CI
Cannon 2007	35	334	21	327	2.8%	1.71 [0.97, 3.00]
I-Chih Chen 2016	47	224	26	224	3.1%	2.02 [1.20, 3.40]
Lars Wallentin 2009	1270	9235	721	9186	93.5%	1.87 [1.70, 2.06]
Laurent Bonello 2014	7	30	5	30	0.6%	1.52 [0.42, 5.47]
Total (95% CI)		**9823**		**9767**	**100.0%**	**1.87 [1.70, 2.05]**
Total events	1359		773			

Heterogeneity: Chi² = 0.29, df = 3 (P = 0.96); I² = 0%
Test for overall effect: Z = 13.16 (P < 0.00001)

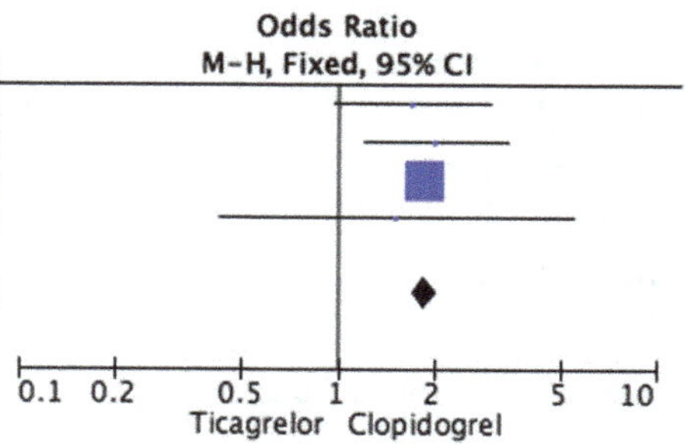

Fig. 5 Pooled analysis of dyspnea events between ticagrelor and clopidogrel

activation and various drug action between individuals, it has potential to be a valid, alternative antiplatelet drug in comparison of clopidogrel. Hence, ticagrelor may be a valid and even more potent antiplatelet drug than clopidogrel, especially as an alternative strategy in treating patients with clopidogrel intolerance or resistance.

Acknowledgements
None.

Funding
No funding was received for this study.

Authors' contributions
DW and X-H Yang have made substantial contributions to conception and design of the study; J-DZ, R-BL and MJ searched literature, extracted data from the collected literature and analyzed the data; DW and X-RC wrote the manuscript; X-HY revised the manuscript; All authors approved the final version of the manuscript.

Competing interests
The authors declare that they have no competing interests.

References

1. Mehta SR, Yusuf S, Peters RJ, et al. Effects of pretreatment with clopidogrel and aspirin followed by long-term therapy in patients undergoing percutaneous coronary intervention: the PCI-CURE study. Lancet. 2001; 358(9281):527–33.
2. Chen ZM, Jiang LX, Chen YP, et al. Addition of clopidogrel to aspirin in 45,852 patients with acute myocardial infarction: randomised placebo-controlled trial. Lancet. 2005;366(9497):1607–21.
3. Matetzky S, Shenkman B, Guetta V, et al. Clopidogrel resistance is associated with increased risk of recurrent atherothrombotic events in patients with acute myocardial infarction. Circulation. 2004;109:3171–5.
4. Wiviott SD, Antman EM. Clopidogrel resistance: a new chapter in a fast-moving story. Circulation. 2004;109:3064–7.
5. Gurbel PA, Bliden KP, Hiatt BL, et al. Clopidogrel for coronary stenting: response variability, drug resistance, and the effect of pretreatment platelet reactivity. Circulation. 2003;107:2908–13.
6. Fox KA, Mehta SR, Peters R, et al. Benefits and risks of the combination of clopidogrel and aspirin in patients under- going surgical revascularization for non- ST-elevation acute coronary syndrome: the Clopidogrel in unstable angina to prevent recurrent ischemic events (CURE) trial. Circulation. 2004; 110:1202–8.
7. Yusuf S, Zhao F, Mehta SR, et al. Effects of clopidogrel in addition to aspirin in pa- tients with acute coronary syndromes without ST-segment elevation. N Engl J Med. 2001;345:494–502 [Errata, N Engl J Med 2001;345:1506, 1716.].
8. Kuliczkowski W, Witkowski A, Polonski L, et al. Interindividual variability in the response to oral antiplatelet drugs: a position paper of the working group on antiplatelet drugs resistance appointed by the section of cardiovascular interventions of the polish cardiac society, endorsed by the working group on thrombosis of the European society of cardiology. Eur Heart J. 2009;30:426–35.
9. Tantry US, Bonello L, Aradi D, et al. Consensus and update on the definition of on-treatment platelet reactivity to adenosine diphosphate associated with ischemia and bleeding. J Am Coll Cardiol. 2013;62(24):2261–73.
10. Storey RF, Husted S, Harrington RA, et al. Inhibition of platelet aggregation by AZD6140, a reversible oral P2Y12 receptor antagonist, compared with clopidogrel in patients with acute coronary syndromes. J Am Coll Cardiol. 2007;50:1852–6.
11. Husted S, Emanuelsson H, Heptin- stall S, et al. Pharmacodynamics, pharmacokinetics, and safety of the oral reversible P2Y12 an- tagonist AZD6140 with aspirin in patients with atherosclerosis: a double-blind comparison to clopidogrel with aspirin. Eur Heart J. 2006;27:1038–47.
12. Husted S, James SK, Bach RG, et al. The efficacy of ticagrelor is maintained in women with acute coronary syndromes participating in the prospective, randomized, PLATelet inhibition and patient Outcomes (PLATO) trial.[J]. Eur Heart J. 2014;35(23):541.
13. Li YH, Hsieh IC, Shyu KG, Kuo FY. What could be changed in the 2012 Taiwan ST-segment elevation myocardial infarction guideline? Acta Cardiol Sin. 2014;30(5):360–4.
14. Amsterdam EA, Wenger NK, Brindis RG, et al. 2014 AHA/ACC guideline for the Management of Patients with non-ST-elevation acute coronary syndromes: a report of the American College of Cardiology/American Heart Association task force on practice guidelines. J Am Coll Cardiol. 2014;64(24):e139–228.
15. Bhatt DL, Pare G, Eikelboom JW, et al. The relationship between CYP2C19 polymorphisms and ischaemic and bleeding outcomes in stable outpatients: the CHARISMA genetics study. Eur Heart J. 2012; 33(17):2143–50.
16. Mehta RH, Parsons L, Peterson ED. National Registry of myocardial infarction I. comparison of bleeding and in-hospital mortality in Asian-Americans versus Caucasian-Americans with ST-elevation myocardial infarction receiving reperfusion therapy. Am J Cardiol. 2012;109(7):925–31.
17. Wells GA, Shea B, O'Connell D, et al. The Newcastle-Ottawa Scale (NOS) for assessing the quality of non randomised studies in meta-analyses. Available at: http://www.ohri.ca/programs/clinical_epidemiology/oxford.asp. Accessed December 27, 2013.
18. Jadad AR, Moore RA, Carroll D, et al. Assessing the quality of reports of randomized clinical trials: is blinding necessary? Control Clin Trials 1996; 17(1):1–12.
19. Higgins JP, Thompson SG. Quantifying heterogeneity in a meta-analysis. Stat Med. 2002;21(11):1539–58.
20. Higgins JP, Thompson SG, Deeks JJ, Altman DG. Measuring inconsistency in meta-analyses. BMJ. 2003;327(7414):557–60.
21. Cannon CP, Husted S, Harrington RA, et al. Safety, tolerability, and initial efficacy of AZD6140, the first reversible oral adenosine diphosphate receptor antagonist, compared with clopidogrel, in patients with non-ST-segment elevation acute coronary syndrome: primary results of the DISPERSE-2 trial. J Am Coll Cardiol. 2007;50(19): 1844–51.
22. Cannon CP, Harrington RA, James S, et al. Comparison of ticagrelor with clopidogrel in patients with a planned invasive strategy for acute coronary syndromes (PLATO): a randomised double-blind study. Lancet. 2010; 375(9711):283–93.
23. Bonello L, Laine M, Kipson N, et al. Ticagrelor increases adenosine plasma concentration in patients with an acute coronary syndrome. J Am Coll Cardiol. 2014;63(9):872–7.
24. Hiasa Y, Teng R, Emanuelsson H. Pharmacodynamics, pharmacokinetics and safety of ticagrelor in Asian patients with stable coronary artery disease. Cardiovasc Interv Ther. 2014;29(4):324–33.
25. Goto S, Huang CH, Park SJ, et al. Ticagrelor vs. clopidogrel in Japanese, Korean and Taiwanese patients with acute coronary syndrome -- randomized, double-blind, phase III PHILO study. Circ J. 2015;79(11):2452–60.
26. Wang H, Wang X. Efficacy and safety outcomes of ticagrelor compared with clopidogrel in elderly Chinese patients with acute coronary syndrome. Ther Clin Risk Manag. 2016;12:1101–5.
27. Xiong R, Liu W, Chen L, Kang T, Ning S, Li J. A randomized controlled trial to assess the efficacy and safety of doubling dose clopidogrel versus ticagrelor for the treatment of acute coronary syndrome in patients with CYP2C19*2 homozygotes. Int J Clin Exp Med. 2015;8(8): 13310–6.
28. Chen IC, Lee CH, Fang CC, et al. Efficacy and safety of ticagrelor versus clopidogrel in acute coronary syndrome in Taiwan: a multicenter retrospective pilot study. J Chin Med Assoc. 2016;79(10):521–30.
29. Lee CH, Cheng CL, Kao Yang YH, Chao TH, Chen JY, Li YH. Cardiovascular and bleeding risks in acute myocardial infarction newly treated with Ticagrelor vs. Clopidogrel in Taiwan. Circ J. 2018;82(3):747–56.
30. Levine GN, Bates ER, Blankenship JC, et al. 2015 ACC/AHA/SCAI focused update on primary percutaneous coronary intervention for patients with ST-

elevation myocardial infarction: an update of the 2011 ACCF/AHA/SCAI guideline for percutaneous coronary intervention and the 2013 ACCF/AHA guideline for the management of ST-elevation myocardial infarction. J Am Coll Cardiol. 2016;67(10):1235–50.

31. Schomig A. Ticagrelor--is there need for a new player in the antiplatelet-therapy field? N Engl J Med. 2009;361(11):1108–11.
32. Wallentin L, Varenhorst C, James S, Erlinge D, Braun OO, Jakubowski JA, et al. Prasugrel achieves greater and faster P2Y12 receptor-mediated platelet inhibition than clopidogrel due to more efficient generation of its active metabolite in aspirin-treated patients with coronary artery disease. Eur Heart J. 2008;29:21–30.
33. Becker RC, Bassand JP, Budaj A, et al. Bleeding complications with the P2Y12 receptor antagonists clopidogrel and ticagrelor in the PLATelet inhibition and patient outcomes (PLATO) trial. Eur Heart J. 2011;32(23):2933–44.
34. Breet NJ, van Werkum JW, Bouman HJ, et al. Comparison of platelet function tests in predicting clinical outcome in patients undergoing coronary stent implantation. JAMA. 2010;303(8):754–62.
35. Wang TY, Chen AY, Roe MT, et al. Comparison of baseline characteristics, treatment patterns, and in-hospital outcomes of Asian versus non-Asian white Americans with non-ST-segment elevation acute coronary syndromes from the CRUSADE quality improvement initiative. Am J Cardiol. 2007; 100(3):391–6.
36. Levine GN, Jeong YH, Goto S, et al. Expert consensus document: world heart federation expert consensus statement on antiplatelet therapy in east Asian patients with ACS or undergoing PCI. Nat Rev Cardiol. 2014;11(10): 597–606.
37. Chiang CE, Zhang S, Tse HF, Teo WS, Omar R, Sriratanasathavorn C. Atrial fibrillation management in Asia: from the Asian expert forum on atrial fibrillation. Int J Cardiol. 2013;164(1):21–32.
38. Chiang CE, Wang KL, Lip GYH. Stroke prevention in atrial fibrillation: an Asian perspective. Thromb Haemost. 2014;111:789–97.
39. Wallentin L, James S, Storey RF, et al. Effect of CYP2C19 and ABCB1 single nucleotide polymorphisms on outcomes of treatment with ticagrelor versus clopidogrel for acute coronary syndromes: a genetic substudy of the PLATO trial. Lancet. 2010;376(9749):1320–8.
40. Kang HJ, Clare RM, Gao R, et al. Ticagrelor versus clopidogrel in Asian patients with acute coronary syndrome: a retrospective analysis from the platelet inhibition and patient outcomes (PLATO) trial. Am Heart J. 2015; 169(6):899–905 e1.
41. Steg PG, Huber K, Andreotti F, et al. Bleeding in acute coronary syndromes and percutaneous coronary interventions: position paper by the working group on thrombosis of the European Society of Cardiology. Eur Heart J. 2011;32:1854–64.
42. Eagle KA, Lim MJ, Dabbous OH, et al. A validated prediction model for all forms of acute coronary syndrome: estimating the risk of 6-month postdischarge death in an international registry. JAMA. 2004;291(22): 2727–33.
43. Granger CB, Goldberg RJ, Dabbous O, et al. Predictors of hospital mortality in the global registry of acute coronary events. Arch Intern Med. 2003; 163(19):2345–53.
44. Lopes RD, Alexander KP. Antiplatelet therapy in older adults with non-ST-segment elevation acute coronary syndrome: considering risks and benefits. Am J Cardiol. 2009;104(5 Suppl):16C–21C.
45. Newby LK. Acute coronary syndromes in the elderly. J Cardiovasc Med (Hagerstown). 2011;12(3):220–2.
46. Belchikov YG, Koenig SJ, Dipasquale EM. Potential role of endogenous adenosine in ticagrelor-induced dyspnea. Pharmacotherapy. 2013; 33(8):882–7.
47. Cattaneo M, Schulz R, Nylander S. Adenosine-mediated effects of ticagrelor: evidence and potential clinical relevance. J Am Coll Cardiol. 2014;63(23):2503–9.
48. Cattaneo M, Faioni EM. Why does ticagrelor induce dyspnea? Thromb Haemost. 2012;108(6):1031–6.

miR-941 as a promising biomarker for acute coronary syndrome

Fuina Bai, Qiaoning Yang, Ruixi Xi, Lizhi Li, Dazhuo Shi* and Keji Chen

Abstract

Background: Circulating miRNAs can function as biomarkers for diagnosis, treatment, and prevention of diseases. However, it is unclear whether miRNAs can be used as biomarkers for acute coronary syndrome (ACS). To this end, we applied gene chip technology to analyze miRNA expression in patients with stable angina (SA), non-ST elevation ACS (NSTE-ACS), and ST-segment elevation myocardial infarction (STEMI).

Methods: We enrolled patients with chest pain who underwent diagnostic coronary angiography, including five patients each with SA, NSTE-ACS, or STEMI, and five controls without coronary artery disease (CAD) but with three or more risk factors. After microarray analysis, differential miRNA expression was confirmed by quantitative real-time reverse transcription polymerase chain reaction (qRT-PCR).

Results: Compared with those in patients with STEMI, differentially expressed microRNAs in controls and patients with SA or NSTE-ACS were involved in inflammation, protein phosphorylation, and cell adhesion. Pathway analysis showed that differentially expressed miRNAs were related to the mitogen-activated protein kinase signaling, calcium ion pathways, and cell adhesion pathways. Compared with their expression levels in patients with STEMI, *miR-941*, *miR-363-3p*, and *miR-182-5p* were significantly up-regulated (fold-change: 2.0 or more, $P < 0.05$) in controls and patients with SA or NSTE-ACS. Further, qRT-PCR showed that plasma *miR-941* level was elevated in patients with NSTE-ACS or STEMI as compared with that in patients without CAD (fold-change: 1.65 and 2.28, respectively; $P < 0.05$). Additionally, *miR-941* expression was significantly elevated in the STEMI group compared with that in the SA ($P < 0.01$) and NSTE-ACS groups ($P < 0.05$). Similarly, *miR-941* expression was higher in patients with ACS (NSTE-ACS or STEMI) than in patients without ACS (without CAD or with SA; $P < 0.01$). There were no significant differences in *miR-182-5p* and *miR-363-3p* expression. The areas under the receiver operating characteristic curves were 0.896, 0.808, and 0.781 for patients in the control, SA, and NSTE-ACS groups, respectively, compared with that for patients with STEMI; that for the ACS group compared with the non-ACS group was 0.734.

Conclusion: *miR-941* expression was relatively higher in patients with ACS and STEMI. Thus, *miR-941* may be a potential biomarker of ACS or STEMI.

Keywords: microRNA, Stable angina, Acute ST-segment elevation myocardial infarction, Acute coronary artery disease

Background

Acute coronary syndrome (ACS) is a major cause of death and disability [1]. Rapid antiplatelet therapy and revascularization could prevent myocardial ischemia and reduce the incidence of cardiovascular events [2]. Thus, the early diagnosis of non-ST elevation ACS (NSTE-ACS) and ST-segment elevation myocardial infarction (STEMI) is essential for improved prognoses. Currently, the clinical diagnosis of ACS relies on assessment of symptoms, ischemia changes in electrocardiogram (ECG), and changes in troponin [2]. However, in elderly individuals and patients with diabetes, typical symptoms are not always observed. Moreover, changes in ECG can be easily influenced by left bundle branch blockage and chronic myocardial infarction. To a certain extent, unstable angina pectoris (UA), non-STEMI (NSTEMI), and STEMI reflect the pathological progress of ACS. Therefore, identification of novel

* Correspondence: shidztcm@163.com
Xiyuan Hospital, China Academy of Chinese Medical Sciences, 1 Xiyuan Caochang, Haidian district, Beijing, China

biomarkers may facilitate the early diagnosis of ACS, particularly in patients with atypical symptoms of ACS.

MicroRNAs (miRNAs) are endogenous, small (22–24-nucleotide) noncoding RNA molecules that regulate the expression of mRNA by combining with the 3′- untranslated region (3′-UTR), subsequently triggering the degradation of mRNA or having negative effects on transcription [3]. miRNAs can regulate nearly 60% of coding genes to exert their biological functions [4, 5]. Recently, many studies have shown that miRNAs can regulate endothelial dysfunction, inflammation, cell autophagy, platelet activation, and aggregation [6–9]. Moreover, miRNA expression can affect the stability of atherosclerotic plaques [10]. miRNAs possess tissue-specific expression and can be secreted into blood or urine.miRNAs of circulartory system can be used as biomarkers of diagnosis, treatment, and prevention of diseases, such as coronary heart disease [11–14]. However, it is still unclear whether miRNAs can be used as biomarkers of ACS and further evaluate the severity of ACS [15].

Therefore, in this study, we applied gene chip technology to analyze the expression of miRNAs in patients with stable angina (SA), NSTE-ACS, and STEMI. We then performed quantitative real-time reverse transcription polymerase chain reaction (qRT-PCR) to determine whether miRNAs could be used as biomarker for the diagnosis of ACS.

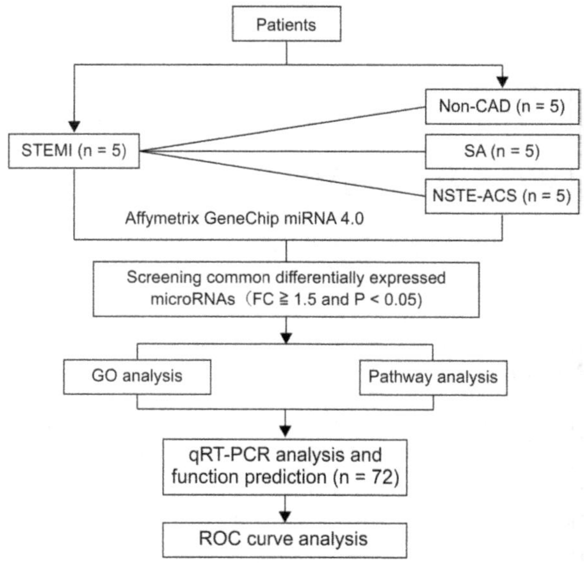

Fig. 1 Schematic of the study design

Methods

Patients and study design

A total of 72 patients with chest pain who underwent diagnostic coronary angiography in Xiyuan Hospital, affiliated hospital of China Academy of Chinese Medical Sciences were enrolled from March 2015 to July 2015. The patients were divided into four groups as follows: 18 patients with STEMI, 18 patients NSTE-ACS, 20 patients with SA, and 16 patients without CAD. Patients in the control group did not have coronary stenosis as confirmed by coronary angiography, but had three or more risk factors for coronary heart disease (see schematic of the study in Fig. 1). Five cases were randomly selected from each group for analysis of gene expression profiles, using an Affymetrix GeneChip miRNA4.0. The differential expression of miRNAs between groups was analyzed according to the following criteria: fold-change (FC), ≥ 1.5 and $P < 0.05$. qRT-PCR was applied to verify the differential expression of miRNAs (FC, ≥ 2; $P < 0.05$). This study was registered in the Chinese Clinical Trial Registry (no. ChiCTR-IPR- 15006336). The study was performed according to the guidelines of the Declaration of Helsinki and was approved by the Xiyuan Hospital Ethics Committee.

Diagnostic criteria

In this study, patients with coronary heart disease were classified as having SA or ACS, including STEMI, NSTE-ACS, and UA. Diagnostic criteria was refered to the 2014 ACC/AHA/AATS/PCNA/SCAI/STS Focused Update of the Guideline for the Diagnosis and Management of Patients With Stable Ischemic Heart Disease [16], 2014 AHA/ACC Guideline for the Management of Patients with Non-ST-Elevation Acute Coronary Syndromes [2], and 2013 ACCF/AHA Guideline for the Management of ST-elevation Myocardial Infarction [17]. In addition, all patients presented stenosis (≥ 50% in at least one main coronary artery) as confirmed by coronary angiography [18].

Inclusion and exclusion criteria

The inclusion criteria were as follows: patients who met the diagnostic criteria, were 35–75 years old, and provided informed consent. The exclusion criteria were as follows: Patients with combined diseases, such as cardiomyopathy, valvular heart disease, severe arrhythmia, heart failure, and other accompanying diseases; patients encountered challenges with data collection, such as religious or language barriers; patients were pregnant or lactating and participating in other clinical studies.

Blood collection and storage

Venous blood samples were collected via antecubital venipuncture from each subject within 3–5 h of the onset of symptoms but before arteriography. Whole blood samples (2 mL) were collected directly into EDTA-containing tubes (BD, Franklin Lakes, NJ, USA), and three volumes of red blood cell lysis buffer (NH4CL2009; Haoyang, Tianjin, China) was added to obtain leukocytes, which were isolated within 2 h by centrifugation at 3000 rpm for 5 min at 4 °C to remove other blood elements. Next, 1 mL TRIzol (15596–026; Invitrogen Life Technologies) was added, and samples were then transferred to RNase/Dnase-free tubes and stored at −80 °C.

RNA isolation and preparation

After collection of all samples, total RNA in leukocytes was isolated using a miRVana RNA Isolation Kit (p/n AM1556; Applied Biosystems, Foster City, CA, USA) according to the manufacturer's specifications. Samples were then subjected to on-column DNase I treatment with RNase-free Dnase (#79254; Qiagen, Valencia, CA, USA). RNA quantity and quality were determined using a NanoDrop 2000 spectrophotometer (Thermo Scientific, USA) and an Agilent 2100 bioanalyzer. The RNA integrity was evaluated by agarose gel electrophoresis with ethidium bromide staining.

miRNA array analysis

Microarray analysis of gene expression was carried out using ELOSA QC Assays prior to array hybridization. Sample labeling, microarray hybridization, and washing were performed based on the manufacturer's standard protocols. Briefly, total RNA was modified with poly A tails and then labeled with biotin. Next, the labeled RNAs were hybridized onto the microarray. Slides were washed and stained, and the arrays were scanned using an Affymetrix Scanner 3000 (Affymetrix).

miRNA microarray analysis was performed to determine differential expression of blood-borne miRNAs among (i) non-CAD individuals and patients with STEMI (n = 5), (ii) patients with SA and STEMI (n = 5), and (iii) patients with NSTE-ACS and STEMI. Bioinformatic determination of downstream predicted targets for candidate miRNAs was performed as described previously by Selbach et al. [19].

Reverse transcription quantitative real-time polymerase chain reaction (RT-qPCR) analysis

Quantification was performed through two-step reaction process: reverse transcription (RT) and qPCR. Each RT reaction consisted of 1 μg RNA, 4 μL miScript HiSpec Buffer, 2 μL Nucleics Mix, and 2 μL miScript Reverse Transcriptase Mix (Qiagen, Germany), in a total volume of 20 μl. Reactions were performed in a GeneAmp PCR System 9700 (Applied Biosystems, USA) for 60 min at 37 °C, followed by heat inactivation of the reverse transcriptase for 5 min at 95 °C. The 20-μL reaction mix was then diluted 5-fold in nuclease-free water and stored at −20 °C.

Real-time PCR was performed using a LightCycler 480II Real-time PCR Instrument (Roche, Switzerland) with 10 μL of the reaction mixture including 1 μL cDNA, 5 μL 2× LightCycler 480 SYBR Green I Master (Roche), 0.2 μL universal primers (Qiagen), 0.2 μL miRNA-specific primer, and 3.6 μL nuclease-free water. Reactions were incubated in a 384-well optical plate (Roche) at 95 °C for 10 min, followed by 40 cycles of 95 °C for 10 s and 60 °C for 30 s. Triplicates were averaged to calculate the expression value for each sample. At the end of the PCR cycling, melt curve analysis was performed to validate the specific generation of the expected PCR product. miRNA-specific primer sequences were designed in the laboratory and synthesized by Generay Biotech (Generay, PRC) based on the miRNA sequences obtained from the miRBase database (Release 20.0) as follows: *hsa-miR-182-5p*, UUUGGCAAUGGUAGAACUCACACU; *hsa-miR-363-3p*, AAUUGCACGGUAUCCAUCUGUA; and *hsa-miR-941*, CACCCGGCUGUGUGCACAUGUGC).

The expression levels of miRNAs were normalized to U6 and were calculated by the $2^{-\Delta\Delta Ct}$ method [20].

Statistical analysis

Affymetrix GeneChip Command Console software (version4.0, Affymetrix) was used to analyze array images to obtain raw data, and RMA normalization was then carried out. Next, Genespring software (version 12.5, Agilent Technologies) was used for subsequent data analysis. Differentially expressed miRNAs were then identified through fold changes, and P-values were calculated using t-tests. The threshold set for up- and downregulated genes was a fold change of 1.5 or more and a P value of less than 0.05. Target genes of differentially expressed miRNAs were the intersection predicted with three databases (Targetscan, PITA, and microRNAorg). Gene ontology (GO) analysis and KEGG analysis were applied to determine the roles of these target genes. Hierarchical clustering was performed to show distinguishable miRNA expression patterns among samples.

Paired and unpaired Student's t tests were performed to compare data as appropriate. Values are expressed as means ± standard deviations (SDs). P values of less than 0.05 (two-sided) were considered significant.

Results

Patient clinicopathological information

Seventy-two patients (18 patients with STEMI, 18 patients with NSTE-ACS, 20 patients with SA, and 16 patients without CAD) were enrolled in this study. The clinicopathological characteristics of the patients are presented in Tables 1 and 2. There were no significant differences in clinical features among groups ($P > 0.05$).

miRNA array analysis

The differential expression of miRNAs among the patient groups was determined by gene chip analysis. The results showed that there exist 13 differentially expressed miRNAs in patients with STEMI comparing with those in patients without CAD and patients with SA and NSTE-ACS. After that, we chose *miR-941*, *miR-363-3p*, and *miR-182-5p* (FC,≥ 2.0; $P < 0.05$) for further analysis by qRT-PCR (Table 3).

Table 1 Baseline clinical characteristics of different patient groups used in microarray analysis

Variable	CAD (*n* = 15)			Without CAD (*n* = 5)
	SA (*n* = 5)	NSTE-ACS (*n* = 5)	STEMI (*n* = 5)	
Age (years, mean ± SD)	55.8 ± 4.15	57.4 ± 11.19	52.8 ± 10.56	52.4 ± 13.28
Sex (male, n)	5	5	5	5
Risk factors (n)				
Hypertension	4	4	2	3
Dyslipidemia	5	3	4	3
Active smoker	4	3	5	1
Medications (*n*)				
Antiplatelet agents	5	5	5	0
β-Blockers	4	3	3	0
CCB	2	1	1	1
ACEI/ARB	4	4	4	2
Statins	5	5	5	1

Abbreviations: *SA* stable angina, *NSTE-ACS* non-ST elevation acute coronary syndrome, *STEMI* ST elevation myocardial infarction, *DM* diabetes mellitus, *CCB* calcium channel blocker, *ACEI* angiotensin-converting enzyme inhibitor, *ARB* angiotensin receptor blocker

Gene ontology (GO) analysis

Differentially expressed miRNAs in patients without CAD and with SA or NSTE-ACS (compared with that in patients with STEMI) were found to be involved in inflammation, protein phosphorylation, RNA polymerase II-dependent transcription, cell adhesion, and other biological processes. Among these, inflammation, cell adhesion, T-cell proliferation, calcium transfer, and apoptosis were closely related to atherosclerosis (Fig. 2).

Table 2 Baseline clinical characteristics of different patient groups used in qRT-PCR analysis

Variable	CAD (*n* = 56)			Without CAD (*n* = 16)
	SA (*n* = 20)	NSTE-ACS (*n* = 18)	STEMI (*n* = 18)	
Age (years, mean ± SD)	55.8 ± 9.15	56.44 ± 8.78	53.50 ± 10.56	52.5 ± 13.50
Sex (male, n)	12	15	16	9
Risk factors (n)				
Hypertension	14	15	13	11
Dyslipidemia	12	13	11	8
DM	9	10	9	7
Active smoker	12	15	14	8
Medications (n)				
Antiplatelet agents	12	16	18	0
β-Blockers	13	11	9	9
Statins	18	16	12	8

Abbreviations: *SA* stable angina, *NSTE-ACS* non-ST elevation acute coronary syndrome, *STEMI* ST elevation myocardial infarction, *DM* diabetes mellitus, *CCB* calcium channel blocker, *ACEI* angiotensin-converting enzyme inhibitor, *ARB* angiotensin receptor blocker

Pathway analysis

The KEGG database was used to analyze target genes of differentially expressed miRNAs. Differentially expressed miRNAs in control and in patients with SA or NSTE-ACS compared with that in patients with STEMI were found to regulate biological processes such as mitogen-activated protein kinase (MAPK) signaling, tumorigenesis, and calcium ion signaling. Among the identified cell signaling pathways, we identified the following pathways involved in the pathological process of atherosclerosis: adhesion molecules, ErbB signaling, metabolism, Wnt signaling, insulin signaling, apoptosis, vascular endothelial growth factor signaling, and cell factor receptor interactions (Fig. 3).

miRNA-pathway network analysis showed that *miR-941* can participate in regulation of T-cell receptor signaling, insulin signaling, and MAPK signaling. Additionally, *miR-182-5p* was related to vascular smooth muscle cell constriction and mammalian target of rapamycin (mTOR) signaling. *miR-363-3p* was involved in Toll-like receptor signaling and actin cytoskeleton regulation. Bioinformatics functional predictions showed that the differential expressed miRNAs could be related to the pathological process of cardiovascular disease (Fig. 4).

qRT-PCR

Next, we performed qRT-PCR to verify the different expression of candidated gene like, *miR-941*, *miR-182-5p*, and *miR-363-3p*.The results showed that *miR-941* expression has no significant difference between the control patients (without CAD) and SA group. However, comparing with control patients, *miR-941* expression was significantly increased by 1.64- and 2.28-fold in patients with NSTE-ACS and STEMI, respectively, ($P < 0.05$; Fig. 5a). There were no significant differences in *miR-182-5p* and *miR-363-3p* among groups ($P > 0.05$; Fig. 5b and c). Additionally, the expression of *miR-941* was increased by 1.66-fold in patients with STEMI compared with that in patients with SA ($P < 0.001$; Fig. 6a-1) and by 1.52-fold in patients with STEMI compared with that in patients with NSTE-ACS ($P < 0.05$; Fig. 6a-2). There were no significant differences in *miR-182-5p* and *miR-363-3p* ($P > 0.05$; Fig. 6b and c).

Since there were no significant differences in *miR-941* expression between patients without CAD and patients with SA, we combined the two groups into the non-ACS group. Compared with that in the non-ACS group, the expression of *miR-941* was upregulated in the ACS group (FC: 1.62; $P < 0.01$; Fig. 7). NSTE-ACS and

Table 3 Differentially expressed miRNAs in patients with ACS versus patients without CAD and patients with SA or NSTE-ACS in microarray analysis

miRNAs	STEMI versus without CAD			STEMI versus SA			STEMI versus NSTE-ACS		
	Fold change	*P* value	Regulation	Fold change	*P* value	Regulation	Fold change	*P* value	Regulation
miR-941	5.305	0.007	Up	4.544	0.003	Up	5.032	0.002	Up
miR-182-5p	2.331	0.013	Down	2.005	0.042	Down	2.121	0.024	Up
miR-363-3p	2.012	0.007	Down	2.016	0.018	Down	2.071	0.048	Up
hsa-mir-941-1	1.895	0.036	Up	2.051	0.001	Up	2.008	0.001	Up
hsa-mir-941-2	1.895	0.036	Up	2.051	0.001	Up	2.008	0.001	Up
hsa-mir-941-3	1.895	0.036	Up	2.051	0.001	Up	2.008	0.001	Up
hsa-mir-941-4	1.895	0.036	Up	2.051	0.001	Up	2.008	0.001	Up
hsa-miR-6798-5p	2.049	0.015	Up	1.866	0.019	Up	2.041	4.32E-04	Up
hsa-miR-4419a	1.737	0.013	Up	1.717	0.006	Up	1.851	9.32E-05	Up
hsa-miR-296-3p	1.811	0.031	Up	2.209	0.012	Up	1.726	0.109	Up
hsa-miR-1227-5p	1.549	0.013	Up	1.629	0.039	Up	1.653	0.147	Up
hsa-miR-4656	1.908	0.005	Up	1.617	0.025	Up	1.232	0.459	Up
hsa-miR-3064-3p	1.765	0.037	Down	1.529	0.001	Down	1.033	0.738	Down

Abbreviations: *SA* stable angina, *NSTE-ACS* non-ST segment elevation acute coronary syndrome, *STEMI* ST segment elevation acute myocardial infarction

STEMI can reflect the degree of disease progression, and *miR-941* was significantly upregulated in patients with STEMI compared with that in patients in the non-ACS group (FC: 1.52; $P < 0.05$; Fig. 6a-2). The differential expression of *miR-941* in the two groups showed that the expression of *miR-941* was associated with the severity of ACS.

Receiver operating characteristic (ROC) curve analysis

Next, we performed ROC curve analysis to test the reliability of *miR-941* as a diagnostic biomarker of STEMI and ACS. Comparing with patients with STEMI, areas under the ROC curves were 0.896, 0.808, and 0.781 for patients in the control, SA, and NSTE-ACS groups, respectively; Comparing with patients in ACS group,the

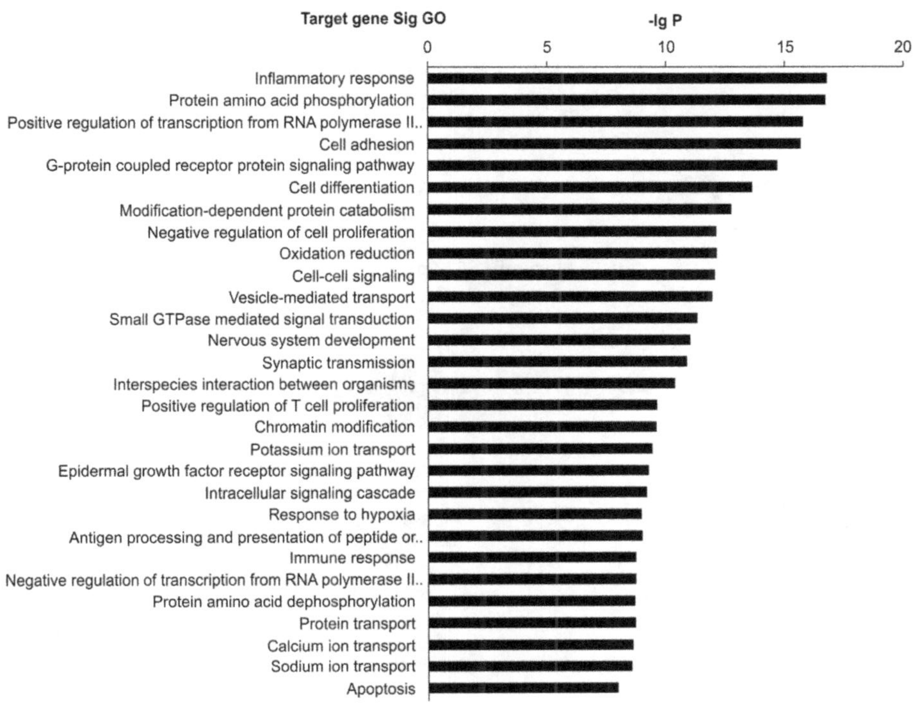

Fig. 2 Gene ontology (GO) analysis

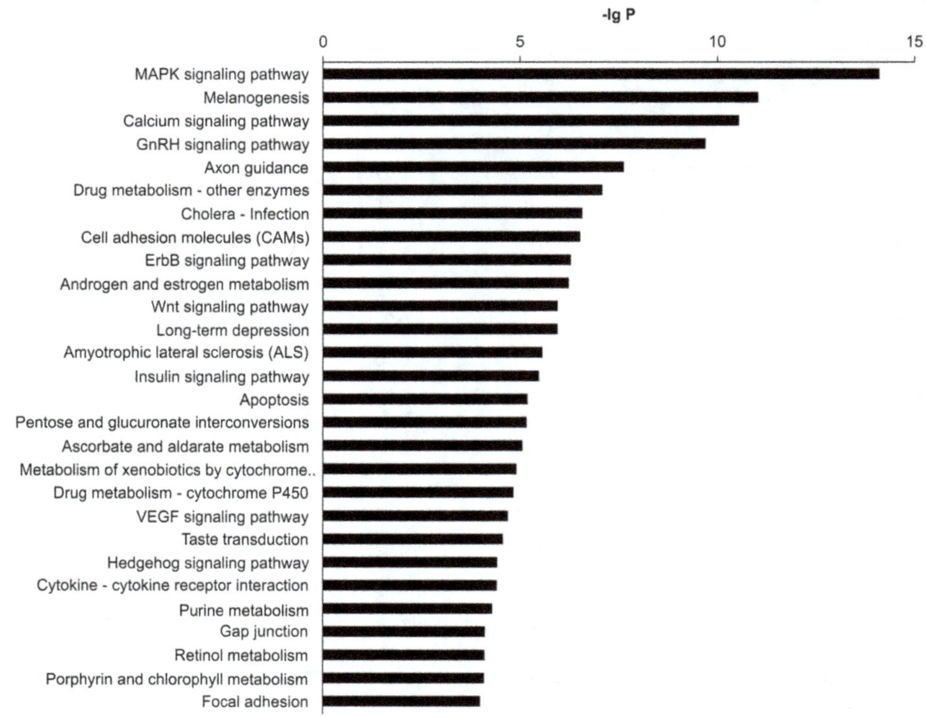

Fig. 3 Pathway analysis

ROC curves of non-ACS group was 0.734 (Fig. 8). Thus, *miR-941* may act as a reliable biomarker of ACS, particularly STEMI. The area under the curve (AUC), 95% confidence intervals (CIs), and *p* values are summarized in Table 4.

Discussion

Aberrant miRNA expression has been involved with a number of human diseases, including cardiovascular diseases [11, 21–23]. ACS has become a major public health problem owing to its high mortality and

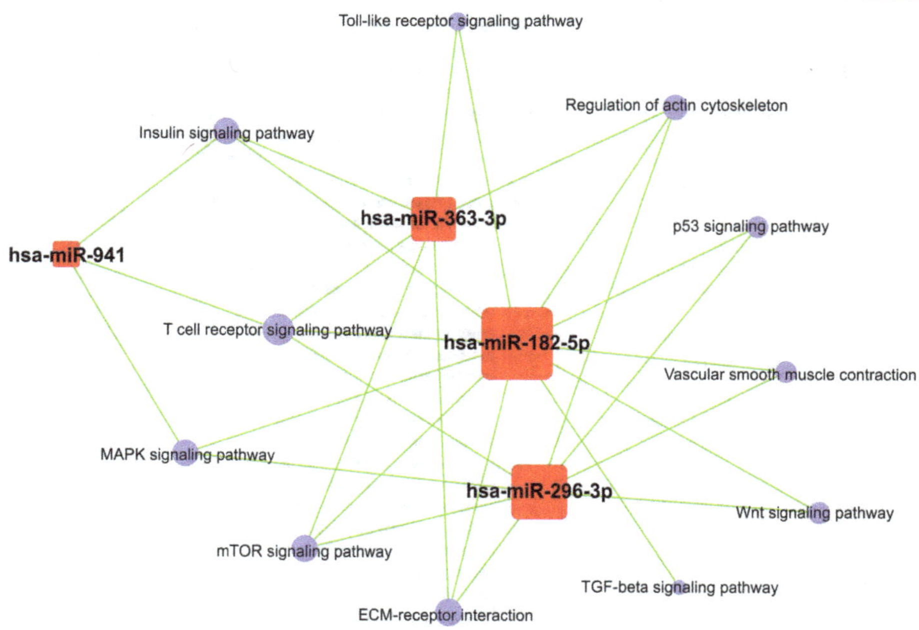

Fig. 4 Microarray pathway network. The red rectangles are miRNAs, the purple circle are pathways, and the green lines represented the regulatory connections between miRNAs and pathways

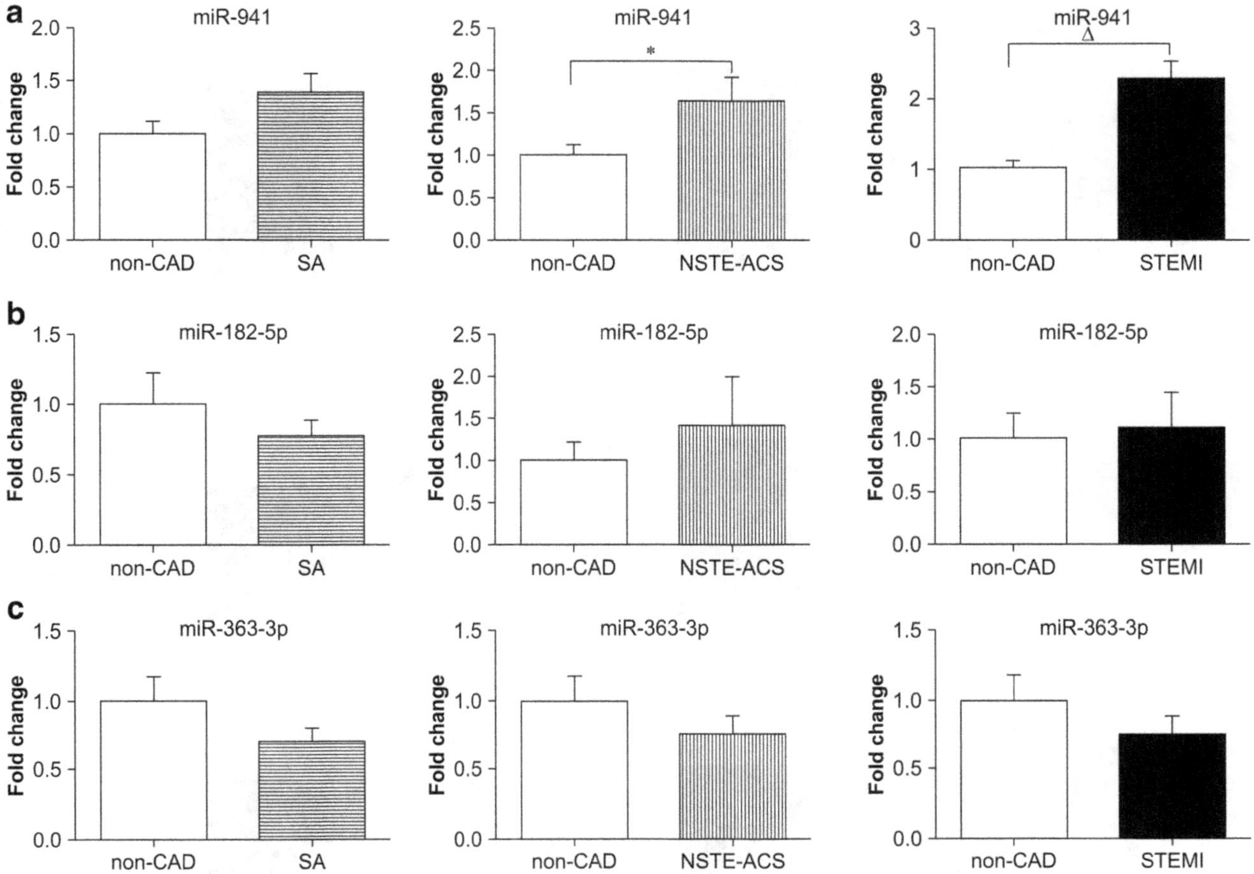

Fig. 5 Expression profiles of candidate miRNAs in patients with and without CAD. The three candidate miRNAs were evaluated with qRT-PCR using 72 samples, including 16 non-CAD, 20 SA, 18 NSTE-ACS, and 18 STEMI samples. *miR-941* was significantly upregulated in the SA, NSTE-ACS, and STEMI groups compared with that in non-CAD patients (**a**). *miR-182-5p* (**b**) and *miR-363-3p* (**c**) were not significantly different in patients with CAD (SA, NSTE-ACS, and STEMI) compared with that in patients without CAD. Abbreviations: CAD: coronary artery disease, SA: stable angina, NSTE-ACS: non-ST elevation acute coronary syndromes, STEMI: ST elevation myocardial infarction. $^{*}P < 0.05$, $^{\Delta}P < 0.001$

morbidity [24–26]. Thus, there is an urgent need to identify new diagnostic and therapeutic biomarkers of ACS; miRNAs may have such applications.

MiRNAs are involved in endothelial dysfunction, inflammation, apoptosis, angiogenesis, atherosclerosis, and other pathological processes involved in cardiovascular diseases [6, 27, 28], and miRNAs of circulartory system may be potential biomarkers of these diseases [7, 29]. *miR-135a*, *miR-31*, *miR-378*, and *miR-147* are biological markers of stable coronary heart disease [30]; *miR-1*, *miR-126*, and *miR-133a* have potential value in the diagnosis of UA [31]; and *miR-208b*, *miR-499*, and *miR-1* play a key role in the diagnosis, progression, and prognosis of acute myocardial infarction (AMI) [15, 32–34]. However, it is unclear whether miRNAs are differentially expressed with changes in the severity of coronary heart disease, including coronary stenosis and myocardial damage. Our findings suggested that *miR-363-3p*, *miR-941*, and *miR-182-5p* were differentially expressed among groups of patients with various types and degrees of coronary heart disease. Additionally, GO and KEGG pathway analysis showed that the differentially expressed miRNAs were involved in inflammatory responses, immune responses, MAPK signal, calcium pathway, ErbB signaling, and other cellular processes. In particular, MAPK signaling and immune responses are involved in the pathogenesis of atherosclerosis and affect the stability of plaques and the formation of blood clots. Furthermore, qRT-PCR analysis verified that *miR-941* was differentially expressed in plasma from patients with CADs (SA, NSTE-ACS, and STEMI) compared with that in patients without CAD. Thus, these data suggested that *miR-941* may have applications as a biomarker of CAD, with the ability to distinguish among ACS and non-ACS groups and to distinguish STEMI from SA and NSTE-ACS. Notably, *miR-941* was gradually upregulated as the degree of coronary artery stenosis and myocardial injury increased (SA < NSTE-ACS < STEMI); thus, *miR-941* was closely associated with the severity of ACS. Accordingly, we concluded that *miR-941* was a

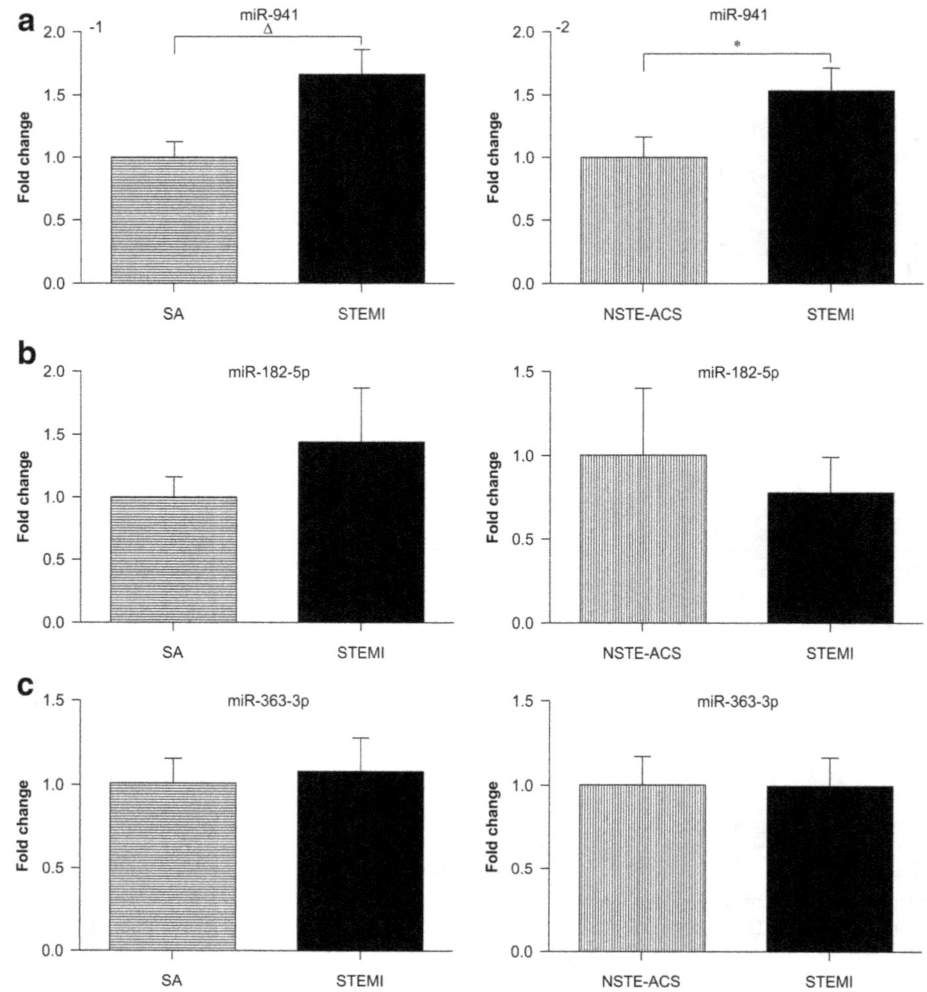

Fig. 6 Expression profiles of candidate miRNAs in patients with SA, NSTE-ACS, and STEMI. The three candidate miRNAs were evaluated by qRT-PCR using 56 samples (20 cases of SA, 18 cases of NSTE-ACS, and 18 cases of STEMI). (**a**) *miR-941*, (**b**) *miR-182-5p*, and (**c**) *miR-363-3p* are shown. Abbreviations: CAD, coronary artery disease; SA, stable angina; NSTE-ACS, non-ST elevation acute coronary syndrome; STEMI, ST elevation myocardial infarction. $^{*}P < 0.05$, $^{\Delta}P < 0.001$

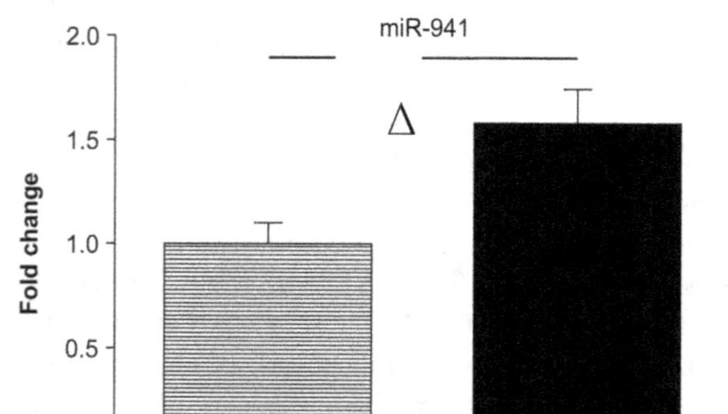

Fig. 7 Expression profiles of *miR-941* in patients with and without ACS. *miR-941* expression was evaluated by qRT-PCR using 72 samples (36 patients without ACS and 36 patients with ACS). Abbreviations: ACS, acute coronary syndrome. $^{\Delta}P < 0.01$

biomarker of ACS, particularly for STEMI, and could predict the severity and progression of coronary heart disease.

Recent bioinformatics analyses have shown that *miR-941* is involved in Wnt signaling, transforming growth factor (TGF)-β signaling, and insulin signaling [35, 36]. However, no research has been reported the role of *miR-941* in atherosclerosis and coronary heart disease. In our study, we found that *miR-941* may be associated with metabolism, inflammation, cell proliferation, and other biological processes through regulation of components involved in insulin signaling, MAPK signaling, T-cell receptor signaling, and other related pathways. However, we were not able to confirm the direct relationship between *miR-941* and the pathogenesis of atherosclerosis. In vitro and in vivo experiments are needed to clarify the biological function of *miR-941* in the pathophysiology of atherosclerosis and to determine

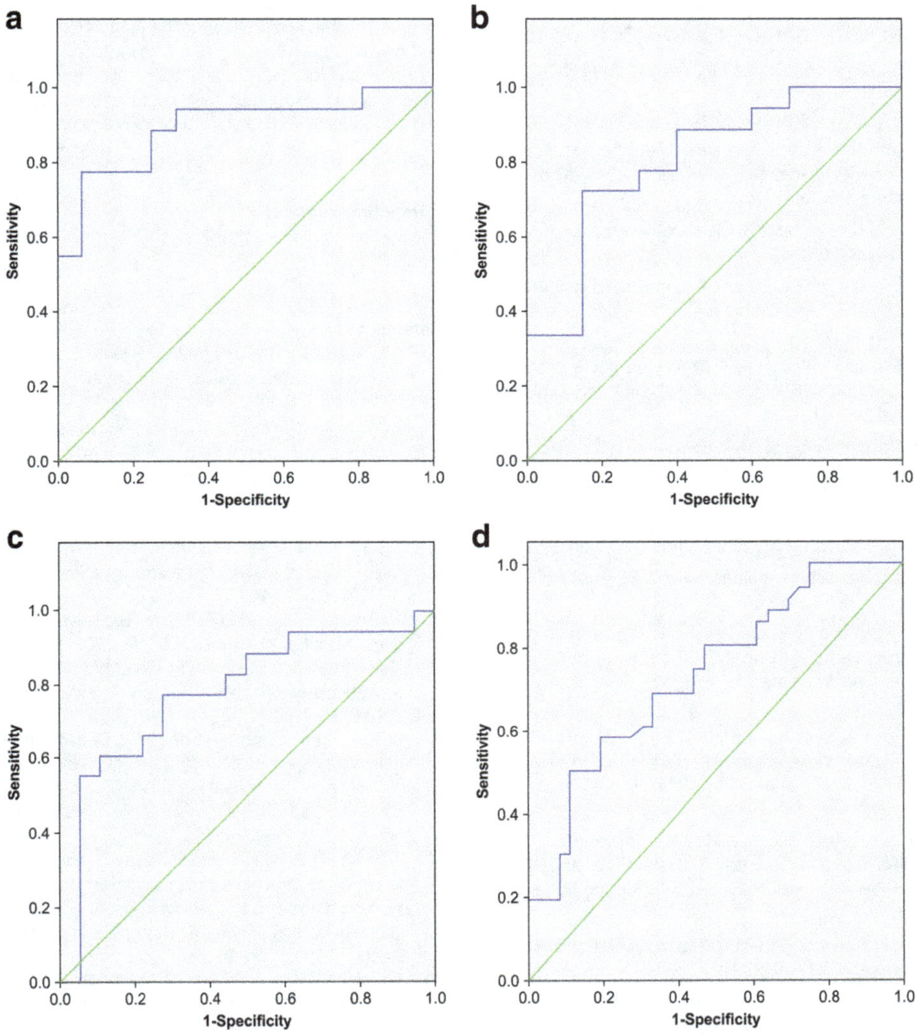

Fig. 8 ROC curve analysis. **a** Expression profiles of *miR-941* in patients with STEMI and without CAD. **b** Expression profiles of *miR-941* in patients with STEMI and SA. **c** Expression profiles of *miR-941* in patients with STEMI and NSTE-ACS. **d** Expression profiles of *miR-941* in patients with and without ACS

whether *miR-941* is involved in pathological processes of inflammation, immunity, metabolism, and platelet activation. Although we found that *miR-941* was differentially expressed between ACS and non-ACS groups, additional studies are needed to establish a rapid, inexpensive method for miRNA analysis. Additionally, greater sample sizes are needed to further confirm the potential applications of this miRNA as a promising diagnostic tool for diagnosis of ACS.

Table 4 ROC curve analysis of *miR-941* expression in patients with ACS and STEMI

miR-941	AUC	95% CI	*P* value
Non-ACS versus ACS	0.734	0.619–0.848	0.001
Without CAD versus STEMI	0.896	0.779–1.000	0.000
SA versus STEMI	0.808	0.670–0.947	0.001
NSTE-ACS versus STEMI	0.781	0.622–0.939	0.004

Abbreviations: *SA* stable angina, *ACS* acute coronary syndrome, *NSTE-ACS* non-ST segment elevation acute coronary syndrome, *STEMI* ST segment elevation acute myocardial infarction, *CAD* coronary artery disease, *ROC* receiver operating characteristic, *AUC* area under the curve

Conclusions

MiR-941 was relatively higher in patients with ACS and STEMI, and could predict the severity and progression of coronary heart disease. Thus, *miR-941* may be a potential biomarker of ACS or STEMI.

Additional files

Additional file 1: The mass detection report of samples. (DOCX 136 kb)

Additional file 1: Baseline Table 1:Original data of Baseline clinical characteristics of different groups used in microarray analysis. (XLSX 10 kb)

Additional file 3: Baseline Table 2:Original data of Baseline clinical characteristics of different groups used in qRT-PCR analysis. (XLSX 11 kb)

Additional file 4: MiRNA-gene-network and miRNA-targets-relation. (XLSX 382 kb)

Additional file 5: Microarray pathway network: Pathway-miRNA-relation and microarray pathway network. The red rectangles are miRNAs, the purple circle are pathways, and the green lines represented the regulatory connections between miRNAs and pathways. (XLSX 137 kb)

Additional file 6: Original data of Table 3: Differentially expressed miRNAs in microarray analysis. (XLSX 19 kb)

Additional file 7: Original data of Fig. 5a: MiR-941 was significantly upregulated in the SA, NSTE-ACS, and STEMI groups compared with that in non-CAD patients. (XLSX 14 kb)

Additional file 8: Original data of Fig. 5b: MiR-182-5p were not significantly different in patients with CAD (SA, NSTE-ACS, and STEMI) compared with that in patients without CAD. (XLSX 17 kb)

Additional file 9: Original data of Fig. 5c: MiR-363-3p were not significantly different in patients with CAD (SA, NSTE-ACS, and STEMI) compared with that in patients without CAD. (XLSX 17 kb)

Additional file 10: Original data of Fig. 6a-1: MiR-941 Expression profiles of candidate miRNAs in patients with SA, NSTE-ACS, and STEMI. The three candidate miRNAs were evaluated by qRT-PCR using 56 samples. (XLSX 13 kb)

Additional file 11: Original data of Fig. 6a-2: MiR-941 Expression profiles of candidate miRNAs in patients with SA, NSTE-ACS, and STEMI. The three candidate miRNAs were evaluated by qRT-PCR using 56 samples. (XLSX 13 kb)

Additional file 12: Original data of Fig. 6b: MiR-182-5p Expression profiles of candidate miRNAs in patients with SA, NSTE-ACS, and STEMI. The three candidate miRNAs were evaluated by qRT-PCR using 56 samples. (XLSX 15 kb)

Additional file 13: Original data of Fig. 6c:MiR-363-3p Expression profiles of candidate miRNAs in patients with SA, NSTE-ACS, and STEMI. The three candidate miRNAs were evaluated by qRT-PCR using 56 samples. (XLSX 15 kb)

Additional file 14: Original data of Fig. 7: Expression profiles of miR-941 in patients with and without ACS. (XLSX 15 kb)

Additional file 15: Table 4-ROC curve: Original data of ROC curve analysis of miR-941 expression in patients with ACS and STEMI. (XLSX 12 kb)

Abbreviations

3′-UTR: 3′-untranslated region; ACS: Acute coronary syndrome; AMI: Acute myocardial infarction; AUC: Area under the curve; CI: Confidence interval; ECG: Electrocardiogram; FC: Fold-change; GO: Gene ontology; MAPK: Mitogen-activated protein kinase; MiRNA: MicroRNA; MTOR: Mammalian target of rapamycin; NSTE-ACS: Non-ST elevation ACS; qRT-PCR: Quantitative real-time reverse transcription polymerase chain reaction; ROC: Receiver operating characteristic; SA: Stable angina; STEMI: ST-segment elevation myocardial infarction; TGF: Transforming growth factor; UA: Unstable angina pectoris

Acknowledgements

We thank Shanghai OE Biotech. Co., Ltd. for technical assistance. We thank all of the patients for agreeing to participate in our study.

Funding

Supported by the Traditional Chinese Medicine Public Welfare Scientific Research Project, State Administration of Traditional Chinese Medicine of People's Republic of China (No. 201007001); and the National Natural Science Foundation of China (No. 81603489).

Authors' contributions

RB and QY were responsible for this manuscript and data analysis; these authors contributed equally to this manuscript. RX was responsible for data collection and follow-up. LL and DS modified the paper and gave constructive suggestions. KC made substantial contributions to conception and design. All authors read and approved the final manuscript.

Competing interests

The authors declare that they have no competing interests.

References

1. Go AS, Mozaffarian D, Roger VL, Benjamin EJ, Berry JD, Blaha MJ, et al. Heart disease and stroke statistics—2014 update: a report from the American Heart Association. Circulation. 2014;129:399–401.
2. Amsterdam EA, Wenger NK, Brindis RG, Casey DE, Ganiats TG, Holmes DR, et al. 2014 AHA/ACC Guideline for the Management of Patients with Non-ST-Elevation Acute Coronary Syndromes: a report of the American College of Cardiology/American Heart Association Task Force on Practice Guidelines. J Am Coll Cardiol. 2014;64:e139–228.
3. Diehl P, Fricke A, Sander L, Stamm J, Bassler N, Htun N, et al. Microparticles: major transport vehicles for distinct microRNAs in circulation. Cardiovasc Res. 2012;93:633–44.
4. Thomson DW, Bracken CP, Goodall GJ. Experimental strategies for microRNA target identification. Nucleic Acids Res. 2011;39:6845–53.
5. Noren Hooten N, Fitzpatrick M, Wood WH 3rd, De S, Ejiogu N, Zhang Y, et al. Age-related changes in microRNA levels in serum. Aging. 2013;5:725–40.
6. Peng Y, Song L, Zhao M, Harmelink C, Debenedittis P, Cui X, et al. Critical roles of miRNA-mediated regulation of TGFβ signalling during mouse cardiogenesis. Cardiovasc Res. 2014;103:258–67.
7. Small EM, Olson EN. Pervasive roles of microRNAs in cardiovascular biology. Nature. 2011;469:336–42.
8. Schroen B, Heymans S. Small but smart—microRNAs in the centre of inflammatory processes during cardiovascular diseases, the metabolic syndrome, and ageing. Cardiovasc Res. 2012;93:605–13.
9. Edelstein LC, Bray PF. MicroRNAs in platelet production and activation. Blood. 2011;117:5289–96.
10. Menghini R, Stohr R, Federici M. MicroRNAs in vascular aging and atherosclerosis. Ageing Res Rev. 2014;17:68–78.
11. Small EM, Frost RJ, Olson EN. MicroRNAs add a new dimension to cardiovascular disease. Circulation. 2010;121:1022–32.
12. Kataoka M, Wang DZ. Non-coding RNAs including miRNAs and lncRNAs in cardio-vascular biology and disease. Cell. 2014;3:883–98.
13. Creemers EE, Tijsen AJ, Pinto YM. Circulating microRNAs: novel biomarkers and extracellular communicators in cardiovascular disease? Circ Res. 2012;110:483–95.
14. van Rooij E. The art of microRNA research. Circ Res. 2011;108:219–34.
15. Li C, Pei F, Zhu X, Duan DD, Zeng C. Circulating microRNAs as novel and sensitive biomarkers of acute myocardial infarction. Clin Biochem. 2012;45:727–32.
16. Fihn SD, Blankenship JC, Alexander KP, Bittl JA, Byrne JG, Fletcher BJ, et al. 2014 ACC/AHA/AATS/PCNA/SCAI/STS focused update of the guideline for the diagnosis and management of patients with stable ischemic heart disease: a report of the American College of Cardiology/American Heart Association Task Force on Practice Guidelines, and the American Association for Thoracic Surgery, Preventive Cardiovascular Nurses Association, Society for Cardiovascular Angiography and Interventions, and Society of Thoracic Surgeons. J Am Coll Cardiol. 2014;64:1929–49.
17. American College of Emergency Physicians, Society for Cardiovascular Angiography and Interventions, O'Gara PT, et al. 2013 ACCF/AHA guideline for the management of ST-elevation myocardial infarction: a report of the American College of Cardiology Foundation/American Heart Association Task Force on Practice Guidelines. J Am Coll Cardiol. 2013;61:e78–140.
18. Libby P, Theroux P. Pathophysiology of coronary artery disease. Circulation. 2005;111:3481–8.
19. Selbach M, Schwanhäusser B, Thierfelder N, Fang Z, Khanin R, Rajewsky N.

Widespread changes in protein synthesis induced by microRNAs. Nature. 2008;455:58–63.
20. Livak KJ, Schmittgen TD. Analysis of relative gene expression data using real-time quantitative PCR and the 2(−Delata Delta C(T)) method. Methods. 2001;25:402–8.
21. Lagos-Quintana M, Rauhut R, Lendeckel W, Tuschl T. Identification of novel genes coding for small expressed RNAs. Science. 2001;294:853–8.
22. Gomes da Silva AM, Silbiger VN. miRNAs as biomarkers of atrial fibrillation. Biomarkers. 2014;19:631–6.
23. Zeller T, Keller T, Ojeda F, Reichlin T, Twerenbold R, Tzikas S, et al. Assessment of microRNAs in patients with unstable angina pectoris. Eur Heart J. 2014;35:2106–14.
24. McManus DD, Lin H, Tanriverdi K, Quercio M, Yin X, Larson MG, et al. Relations between circulating microRNAs and atrial fibrillation: data from the Framingham Offspring Study. Heart Rhythm. 2014;11:663–9.
25. Pagidipati NJ, Gaziano TA. Estimating deaths from cardiovascular disease: a review of global methodologies of mortality measurement. Circulation. 2013;127:749–56.
26. Arbab-Zadeh A, Nakano M, Virmani R, Fuster V. Acute coronary events. Circulation. 2012;125:1147–56.
27. Dangwal S, Bang C, Thum T. Novel techniques and targets in cardiovascular microRNA research. Cardiovasc Res. 2012;93:545–54.
28. Fichtlscherer S, Zeiher AM, Dimmeler S. Circulating microRNAs: biomarkers or mediators of cardiovascular diseases? Arterioscler Thromb Vasc Biol. 2011; 31:2383–90.
29. Sayed AS, Xia K, Salma U, Yang T, Peng J. Diagnosis, prognosis and therapeutic role of circulating miRNAs in cardiovascular diseases. Heart Lung Circ. 2014;23:503–10.
30. D'Alessandra Y, Carena MC, Spazzafumo L, Martinelli F, Bassetti B, Devanna P, et al. Diagnostic potential of plasmatic MicroRNA signatures in stable and unstable angina. PLoS One. 2013;8:e80345.
31. Long G, Wang F, Duan Q, Chen F, Yang S, Gong W, et al. Human circulating microRNA-1 and microRNA-126 as potential novel indicators for acute myocardial infarction. Int J Biol Sci. 2012;8:811–8.
32. Sayed AS, Xia K, Yang TL, Peng J. Circulating microRNAs: a potential role in diagnosis and prognosis of acute myocardial infarction. Dis Markers. 2013;35:561–6.
33. Liu P, Qiu C, Li B, Ding X, Wang Z, Li Y, et al. Clinical impact of circulating miR-133, miR-1291 and miR-663b in plasma of patients with acute myocardial infarction. Diagn Pathol. 2014;9:89.
34. Liebetrau C, Mollmann H, Dorr O, Szardien S, Troidl C, Willmer M, et al. Release kinetics of circulating muscle-enriched microRNAs in patients undergoing transcoronary ablation of septal hypertrophy. J Am Coll Cardiol. 2013;62:992–8.
35. Zhang PP, Wang XL, Zhao W, Qi B, Yang Q, Wan H, et al. DNA methylation-mediated repression of miR-941 enhances lysine (K)-specific demethylase 6B expression in hepatoma cells. J Biol Chem. 2014;289:24724–35.
36. Hu HY, He L, Fominykh K, Yan Z, Guo Sm Zhang X, et al. Evolution of the human-specific microRNA miR-941. Nat Commun. 2012;3:1145.

Permissions

All chapters in this book were first published in CD, by BioMed Central; hereby published with permission under the Creative Commons Attribution License or equivalent. Every chapter published in this book has been scrutinized by our experts. Their significance has been extensively debated. The topics covered herein carry significant findings which will fuel the growth of the discipline. They may even be implemented as practical applications or may be referred to as a beginning point for another development.

The contributors of this book come from diverse backgrounds, making this book a truly international effort. This book will bring forth new frontiers with its revolutionizing research information and detailed analysis of the nascent developments around the world.

We would like to thank all the contributing authors for lending their expertise to make the book truly unique. They have played a crucial role in the development of this book. Without their invaluable contributions this book wouldn't have been possible. They have made vital efforts to compile up to date information on the varied aspects of this subject to make this book a valuable addition to the collection of many professionals and students.

This book was conceptualized with the vision of imparting up-to-date information and advanced data in this field. To ensure the same, a matchless editorial board was set up. Every individual on the board went through rigorous rounds of assessment to prove their worth. After which they invested a large part of their time researching and compiling the most relevant data for our readers.

The editorial board has been involved in producing this book since its inception. They have spent rigorous hours researching and exploring the diverse topics which have resulted in the successful publishing of this book. They have passed on their knowledge of decades through this book. To expedite this challenging task, the publisher supported the team at every step. A small team of assistant editors was also appointed to further simplify the editing procedure and attain best results for the readers.

Apart from the editorial board, the designing team has also invested a significant amount of their time in understanding the subject and creating the most relevant covers. They scrutinized every image to scout for the most suitable representation of the subject and create an appropriate cover for the book.

The publishing team has been an ardent support to the editorial, designing and production team. Their endless efforts to recruit the best for this project, has resulted in the accomplishment of this book. They are a veteran in the field of academics and their pool of knowledge is as vast as their experience in printing. Their expertise and guidance has proved useful at every step. Their uncompromising quality standards have made this book an exceptional effort. Their encouragement from time to time has been an inspiration for everyone.

The publisher and the editorial board hope that this book will prove to be a valuable piece of knowledge for researchers, students, practitioners and scholars across the globe.

List of Contributors

Ying-Hsin Chen, Sheng-Chuan Hu and Jing-Ren Jeng
Institute of Medical Sciences, Tzu-Chi University, Hualien, Taiwan

Ying-Hsin Chen
Department of Emergency Medicine, Tri-Service General Hospital, National Defense Medical Center, Taipei, Taiwan

Jui-Ming Liu
Division of Urology, Department of Surgery, Chang Gung Memorial Hospital and Graduate Institute of Clinical Medical Sciences, Taoyuan, Taiwan

Ren-Jun Hsu, Chieh-Lin Wu and Cheng-Ping Yu
Department of Pathology and Graduate Institute of Pathology and Parasitology, Tri-Service General Hospital, National Defense Medical Center, Taipei, Taiwan

Ren-Jun Hsu, Chieh-Lin Wu and Cheng-Ping Yu
Biobank Management Center of Tri- Service General Hospital, National Defense Medical Center, Taipei, Taiwan

Sheng-Chuan Hu
Department of Emergency Medicine, Buddhist Tzu-Chi General Hospital, Tzu-Chi University, Hualien, Taiwan

Horng-Jyh Harn
Department of Pathology, China Medical University Hospital, China Medical University, Taichung, Taiwan

Shee-Ping Chen
Tzu-Chi Stem Cell Centre, Buddhist Tzu-Chi General Hospital, Hualien, Taiwan

Jing-Ren Jeng
Division of Cardiology, Buddhist Tzu-Chi General Hospital, Tzu-Chi University, Hualien, Taiwan

Jar-Yi Ho
Graduate Institutes of Life Sciences, National Defense Medical Center, Taipei, Taiwan

Jar-Yi Ho and Cheng-Ping Yu
Department of Pathology, Tri-Service General Hospital, 114 No.161, Sec. 6, Minquan E. Rd, Neihu Dist, Taipei City 114, Taiwan

Yuji Nishizaki, Kazunori Shimada, Tetsuro Miyazaki, Katsumi Miyauchi and Hiroyuki Daida
Department of Cardiology, Juntendo University Graduate School of Medicine, 2-1-1 Hongo Bunkyo-ku, Tokyo 113-8421, Japan

Shigemasa Tani and Ken Nagao
Department of Cardiology, Nihon University Hospital, 1-6 Kanda Surugadai Chiyoda-ku, Tokyo 101-8309, Japan

Takayuki Ogawa and Michihiro Yoshimura
Divison of Cardiology, Department of Internal Medicine, The Jikei University School of Medicine, 3-25-8, Nishi-Shimbashi Minato-ku, Tokyo 105-8461, Japan

Jiro Ando, Masao Takahashi and Issei Komuro
Department of Cardiovascular Medicine, Graduate School of Medicine, The University of Tokyo, 7-3-1 Hongo Bunkyo-ku, Tokyo 113-8655, Japan

Masato Yamamoto
Department of Internal Medicine, Tokyo Takanawa Hospital, 3-10-11, Takanawa Minato-ku, Tokyo 108-8606, Japan

Tomohiro Shinozaki
Department of Biostatistics, School of Public Health, The University of Tokyo, 7-3-1 Hongo Bunkyo-ku, Tokyo 113-0033, Japan

Atsushi Hirayama
Division of Cardiology, Department of Medicine, Nihon University School of Medicine, 30-1 Ohyaguchi Kamichou Itabashi-ku, Tokyo 173-8610, Japan

Ryozo Nagai
Jichi Medical University, 3311-1 Yakushiji, Shimotsuke-shi, Tochigi-ken 329-0498, Japan

Arjuna Medagama, Chinthani De Silva and Manoj Prasanna Galgomuwa
Department of Medicine, Faculty of Medicine, University of Peradeniya, Galaha Rd, Peradeniya 20400, Sri Lanka

Ruwanthi Bandara
Professorial Medical Unit, Teaching Hospital, Peradeniya, Sri Lanka

Jorge Alfonso Ross Terres
Glaxo Smith Kline, Mississauga, ON, Canada

Jorge Alfonso Ross Terres, G. Lozano-Ortega and R. Kendall
GlaxoSmithKline, 2301 Renaissance Boulevard, King of Prussia, PA 19406, USA

M. J. Sculpher
Oxford Outcomes Ltd, Vancouver, Canada

Jorge Alfonso Ross Terres, G. Lozano-Ortega, R. Kendall and M. J. Sculpher
Center of Helth Economics, University of York, York, UK

Julija Brozaitiene, Narseta Mickuviene, Aurelija Podlipskyte, Julius Burkauskas and Robertas Bunevicius
Behavioral Medicine Institute, Lithuanian University of Health Sciences, Palanga, Lithuania

Moustapha Sarr, Djibril Mari Ba, Mouhamadou Bamba Ndiaye, Malick Bodian, Modou Jobe, Adama Kane, Maboury Diao, Mouhamadoul Mounir Dia, Soulemane Pessinaba and Serigne Abdou Ba
Service de Cardiologie, CHU Aristide Le Dantec University Hospital, Dakar étoile, Avenue Pasteur, Dakar, Senegal

Alassane Mbaye and Abdoul Kane
Service de Cardiologie, Hôpital Général de Grand Yoff, Dakar, Senegal

Matias B. Yudi, David J. Clark, Katie Kalten and Omar Farouque
Department of Cardiology, Austin Health, Melbourne, Australia

Matias B. Yudi, David J. Clark, Omar Farouque and Michael Jelinek
Department of Medicine, University of Melbourne, Melbourne, Australia

David Tsang
Department of Cardiology, Western Health, Melbourne, Australia

Michael Jelinek and Sandeep Arunothayaraj
Department of Cardiology, St Vincent's Hospital, Melbourne, Australia

Michael Jelinek
Department of Heart and Mind, Australian Catholic University, Melbourne, Australia

Subodh Joshi and Khoa Phan
Monash Heart, Monash Health, Melbourne, Australia

Arthur Nasis
Department of Cardiology, Royal Melbourne Hospital, Melbourne, Australia

John Amerena
Department of Cardiology, Barwon Health, Geelong, Australia

Chris Reid
School of Public Health, Curtin University, Perth, Western Australia, Australia

Pei Ma, Lu Han, Zhihua Lv, Wei Chen, Hanning Hu, Jiancheng Tu, Xin Zhou and Song-Mei Liu
Center for Gene Diagnosis, Zhongnan Hospital of Wuhan University, Donghu Road 169#, Wuhan 430071, Hubei, PR China

Chung-Lieh Hung
Department of Internal Medicine, Division of Cardiology, MacKay Memorial Hospital, Taipei, Taiwan

Chung-Lieh Hung, Wen-Han Chang and Shou-Chuan Shih
Department of Medicine, Mackay Medical College, New Taipei city, Taiwan

Ding-Kuo Chien and Wen-Han Chang
Emergency Department, MacKay Memorial Hospital, Taipei, Taiwan

Ding-Kuo Chien, Wen-Han Chang and Shou-Chuan Shih
Department of Nursing, Mackay Junior College of Medicine, Nursing and Management, Taipei, Taiwan

Ding-Kuo Chien and Wen-Han Chang
Graduate Institute of Injury Prevention and Control, Taipei Medical University, Taipei, Taiwan

Ding-Kuo Chien
Institute of Mechatronic Engineering, National Taipei University of Technology, Taipei, Taiwan

Shou-Chuan Shih
Department of Internal Medicine, Division of Gastroenterology, MacKay Memorial Hospital, Taipei, Taiwan

Wen-Han Chang
School of Medicine, Taipei Medical University, Taipei, Taiwan

Pamela J. Bradshaw, Frank M. Sanfilippo, Michael S. T. Hobbs and Peter L. Thompson
School of Population Health, University of Western Australia, M431, 35 Stirling Highway, Crawley, WA 6009, Australia

Pamela J. Bradshaw, Judith M. Katzenellenbogen and Sandra C. Thompson
Western Australian Centre for Rural Health, University of Western Australia, M706, 35 Stirling Highway, Crawley, WA 6009, Australia

Peter L. Thompson
Department of Research, 2nd Floor A Block (Mailbox 26), Sir Charles Gairdner Hospital, Hospital Avenue, Nedlands 6009WA, Australia

Hou Tee Lu and Rusli Bin Nordin
Clinical School Johor Bahru, Jeffrey Cheah School of Medicine and Health Sciences, Monash University Sunway campus, 8 Jalan Masjid Abu Bakar, 80100, Johor Bahru, Johor, Malaysia

Hou Tee Lu
Department of Cardiology, Sultanah Aminah Hospital, Jalan Abu Bakar, 80100, Johor Bahru, Johor, Malaysia

Abdelkader Chalghoum, Yosri Noichri, Azza Dandana, Abdelhédi Miled and Salima Ferchichi
Laboratory of Biochemistry, Farhat HACHED Hospital, Street Doctor Moreau, 4000 Sousse, Tunisia

Abdelkader Chalghoum
Valorization and Technology Transfer Space, Center of Biotechnology of Borj Cedria, 2050 HamamLif, Tunisia

Bruno Baudin
Department of Biochemistry, Saint-Antoine Hospital, 184 Street Faubourg Saint-Antoine, 75571 Paris, Cedex 12, France

Hadeel Alkofide, Madhab Ray and Jayanta T. Mukherjee
Clinical and Translational Science Graduate Program, Sackler School of Biomedical Sciences, Tufts Clinical and Translational Science Institute, Tufts University, Boston, MA, USA

Hadeel Alkofide
Department of Clinical Pharmacy, College of Pharmacy, King Saud University, Riyadh, Saudi Arabia

Gordon S. Huggins
MCRI Center for Translational Genomics, Molecular Cardiology Research Institute, Tufts Medical Center, Boston, MA, USA

Joni R. Beshansky, Robin Ruthazer and Harry P. Selker
Center for Cardiovascular Health Services Research, Institute for Clinical Research and Health Policy Studies, Tufts Medical Center, Boston, MA, USA

Joni R. Beshansky
Regulatory and Clinical Research Management, Department of Health Sciences, Regis College, Weston, MA, USA

Robin Ruthazer, Jayanta T. Mukherjee and Harry P. Selker
Tufts Clinical and Translational Science Institute, Tufts University, Boston, MA, USA

Inga Peter
Department of Genetics and Genomic Sciences, Icahn School of Medicine at Mount Sinai, New York, NY, USA

Pei-Yin Jin, Xiao-Yan Guo, Wei-Fang Liang and Qin-Fu Han
Department of Cardiovascular Medicine, The People's Hospital of Anyang, Anyang, Henan, China

Hai-San Zhang
The Second Affiliated Hospital of Xinxiang Medical University, Xinxiang 453002, Henan, China

Youqin Zhan, Tan Xu and Xuerui Tan
Department of Cardiology, First Affiliated Hospital of Shantou University Medical College, Shantou, Guangdong 515041, China

Luís Leite, Rui Baptista and Luís Elvas
Departament of Cardiology, Centro Hospitalar e Universitário de Coimbra, Praceta Prof. Mota Pinto, Coimbra 3000-075, Portugal

Jorge Leitão, Joana Cochicho, Filipe Breda, Armando Carvalho and José Nascimento Costa
Department of Internal Medicine, Centro Hospitalar e Universitário de Coimbra, Praceta Prof. Mota Pinto, Coimbra 3000-075, Portugal

Isabel Fonseca
Emergency Department, Centro Hospitalar e Universitário de Coimbra, Praceta Prof. Mota Pinto, Coimbra 3000-075, Portugal

Jinjin Zhang and Pingping Yan
Department of Cardiology, North Huashan Hospital of Fudan University, Shanghai 201907, People's Republic of China

Xianhao Wu
Department of Cardiology, Tongren Hospital, Shanghai 200050, People's Republic of China

Peizhen Gao
Department of Beixinjing Community Health Center, Shanghai 200335, People's Republic of China

Stephen Jan
The George Institute for Global Health, Sydney Medical School, University of Sydney, King George V Building, 83–117 Missenden Rd, Camperdown, NSW 2050, Australia

Stephen W-L. Lee
Queen Mary Hospital, Hong Kong, SAR, China

Jitendra P. S. Sawhney
Sir Ganga Ram Hospital, New Delhi, India

Tiong K. Ong
Sarawak General Hospital, Kuching, Malaysia

Chee Tang Chin
National Heart Centre Singapore, Singapore, Singapore

Hyo-Soo Kim
Seoul National University Hospital, Seoul, South Korea

Rungroj Krittayaphong
Siriraj Hospital, Bangkok, Thailand

Vo T. Nhan
Cho Ray Hospital, Ho Chi Minh City, Vietnam

Stuart J. Pocock
London School of Hygiene and Tropical Medicine, London, UK

Ana M. Vega
Observational Research Centre, Global Medical Affairs, AstraZeneca, Madrid, Spain

Nobuya Hayashi
AstraZeneca, Osaka, Japan

Yong Huo
Peking University First Hospital, Beijing, China

Pravesh Kumar Bundhun
Institute of Cardiovascular Diseases, the First Affiliated Hospital of Guangxi Medical University, Nanning, Guangxi 530027, People's Republic of China

Musaben Shaik
Department of Paediatrics, Pragati Children's Hospital, Ch Pet andhra Pradesh, India

Jun Yuan
Department of Cardiology, The People's Hospital of Guangxi Zhuang Autonomous Region, Nanning, Guangxi 530021, China

Michelle M. A. Kip, Hendrik Koffijberg, Marco J. Moesker, Maarten J. IJzerman and Ron Kusters
Department of Health Technology and Services Research, MIRA institute for Biomedical Technology and Technical Medicine, University of Twente, Enschede, the Netherlands

Ron Kusters
Laboratory for Clinical Chemistry and Haematology, Jeroen Bosch Ziekenhuis, Den Bosch, the Netherlands

Jing Li, Jingang Zheng, Yifeng Zhou, Xiaofei Liu and Wenhua Peng
Department of Cardiology, China-Japan Friendship Hospital, No. 2, Yinghua Road, Beijing 100029, China

Nilukshana Yogendranathan, H. M. M. T. B. Herath, S.P. Pahalagamage and Aruna Kulatunga
National Hospital, Colombo, Sri Lanka

Dong Wang, Xiao-Hong Yang, Ji-Dong Zhang, Rui-Bin Li, Min Jia and Xiao-Ran Cui
Department of Sixth Cardiovascular Medicine, Second Hospital of Hebei Medical University, No. 309 North Zhonghua Street, Shijiazhuang 05400, Hebei, China

Ruina Bai, Qiaoning Yang, Ruixi Xi, Lizhi Li, Dazhuo Shi and Keji Chen
Xiyuan Hospital, China Academy of Chinese Medical Sciences, 1 Xiyuan Caochang, Haidian district, Beijing, China

Index

www.ingramcontent.com/pod-product-compliance
Lightning Source LLC
LaVergne TN
LVHW080653210926
848485LV00003B/368